Treatment and Management of Tropical Liver Disease

Edited by

JOSE DEBES, MD, PhD
University of Minnesota
Minneapolis, Minnesota
United States

ELSEVIER

Elsevier
1600 John F. Kennedy Blvd.
Ste 1800
Philadelphia, PA 19103-2899

TREATMENT AND MANAGEMENT OF TROPICAL LIVER DISEASE
ISBN: 978-0-323-87031-3

Content Strategist: Nancy Tuffy
Content Development Specialist: Kevin Travers
Content Development Manager: Ellen Wurm-Cutter
Publishing Services Manager: Shereen Jameel
Project Manager: Haritha Dharmarajan
Design Direction: Ryan Cook

Printed in the United States of America

Last digit is the print number: 9 8 7 6 5 4 3 2 1

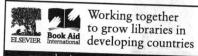

CONTRIBUTORS

Elizabeth Aby, MD
Department of Medicine
Division of GI
University of Minnesota
Minneapolis, Minnesota
United States

Vineet Ahuja, MD, DM
Gastroenterology
All India Institute of Medical Sciences
New Delhi
India

Mohammed Alizzi, MBBS, MPH
Townsville University Hospital
Townsville, Queensland
Australia

Pravin Amin, MD, FCCM, FNCS
Critical Care Medicine
Bombay Hospital Institute of Medical Sciences
Mumbai, Maharashtra
India

Vinay Amin, MBBS
Bombay Hospital
Mumbai, Maharashtra
India

Chimaobi M. Anugwom, MBBS
Digestive Care
Health Partners
Saint Paul, Minnesota
United States
Division of Gastroenterology, Hepatology and Nutrition
University of Minnesota
Minneapolis, Minnesota
United States

Juan Pablo Arab, MD
Departamento de Gastroenterología
Escuela de Medicina
Pontificia Universidad Católica de Chile
Santiago
Chile
Division of Gastroenterology
Department of Medicine
Western University & London Health Sciences Centre
London, Ontario
Canada

Marco Arrese
Departamento de Gastroenterología
Escuela de Medicina
Pontificia Universidad Católica de Chile
Santiago
Chile

Domingo Balderramo, MD, PhD
Hospital Privado Universitario de Cordoba
Cordoba
Argentina

Abate Bane, MD
Division of Gastroenterology & Hepatology
Department of Internal Medicine
Addis Ababa University
Ethiopia

Luciano Beltrão Pereira, MD
Liver and Transplant Institute of Pernambuco
Pernambuco
Brazil

Joerg Boecker, MD
Department of Surgery Division of HPB Surgery
Asklepios Klinik Barmbek
Hamburg, Hamburg
Germany

Karl J. Oldhafer
Department of Surgery Division of HPB Surgery
Asklepios Klinik Barmbek
Hamburg
Germany

Enrico Brunetti
Surgical, Clinical, Diagnostic and Pediatric Sciences
University of Pavia
Pavia
Italy

Miguel Mauricio Cabada, MD, MSc, FASTMH
Internal Medicine
University of Texas Medical Branch
Galveston, Texas
United States
UPCH-UTMB Collaborative Research Center
Universidad Peruana Cayetano Heredia
Cusco
Peru

Francesca Cainelli, MD
Faculty of Medicine
University of Puthisastra
Phnom Penh
Cambodia

Wanessa Trindade Clemente, MD, PhD
Department of Laboratory Medicine
Faculdade de Medicina da Universidade Federal de Minas Gerais (UFMG)
Transplant Infectious Disease, Liver Transplant Program
Hospital das Clínicas da UFMG
Belo Horizonte, Minas Gerais
Brazil

Bart J. Currie, MBBS, FRACP, FAFPHM, DTM+H
Northern Territory Medical Program and Menzies School of Health Research
Royal Darwin Hospital
Darwin
Northern Territory
Australia

Jose Debes, MD, PhD
University of Minnesota
Minneapolis, Minnesota
United States

Hailemichael Desalegn, MD, PhD
Internal Medicine
St. Paul's Hospital Millennium Medical College
Addis Ababa
Ethiopia

Luis Antonio Diaz, MD
Departamento de Gastroenterología
Escuela de Medicina
Pontificia Universidad Católica de Chile
Santiago
Chile

C. E. Eapen, MD, DM
Hepatology Department
Christian Medical College
Vellore, Tamil Nadu
India

Axel Eickhoff, MD
Department of Internal Medicine II
Division of Gastroenterology and Hepatology
Klinikum Hanau
Academic Teaching Hospital of the Medical Faculty
Goethe University Frankfurt/ Main
Frankfurt/Main
Germany

Siobhan M. Flanagan, MD
Vascular and Interventional Radiology
University of Minnesota Medical Center
Minneapolis, Minnesota
United States

James Ford, MD
Emergency Medicine
UCSF
San Francisco, California
United States

Ashish Goel, MD, DM, PhD
Hepatology
Christian Medical College
Vellore
India

Victor R. Gordeuk, BS, MD
Medicine
University of Illinois at Chicago
Chicago
Illinois
United States

Eduardo Gotuzzo, MBBS
School of Medicine
Universidad Peruana Cayetano Heredia
Lima
Peru

Francisco Idalsoaga, MD
Departamento de Gastroenterología
Escuela de Medicina
Pontificia Universidad Católica de Chile
Santiago
Chile

Ifeorah M. Ijeoma, BMLS, MSc, PhD
Medical Microbiology Unit Department of Medical Laboratory Sciences
University of Nigeria Nsukka
Enugu
Nigeria

Carol A. Kauffman, MD
Infectious Diseases/Internal Medicine
University of Michigan
Ann Arbor, Michigan
United States

Mandip K.C., MD
Department of Medicine Division of Gastroenterology, Hepatology, and Nutrition
University of Minnesota
Minneapolis, Minnesota
United States

John Lake, MD
Medicine
University of Minnesota Medical School
Minneapolis, Minnesota
United States

Thomas M. Leventhal, MD
Gastroenterology, Hepatology and Nutrition
University of Minnesota
Minneapolis, Minnesota
United States

Kathleen Linder, MD
Internal Medicine
University of Michigan
Staff Physician
Infectious Diseases Section
LTC Charles S. Kettles VAMC
Ann Arbor, Michigan
United States

Tommaso Manciulli, MD, PhD
WHO Collaborating Center for the Clinical Management of Cystic Echinococcosis
University of Pavia
Pavia
Italy
Department of Experimental and Clinical Medicine
University of Florence
Florence
Italy

Mariana Martel, MBBS
School of Medicine
Universidad Peruana Cayetano Heredia
Lima
Peru

Ângelo Z. Mattos, MD, MSc, PhD
Graduate Program in Medicine: Hepatology Federal University of Health Sciences of Porto Alegre
Gastroenterology and Hepatology Unit
Irmandade Santa Casa de Misericórdia
Porto Alegre
Brazil

Yusuf Musa, MBBS, MD, FMCP
Gastroenterology Unit
Department of Internal Medicine
Federal Teaching Hospital Katsina
Katsina
Nigeria

Robert Norton, FRCPA, MD
Faculty of Medicine
University of Queensland
Brisbane
Pathology
Townsville University Hospital
Townsville, Queensland
Australia

Karl Jürgen Oldhafer
Department of Surgery
Asklepios Hospital Barmbek
Hamburg
Germany

Opeyemi Owoseni, MBBS, FMCP
Internal Medicine
Federal Medical Center
Abeokuta, Ogun State
Nigeria

Francisco Guilherme Cancela Pena
Division of Gastroenterology
Hepatology and Liver Transplantation
Hospital das Clínicas EBSERH/UFMG - Universidade Federal de Minas Gerais (UFMG)
Instituto de Previdência dos Servidores do Estado de Minas Gerais - IPSEMG
Belo Horizonte, Minas Gerais
Brazil

Leila Moreira Beltrão Pereira, MD, PhD
Gastrohepatology Unit
Oswaldo Cruz University Hospital
Sao Paulo
Brazil

Kittiyod Poovorawan, MD
Clinical Tropical Medicine
Mahidol University
Bangkok
Thailand

Xinshun Qi, MD
Department of Gastroenterology
General Hospital of Northern Theater Command
Shenyang
Liaoning Province
China

Lewis R. Roberts, MB ChB, PhD
Division of Gastroenterology and Hepatology
Mayo Clinic College of Medicine and Science
Rochester, Minnesota
United States

Prasert Saichua, MD
Department of Tropical Medicine
Faculty of Medicine
Khon Kaen University
Thailand

Amir Sultan Seid, MD
Division of Gastroenterology, Department of Internal Medicine
Addis Ababa University, Addis Ababa
Ethiopia

Vishal Sharma, MD, DM
Gastroenterology
PGIMER, Chandigarh
India

Ananta Shrestha, MBBS, MD
Hepatology
Alka Hospital, Kathmandu
Bagmati
Nepal

Ashwani K. Singal, MD, MS, FACG, FAASLD, AGAF
Gastroenterology and Hepatology
University of South Dakota
Chief Clinical Research and Transplant Hepatologist
Transplant Hepatology
Avera Transplant Institute
Health Research Scientist
VA Medical Center
Sioux Falls, South Dakota
United States

Pirathaban Sivabalan, MBBS, MPHTM
Microbiology
Townsville University Hospital
Townsville, Queensland
Australia

Leila Maria Soares Tojal de Barros Lima, MD
Department of Internal Medicine
Federal University of Alagoas
Maceio
Brazil

Mark W. Sonderup, B Pharm, MBChB, FCP(SA), MMED, FRCP(UK)
Division of Hepatology
Department of Medicine
Faculty of Health Sciences
University of Cape Town and Groote Schuur Hospital
Cape Town, Western Cape
South Africa

C. Wendy Spearman, MBChB, MMed, PhD, FCP(SA) and FRCP(London)
Division of Hepatology
Department of Medicine
University of Cape Town
Cape Town
Western Province
South Africa

Banchob Sripa, PhD
Pathology
Khon Kaen University
Khon Kaen
Thailand

Manaswita Tappata, MD
Department of Medicine
University of Minnesota
Minneapolis, Minnesota
United States

Rolf Teschke, MD
Department of Internal Medicine II
Division of Gastroenterology and Hepatology
Klinikum Hanau
Academic Teaching Hospital of the Medical Faculty
Goethe University Frankfurt/ Main
Frankfurt/Main
Germany

Perry J.J. van Genderen, MD, PhD
Consultant Physician and Associate
Medical Microbiology and Infectious Diseases
Erasmus MC University Hospital
Rotterdam
Netherlands

Sandro Vento, MD
Faculty of Medicine
University of Puthisastra
Phnom Penh
Cambodia

Tran Dang Xuan, PhD
Center for the Planetary Health and Innovation Science
The IDEC Institute
Laboratory of Plant Physiology and Biochemistry
Graduate School of Advanced Science and Engineering
Smart Agriculture Faculty, Graduate School of Advanced Science and Engineering
Hiroshima University
Hiroshima
Japan

Mirghani Abd El Rahman Yousif Sr, MPharm, PhD
Clinical Pharmacy
University of Gezira
Wad Medani, Gezira
Sudan

CONTENTS

SECTION I Viral Hepatitides

SECTION II Liver Masses

SIOBHAN M. FLANAGAN, MD

SECTION III Tropical Infectious Liver Disease

SECTION I

Viral Hepatitides

CHAPTER 1

Hepatitis A

Domingo Balderramo

KEY POINTS

- HAV infection accounts for about 1.5 million clinical cases of hepatitis each year.
- HAV transmission is related to ingestion of contaminated water or food or direct contact with an infectious patient.
- HAV infection usually presents a mild course and only a small proportion of patients may present a severe course including fulminant hepatitis.
- HAV can occur sporadically or in an epidemic form.
- Nearly all patients infected recover fully from HAV infection and develop lifelong protective immunity.
- A safe and effective vaccine is available worldwide to prevent HAV infection.

Introduction

Hepatitis A infection represents the most common form of acute viral hepatitis globally. This infection is caused by the hepatitis A virus (HAV), a member of the genus *Hepatovirus* in the family Picornaviridae.[1] HAV infection is usually a self-limited illness that never becomes chronic. Infection confers lifelong immunity and it is preventable via vaccination.[1]

EPIDEMIOLOGY

HAV is generally transmitted via the fecal-oral route. Risk factors for HAV transmission are summarized in Table 1.1. Maternal-fetal transmission has not been described.

Although the incidence of HAV has declined substantially since the implementation of vaccination, the World Health Organization (WHO) estimates more than 150 million HAV infections, causing approximately 1.5 million clinical cases of hepatitis A each year.[2] China and India witness about one-third of the global incident cases in a single year.[3]

Hepatitis A can occur sporadically or in an epidemic form. Endemic regions have varied in the last few decades and include Qatar, Afghanistan, sub-Saharan Africa, and some countries in South America (Figure 1.1). Other regions with high-income countries such as Asia-Pacific, Oceania, and Australasia have shown the highest increasing trend of HAV infection from 1990 to 2019.[3] Previous endemic regions such as Belarus, China, Brazil, Argentina, and Romania have shown a significant decrease after the introduction of the HAV vaccine and improvement in living conditions. This changing epidemiologic situation is likely associated with an increasing number of adults without protective antibodies acquired at an early age in life and therefore an associated risk for outbreaks.[4]

Sporadic outbreaks in non-endemic countries can occur in a variety of settings, including the presence of contaminated frozen produce and through infected travelers from endemic regions.

TABLE 1.1 ■ **Risk Factors for HAV Infection**

• Person-to-person contact: Transmission within households Sexual transmission (men who have sex with men) Residential institution transmission
• Contact with contaminated food or water: Raw or undercooked shellfish, vegetables, or other kinds of foods Foods contaminated by infected food handlers
• Users of illicit drugs
• Travelers from non-endemic to HAV-endemic countries

HAV, hepatitis A virus.

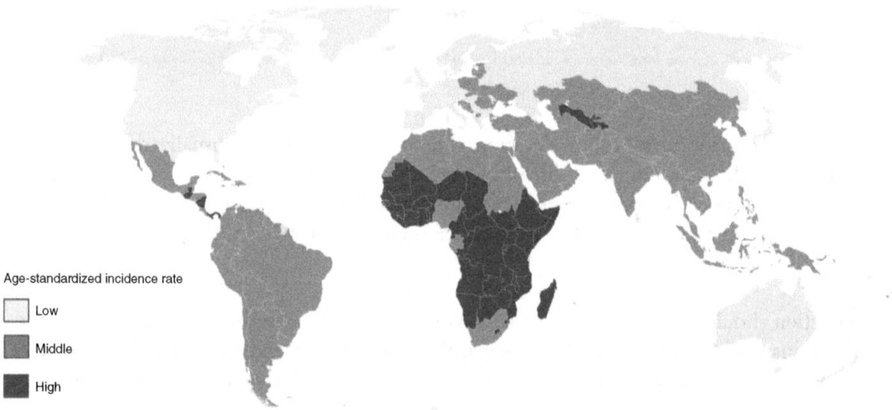

Figure 1.1 Age-adjusted incidence rate of hepatitis A in 2019. (Adapted from Ref. 3.)

In addition, outbreaks in healthcare settings and among homeless individuals have also been described. Over the last decade, outbreaks among individuals who had reported drug use or among men who have sex with men have been reported.[5-7]

Clinical Presentation

Acute HAV infection in adults is usually a self-limited illness. The incubation period of HAV infection ranges from 15 to 50 days.[1] Symptoms are more frequent in adults and less common in children. Nausea and vomiting, anorexia, fever, malaise, and abdominal pain are the most frequent initial manifestations[8] (Table 1.2). After the initial manifestations, dark urine, acholia (pale stools), and jaundice develop in a great proportion of symptomatic cases. Jaundice peaks approximately 2 weeks after the initial manifestations, while initial symptoms tend to resolve at the same time. Findings on physical exam include jaundice, hepatomegaly, and right upper quadrant tenderness.[9] A small proportion of patients develop splenomegaly, skin rash, and arthralgias. In pregnant women, HAV infection has been associated with higher rates of preterm labor and gestational complications.[10]

Laboratory abnormalities include significant elevations of serum aminotransferases and bilirubin.[11] Serum aminotransferase levels may exceed 10,000 mIU/mL, and this alteration

TABLE 1.2 ■ **Symptoms and Signs in Patients With HAV Infection**

Symptom	**% of Patients**
Nausea/vomiting	>75
Anorexia	>75
Dark urine/acholia	>75
Malaise	50–75
Fever	50–75
Abdominal pain	50–75
Headache	25–50
Sign	
Jaundice	>75
Hepatomegaly	50–75
Abdominal tenderness	50–75
Splenomegaly	<25

HAV: hepatitis A virus.

frequently occurs prior to bilirubin elevation. These abnormal values usually decline within 2 weeks of peak levels and return to normal in a great proportion of patients within 3 months of initial manifestations.[11] Importantly, infected individuals are contagious from the incubation period (presymptomatic) to 1 month after jaundice presentation.[12]

Diagnosis

HAV infection should be suspected in patients with jaundice in the setting of known risk factors for HAV transmission (Table 1.1). Since hepatitis A is clinically indistinguishable from other hepatitis viruses, specific serum markers and nucleic acid detection techniques are required to make the diagnosis.[3]

The diagnosis is established by detection of serum IgM anti-HAV antibodies.[8] These antibodies are detectable from symptom onset and remain detectable for approximately 3 to 6 months. The presence of serum IgM antibodies in the absence of clinical symptoms may reflect prior HAV infection with prolonged persistence of antibodies, a false-positive result, or asymptomatic infection (more frequent in children than in adults).[9] Serum IgG anti-HAV antibodies appear early in the convalescent period of the infection and persist during follow-up and are associated with lifelong immunity.[11] The presence of serum IgG antibodies for HAV in the absence of anti-HAV IgM is associated generally with past infection or vaccination. Imaging studies are not indicated for diagnosis of HAV infection, although the use of ultrasonography may sometimes be appropriate to rule out alternative diagnoses such as biliary complications in patients with persistent abdominal pain and jaundice.[13]

Differential Diagnosis

The differential diagnosis of HAV infection includes other viruses that can cause hepatitis, and only serology tests can clarify the final diagnosis. These viruses include hepatitis B, C, D, and E virus, less likely Epstein-Barr virus and cytomegalovirus, yellow fever virus, herpes simplex virus, and adenovirus (most commonly in immunocompromised hosts). HIV infection is associated with gastrointestinal symptoms, but hepatitis is rarely present.

Other infectious causes of fever and jaundice include malaria, leptospirosis, syphilis, and Q fever.

Management

HAV infection usually presents a self-limited course, and treatment consists only of supportive care.[11] Medications that might cause liver damage should be avoided during the period of jaundice including acetaminophen, nonsteroidal anti-inflammatory drugs, antibiotics, and antiemetic drugs.[8] Full clinical and biochemical recovery is observed within 3 months in the majority of patients.[9]

Complications

The main complications of HAV infection include fulminant hepatic liver failure, cholestatic hepatitis, relapsing hepatitis, and autoimmune hepatitis.

- *Fulminant hepatic failure*: impaired synthetic function and encephalopathy develops in less than 1% of patients with HAV infection, especially in adult patients older than 50 years and with underlying liver disease.[14] Treatment in this severe clinical situation includes intensive care admission and liver transplant evaluation.
- *Cholestatic hepatitis*: it is characterized by jaundice, pruritus, fever, weight loss, diarrhea, and malaise persisting for a long period (≥3 months) and is observed in less than 5% of cases. Laboratory findings include elevated serum bilirubin and alkaline phosphatase values as well as moderate elevation of serum aminotransferases.[15] This complication resolves spontaneously without consequences, and identification is important to avoid unnecessary testing or treatments.
- *Relapsing hepatitis*: the clinical course of this complication includes an apparent clinical recovery after acute infection with a tendency toward normalization of the serum aminotransferases, followed by biochemical and clinical relapse. Symptoms of the clinical relapse often are milder than the initial manifestations and usually occur within 3 weeks to 6 months following resolution of acute HAV infection.[16,17] Duration of clinical relapse is generally less than 3 weeks following complete recovery.[16] This complication could be expected in up to 11% of patients according to some studies.[18] The cause of relapsing hepatitis is unknown, and no risk factors for relapse have been described. HAV can be present in stools during the period of relapse, so these patients can transmit the infection.[19] Similar to cholestatic hepatitis, identification is important to avoid unnecessary testing or treatments.
- *Autoimmune hepatitis*: HAV infection has been mentioned in a few reports as a trigger for development of autoimmune hepatitis in susceptible individuals.[20]

Prevention and Vaccine

Actions for prevention of HAV infection according to the WHO include improved sanitation, vaccination, and attention to hygienic practices such as regular handwashing before meals and after going to the bathroom, safe drinking water, and proper disposal of sewage within communities.[8]

Several injectable inactivated hepatitis A vaccines are available worldwide with similar protection ranging from 95% to 100% and a few side effects. No vaccine is licensed for children younger than 1 year of age.[8] Indications of vaccination include children more than 12 months of age and adults at increased risk. Risk factors include individuals traveling to or working in countries with high or intermediate rates of HAV, men who have sex with men, individuals who use injection or non-injecting illicit drugs, individuals with occupational risk for exposure, or who anticipate a close contact with individuals at high risk for HAV infection (Table 1.1). Other subgroups include individuals with chronic liver disease or HIV infection and pregnant women at risk for HAV infection or severe disease from HAV infection based on previous liver disease. For individuals at risk for hepatitis A exposure who are allergic to the HAV vaccine or are <12 months of age, passive immunization via immune globulin could be considered.

In 2019, the HAV vaccine was introduced as a routine immunization for children in only 34 countries worldwide.[3] Israel became in 1999 the first country to introduce an inactivated hepatitis A vaccine into its national childhood vaccination program. Age-adjusted seroprevalence rates of HAV antibodies significantly increase 12 years after the implementation.[21]

Prevaccine serology: there is no indication for serologic testing of children prior to vaccination. Individuals for whom prevaccination serologic testing is most cost-effective include adults from areas with high or intermediate HAV endemicity.

Dosing and safety: immunization with single-antigen inactivated hepatitis A vaccine consists of two doses for children and adults. The combination inactivated vaccine consists of three doses only for adults. There is no need for HAV booster vaccination after completion of the primary two-dose vaccination series and it confers lifelong protection.[1]

Single-dose strategy: universal and mandatory single-dose HAV vaccination to children from age 1 year was introduced in Argentina in 2005 according to a cost-saving strategy. Early evaluation of this strategy showed a significant impact without new pediatric fulminant hepatitis cases due to HAV reported since 2007.[22] Comparable results were also described in other countries including Nicaragua, Korea, India, and China using a similar strategy.[1]

Vaccine adverse events: the most common adverse events are fever, injection site reaction, rash, and headache. Serious adverse events are very infrequent. Data on the safety of hepatitis A vaccination during pregnancy are limited, with a probably low risk for the fetus. The indication of vaccination should be weighed against the risk for hepatitis A exposure.

References

1. Lemon SM, Ott JJ, Van Damme P, Shouval D. Type A viral hepatitis: a summary and update on the molecular virology, epidemiology, pathogenesis and prevention. *J Hepatol.* 2018;68:167.
2. WHO. WHO position paper on hepatitis A vaccines. *Wkly Epidemiol Rec.* 2012;87(28-29):261-276.
3. Cao G, Jing W, Liu J, Liu M. The global trends and regional differences in incidence and mortality of hepatitis A from 1990 to 2019 and implications for its prevention. *Hepatol Int.* 2021;5(5):1068-1082.
4. Wang Z, Chen Y, Xie S, Lv H. Changing epidemiological characteristics of hepatitis A in Zhejiang Province, China: increased susceptibility in adults. *PLoS One.* 2016;11(4):e0153804.
5. Mariojoules J, Castro G, Pisano MB, et al. Hepatitis A outbreak affecting men who have sex with men (MSM) in central Argentina, occurred in July 2017–April 2018, later than the European outbreak. *J Clin Virol.* 2019;117:49-53.
6. Foster MA, Hofmeister MG, Albertson JP, et al. Hepatitis A virus infections among men who have sex with men—Eight U.S. states, 2017–2018. *MMWR.* 2021;70(24):875-878.
7. Figgatt M, Hildick-Smith J, Addish E, et al. Susceptibility to hepatitis A and B virus among clients at a syringe services program in Philadelphia, 2018. *Public Health Rep.* 2020;135(5):691-699.
8. WHO. *Hepatitis A.* 27 July 2021. Available at: https://www.who.int/news-room/fact-sheets/detail/hepatitis-a. Accessed February 10, 2022.
9. Cuthbert JA. Hepatitis A: old and new. *Clin Microbiol Rev.* 2001;14(1):38-58.
10. Elinav E, Ben-Dov IZ, Shapira Y, et al. Acute hepatitis A infection in pregnancy is associated with high rates of gestational complications and preterm labor. *Gastroenterology.* 2006;130(4):1129.
11. Brundage SC, Fitzpatrick AN. Hepatitis A. *Am Fam Physician.* 2006;73(12):2162-2168.
12. Richardson M, Elliman D, Maguire H, Simpson J, Nicoll A. Evidence base of incubation periods, periods of infectiousness and exclusion policies for the control of communicable diseases in schools and preschools. *Pediatr Infect Dis J.* 2001;20(4):380.
13. Bura M, Michalak M, Chojnicki MK, Kowala-Piaskowska A, Mozer-Lisewska I. Viral hepatitis A in 108 adult patients during an eight-year observation at a single center in Poland. *Adv Clin Exp Med.* 2015;24(5):829-836.
14. Kemmer NM, Miskovsky EP. Hepatitis A. *Infect Dis Clin North Am.* 2000;14(3):605-615.
15. Jung YM, Park SJ, Kim JS, et al. Atypical manifestations of hepatitis A infection: a prospective, multicenter study in Korea. *J Med Virol.* 2010;82(8):1318-1326.

16. Glikson M, Galun E, Oren R, Tur-Kaspa R, Shouval D. Relapsing hepatitis A. Review of 14 cases and literature survey. *Medicine (Baltimore).* 1992;71(1):14-23.
17. Ma M, Golfeyz S, Chen C, Naik J. Relapsing hepatitis A: an asymptomatic recurrence of elevated liver chemistries. *Am J Gastroenterol.* 2018;113:S1342-S1343.
18. Tong MJ, el-Farra NS, Grew MI. Clinical manifestations of hepatitis A: recent experience in a community teaching hospital. *J Infect Dis.* 1995;171 (suppl 1):S15-S18.
19. Sjogren MH, Tanno H, Fay O, et al. Hepatitis A virus in stool during clinical relapse. *Ann Intern Med.* 1987;106(2):221-226.
20. Tagle Arrospide M, León Barúa R. Viral hepatitis A as a triggering agent of autoimmune hepatitis report of a case and review of literature. *Rev Gastroenterol Peru.* 2003;23(2):134-137.
21. Bassal R, Weil M, Cohen D, Sofer D, Mendelson E, Shohat T. Seroprevalence of hepatitis A twelve years after the implementation of Toddlers' vaccination: a population-based study in Israel. *Pediatr Infect Dis J.* 2017;36(10):e248-e251.
22. Cervio G, Trentadue J, D'Agostino D, et al. Decline in HAV-associated fulminant hepatic failure and liver transplant in children in Argentina after the introduction of a universal hepatitis A vaccination program. *Hepat Med.* 2011;3:99-106.

CHAPTER 2

Hepatitis B Virus

James S. Ford ■ Jose D. Debes

KEY POINTS

- Hepatitis B virus (HBV) is the most common cause of liver cancer worldwide
- Chronic hepatitis B (CHB) is defined as the presence of the HBsAg for >6 months
- Transmission occurs via pregnancy, sexual intercourse, and contact with infected blood
- CHB is rarely symptomatic; therefore a high index of suspicion is needed and routine screening should be employed, especially in high-risk populations
- Risk of developing CHB is highly dependent on age of exposure (>90% if exposed as a newborn, ~5% if exposed as an adult)
- Most treatments for HBV aim to control but not cure the infection. Treatment is indicated in the presence of cirrhosis or in the presence of active viral replication plus evidence of liver inflammation or fibrosis
- HBV is vaccine preventable. While all patients will benefit from vaccination, newborns, children, and pregnant woman should be prioritized.

Overview

Hepatitis B virus (HBV), a viral pathogen with an affinity for human hepatocytes, is a major cause of morbidity and mortality worldwide. Acute HBV infections can be asymptomatic or can cause fulminant liver failure. Chronic HBV infection (CHB) is associated with serious downstream sequelae including cirrhosis and hepatocellular carcinoma (HCC).[1] While HBV infection is vaccine preventable, there are over 350 million people with chronic infection, a global prevalence of 3.9%.[2]

EPIDEMIOLOGY

HBV accounts for 29% of all liver diseases in the world.[3] There are approximately 1.5 million new cases of HBV infection every year worldwide.[2,4] It is estimated that less than 10% of individuals with CHB know their infection status, and this lack of awareness contributes to transmission of the disease. The largest burden of HBV occurs in low- and middle-income countries. Limited HBV screening and treatment in these regions leads to large geographic disparities in morbidity and mortality.[2]

Over 820,000 individuals with CHB die every year from its downstream complications, such as cirrhosis and HCC.[2] HBV is the most common etiology of liver disease in men who die of cirrhosis (31.5%) and the second most common in women who die of cirrhosis (24.5%).[5] HBV is the leading cause of HCC in the world.[6]

Due to global efforts to prevent the transmission of viral hepatitis, liver disease-associated mortality fell substantively in many low-, middle- and high-income countries between 1980 and 2010.[7] In 1992, the World Health Organization (WHO) recommended inclusion of HBV vaccination into universal childhood immunization programs, and since then, childhood rates of chronic HBV have declined by over 3.5-fold (4.7% to 1.3%).[8] The global rate of HBV vaccination is estimated to be 84%.[5] The Americas and the Western Pacific have achieved 90% vaccine coverage in children <1 year, whereas Europe, Africa, Southeast Asia, and the Eastern Mediterranean have yet to reach this benchmark.[5] In many regions, however, vaccination rates are lower in rural areas, as many births occur outside of hospital settings. Rural populations typically have limited access to traditional healthcare facilities and thus are poorly represented in national statistics, which leads to an overestimation of vaccination coverage[5] (Figure 2.1).

Virology

HBV is a partially double-stranded, circular DNA virus that is a member of the *Hepadnaviridae* family.[9] There are 10 HBV genotypes (A–J), which are endemic to distinct geographic territories.[10] The infectious HBV particle is a spherical, double-shelled virion whose structural components are composed of proteins (antigens) that are important for HBV replication as well as clinical diagnosis. Hepatitis B surface antigen (HBsAg) combines with a lipid envelope to create the external virion shell, and hepatitis B core antigen (HBcAg) is complexed with virally encoded polymerase to form the internal virion shell that houses the viral genome.[9] Hepatitis B e antigen (HBeAg) is another important viral antigen that may have a role in evading the host immune system.[11] In order to infect its host, HBsAg binds the hepatocyte membrane and the virion is disassembled and transported across the membrane, where the virion reassembles and begins replication.[9] Once the HBV genome is released, it can undergo a series of modifications that lead to the formation of the stable, covalently closed circular DNA (cccDNA), which can occasionally integrate into the host's genome.[9] The stable cccDNA is used for viral replication and acts as a transcriptional template for HBV protein synthesis.

Once CHB is established, infection is characterized by the presence of different clinical phases in which viral replication and liver damage fluctuate. Four distinct clinical phases are

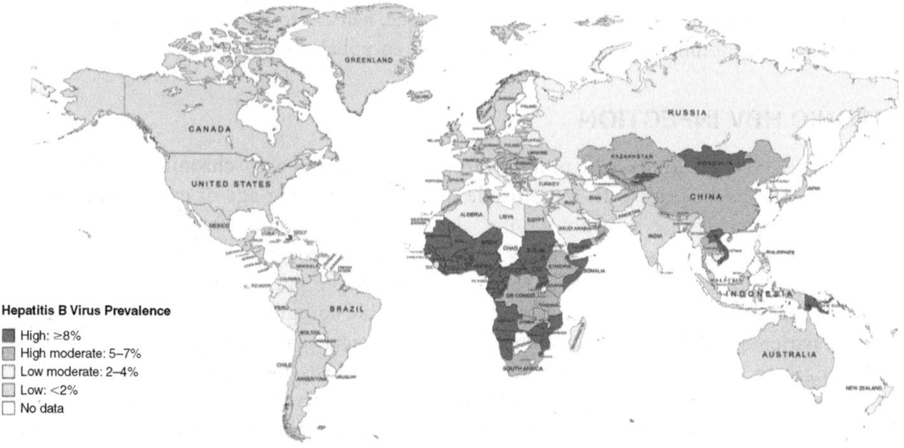

Figure 2.1 Map of global seroprevalence of hepatitis B virus. (Based on: Schweitzer A, Horn J, Mikolajczyk R, Krause G, Ott J. Estimations of worldwide prevalence of chronic hepatitis B virus infection: a systematic review of data published between 1965 and 2013. *Lancet*. 2015;386(10003):1546-1555.)

generally defined in patients and have been described on the basis of serum alanine aminotransferase (ALT) levels, HBV DNA levels, and the presence or absence of the viral antigen HBeAg in serum.[9,12] Overall, these phases reflect the natural history of CHB and are termed HBeAg-positive chronic infection (i.e., Immune Tolerant; IT), HBeAg-positive chronic hepatitis (i.e., Immune Active; IA), HBeAg-negative chronic infection (i.e., Inactive Carrier; IC), and HBeAg-negative chronic hepatitis (i.e., ENEG). Caution should be used when assessing these phases, as recent research shows differential immune and inflammatory patterns across phases.[13-15] Moreover, these phases fluctuate over the lifetime of a patient.

TRANSMISSION

Age of exposure to HBV is critical in influencing the progression to chronic infection. Exposure to the virus during birth or in the early years of life leads to chronic infection in approximately 90% of cases, while exposure during adulthood leads to chronicity in less than 5% of cases. Vertical transmission (infected mother to fetus or newborn) is the most common mechanism of HBV infection in children, occurring in 1% to 28% of pregnancies in endemic regions where HBeAg is prevalent, such as Asia.[16] Vertical transmission can occur in utero or at the time of birth, and when this occurs, the likelihood that the infected child will develop CHB is high (depending on the HBeAg status of the mother).[16] HBV can also be transmitted by coming into contact with infected bodily fluids such as blood (needle stick injuries, intravenous drug needle sharing) or through sexual contact. These forms of transmission are more frequent in areas of the world such as Latin America and Africa, where a large number of infected individuals are HBeAg negative.[17] Since infection is often asymptomatic, transmission is often propagated by individuals who are unaware of their HBV-positive status.[2]

Clinical Presentation

ACUTE HBV INFECTION

After exposure to HBV, the typical incubation period is 2 to 3 months but can range from 1 to 6 months.[18] Approximately two-thirds of patients with acute HBV infection are asymptomatic, while one-third will develop clinical signs and symptoms of acute hepatitis.[9] These symptoms range from mild constitutional symptoms (fever, fatigue, nausea) to fulminant liver failure (1%), characterized by abdominal pain, severe jaundice, and encephalopathy/coma.

CHRONIC HBV INFECTION

Approximately 5% of adults will progress from acute infection to chronic infection. The overall disease course varies with a multitude of factors including age of exposure, presence of underlying liver disease, consumption of alcohol, and other comorbid factors, including other co-infections such as HIV or HCV.[18] It is important to emphasize that chronic HBV rarely leads to symptoms until late in the disease. Therefore patients will be asymptomatic for years to decades, until the development of irreversible complications such as cirrhosis or HCC. In patients with HBV-associated cirrhosis the clinical syndrome is often characterized by the stigmata of cirrhosis. In early, compensated cirrhosis findings may include spider angiomas, palmar erythema, splenomegaly, and gynecomastia. In advanced or decompensated cirrhosis, ascites, jaundice, peripheral edema, encephalopathy, and gastrointestinal bleeding (gastric/esophageal varices, portal hypertensive gastropathy) are possible. A number of extrahepatic manifestations such as arthralgias, glomerulonephritis, and polyarteritis nodosa can occur as well.

Diagnosis

Laboratory assessment of HBV can be nuanced, as the serologic presence of certain antigens and antibodies changes over time. Broadly speaking, HBsAg is a marker of infection, "surface" antibody (anti-HBs) is a marker of immunity against HBV, and "core" antibody (anti-HBc) is a marker of exposure to HBV (IgM indicates acute exposure, IgG indicates previous exposure). During an acute infection, detection of HBsAg can occur as early as 2 weeks after exposure (in a previously negative individual). However, in some patients the incubation period can be as long as 6 months.

In patients who go on to clear the virus HBsAg levels typically fall and become undetectable by approximately 24 weeks. This period is referred to as the "window" period. During this period, it is difficult to establish the diagnosis of chronic HBV.[18] In general, chronic HBV infection is defined by patients with HBsAg levels that remain detectable for ≥6 months. Generally, these patients will express anti-HBc IgG. Acute HBV infection can be diagnosed by the presence of anti-HBc IgM in an individual with biochemical evidence of hepatitis (of note: anti-HBc IgM can also be positive during a flare). The presence of HBV DNA in a new acute hepatitis in the absence of anti-HBc IgM can aid in the diagnosis of acute HBV (as long as anti-hepatitis B core IgG is negative). Table 2.1 describes the different scenarios of HBV based on serological markers.

APPROACH TO INDIVIDUALS INFECTED WITH HBV

Due to the lack of symptoms, as detailed above, individuals diagnosed with chronic HBV should be evaluated with a thorough physical examination and undergo laboratory and imaging testing, depending on the resources available, to determine the need for treatment, screening, and prevention of complications. Moreover, immediate family members (significant others and children) and/or household contacts should also be screened for HBV. If a clear point of infection is not found in the history, screening of parents and siblings is also recommended.

Whenever possible, HBV-infected patients should be screened for HIV and HCV and, if available, HDV. Liver enzymes (ALT-GPT, AST-GOT, total bilirubin and alkaline phosphatase) should be obtained to evaluate for the presence of liver inflammation. Liver fibrosis scores, such as Fibrosis-4 (FIB4) and AST to Platelet Ratio Index (APRI), can be calculated using readily available laboratory testing such as ALT, AST, and platelet count.[19] It is also important to measure HBeAg or HBe antibody (anti-HBe) levels, as well as HBV DNA levels, to determine viral replication. Unfortunately, HBV DNA levels are often expensive and difficult to obtain in resource-limited settings. However, HBeAg and anti-HBe are easily measured via rapid testing kits, which are relatively inexpensive and are more available worldwide.[20] Liver ultrasonography can be helpful in identifying liver masses (concerning for HCC) and the presence of ascites (concerning for decompensated cirrhosis). Finally, a thorough physical examination should be performed to assess for stigmata of cirrhosis, such as spider angiomas, palmar erythema, abdominal distention, and jaundice.

TABLE 2.1 ■ **Serologic Markers During Different Stages of HBV Infection or Vaccination**

Stage of Infection	HBsAg	Anti-HBc IgM	Anti-HBc IgG	Anti-HBs
Acute Infection	+	+	-	-
"Window" Period	-	+	-	-
Chronic Infection	+	-	+	-
Resolved Infection	-	-	+	+
Vaccinated	-	-	-	+

While evaluation of CHB will vary by region and resource availability, at the very minimum, we recommend performing a liver ultrasound and checking ALT-GPT and bilirubin levels, some measure of replication marker (ideally HBV DNA, otherwise HBeAg or anti-HBe), and HIV serologies. We also advise obtaining platelet counts and calculating fibrosis scores. If resources allow, testing should be conducted for other co-infections (i.e., hepatitis C virus [HCV], hepatitis D virus [HDV] etc.), and more advanced liver fibrosis studies (such as elastography) should be performed.

In individuals with normal liver enzymes, and negative or very low HBV DNA, it is reasonable to defer antiviral therapy and to monitor AST/ALT every 6 to 12 months and HBV DNA levels every 12 months, if possible. Depending on patient age and HBV DNA levels, individuals will benefit from HCC surveillance using ultrasound.[21]

Finally, every patient should undergo HBV education, with emphasis on the deleterious effects of alcohol on the liver and the need to prevent transmission (using barrier protection during intercourse, vaccinating family members and significant others, informing their healthcare provider and dentist about their status, and not sharing nail clippers, razors, etc.).[2]

Treatment

ANTIVIRAL THERAPY

Current HBV treatments can control but usually do not cure the infection. Discussion with patients should stress the concept that treatment with oral medications should be undertaken for several years, if not for life. The two primary treatment options are nucleotide/nucleoside analogues and interferon (IFN) therapy. IFN therapy (injectable) can be curative in rare cases, but its complex side effect profile makes it a non-preferred option that should only be used in select cases and under the supervision of experienced providers.[22]

The decision-making process regarding which patients with CHB should receive treatment should be determined on a case-by-case basis, taking into account geographic location and available resources. Treatment of acute hepatitis B should be done only if needed (rarely) and in consultation with a specialist. Treatment guidelines differ subtly between the WHO and the American Association for the Study of Liver Diseases (AASLD), among others. Most guidelines recommend treatment when there is the presence of cirrhosis or when HBV DNA levels are high and there is evidence of active liver injury. Moreover, a large number of patients will fall into a category with either high viral replication or inflammation, but not both. Of note, most studies have assessed the benefit of treatment in North American, European, or Asian populations; data are lacking in African populations, making treatment decisions in this region complex and difficult.[23] Finally, the necessary resources for monitoring HBV treatment are often limited in multiple areas of the world. Initiation of treatment of any patient with HBV should be made in consultation with an experienced provider. Treatment duration is a complex decision, but most patients will need life-long antiviral therapy. However, approximately 5% of patients with CHB will clear the virus and may be able to discontinue treatment. Treatment recommendations for the WHO and the AASLD are provided below.

WHO HBV ANTIVIRAL TREATMENT INDICATIONS (2015)[24]

1. Individuals with evidence of cirrhosis, regardless of age or other testing characteristics
2. Individuals ≥ 30 years with abnormal liver function tests (LFTs) on three separate occasions during a 6- to 12-month period *and* HBV DNA>20,000 IU/mL (this condition is not needed in settings without access to HBV DNA testing)[25]
3. Individuals with HIV and a CD4 count ≤500 (cells/mm^2) (most experts recommend treatment in HIV co-infected patients, regardless of CD4 count)

AASLD HBV ANTIVIRAL TREATMENT INDICATIONS (2016, 2018)[10,21]

1. Adults with immune-active CHB, as defined below:
   a. ALT>2× upper limit of normal
   b. Significant histological disease + HBV DNA>2000 IU/mL if HBeAg negative *or* HBV DNA >20,000 IU/mL if HBeAg positive
2. Adults >40 years with immune-tolerant CHB (HBV DNA ≥1,000,000 IU/mL *and* biopsy showing significant necroinflammation or fibrosis)
3. Adults with CHB and cirrhosis
4. Children (2–18 years) with elevated ALT and measurable HBV DNA levels

A summary of recommended HBV antiviral therapies is provided in Table 2.2. Generic and relatively affordable versions of these drugs are now available in low- and middle-income countries ($50–350/patient/year).[24] Overall entecavir and tenofovir (either form) are preferred based on low resistance and good tolerability. Lamivudine may be effective for short treatment durations if there are no other local alternatives, but its resistance index is unfavorably high.[26] Prior to initiation of therapy, patients should be counseled on the potential benefits and side effects of treatment, the need for follow-up monitoring, and the importance of committing to long-term treatment.

Complications

HBV leads to the development of cirrhosis, which can lead to ascites and spontaneous bacterial peritonitis, esophageal varices and gastrointestinal bleeding, hepatic encephalopathy, coagulopathy, and other stigmata of cirrhosis. HBV can cause HCC indirectly through the induction of cirrhosis and directly via HBV genome integration.[27] HBV has also been implicated in a variety of autoimmune disorders such as membranoproliferative glomerulonephritis, cutaneous vasculitis, essential mixed cryoglobulinemia, and polyarteritis nodosa and has been associated with rheumatoid arthritis, polymyalgia rheumatica, and polymyositis in certain patients (although at a much lower rate than HCV).[28] Lastly, HBV predisposes individuals to co-infection with HDV, as HDV is dependent on HBV for viral replication. Co-infection with both viruses confers a greater risk of cirrhosis and HCC (cirrhosis, HCC, and HDV are all discussed separately in other chapters of the book).

HCC AND SURVEILLANCE

HBV is the leading cause of HCC in the world.[6,29] In the African continent HCC is a more dreaded complication of HBV than cirrhosis. The incidence of HCC in CHB is associated with

TABLE 2.2 ■ **Summary of Antiviral Therapy Guidelines**

1st-Line Antiviral Therapy	Treatment Population
Tenofovir disoproxil fumarate (TDF)	All adults and children ≥12 years
Tenofovir alafenamide (TAF)	Adults
Entecavir	Adults and children 2–11 years
PEG-IFN-α-2a	Adults
PEG-IFN-α-2b	Adults and children ≥1 year
2nd-line Antiviral Therapy	**Treatment Population**
Lamivudine	Adults and children ≥2 years
Adefovir	Adults and children ≥12 years
Telbivudine	Adults

the male sex, advanced age, early age of infection, HBV DNA viral load, family history of HCC, alcohol use, smoking use, and exposure to environmental toxins such as aflatoxins.[30,31] HBV is one of the few causes of HCC that can lead to cancer without first leading to cirrhosis (non-cirrhotic HCC), which occurs in approximately 20% of cases.[32] Therefore patients with HBV (age depending on region of the world) should be screened for HCC even in the absence of cirrhosis.[24,31]

Prevention

Given that HBV is rarely curable, prevention remains the most important tool in preventing the downstream complications of infection. HBV screening and vaccination of reproductive-age women who are planning to conceive is important.[16] In cases where a pregnant mother is not immune to HBV and does not have an active HBV infection, vaccination during pregnancy is safe and should be performed to prevent infection of the mother during her pregnancy. HBV screening should occur in the first trimester of pregnancy.

Without prophylaxis, the risk of vertical transmission of an infected mother to her newborn ranges from 20% to 85%.[33] This is variable depending on HBeAg positivity (HBeAg+ individuals have much higher rate of transmission) and HBV DNA levels. Newborns of infected mothers should be offered HBV vaccination at birth (or within 24 hours of birth) because this can reduce risk of infection by 80%.[34] Administering hepatitis B immunoglobulin (HBIG) in conjunction with the HBV vaccine has also been shown to reduce infection rates in newborns even further and is currently recommended, if available.[35] In addition to HBV vaccination at birth, the WHO also recommends antiviral (i.e., tenofovir) prophylaxis for pregnant women with active HBV and with a DNA viral load (VL) ≥200,000 IU.[36] Treatment of this population should be considered after 20 weeks and done in consultation with an expert in the field.

In adults the risk of chronic infection is much lower; however, given the serious downstream clinical sequelae of infection, and the absence of a definitive cure, prevention is essential to reduce global morbidity and mortality.[37] All children and adults should be fully vaccinated (two or three doses depending on the vaccine brand and type). Table 2.3 shows a summary of important preventive measures against HBV infection.

TABLE 2.3 ■ **Summary of Preventive Measures Against Hepatitis B Virus Infection**

Preventive Modality	Comment
Prevention of Vertical Transmission	
Newborn HBV Vaccination	First dose at birth or in first 24 hours of life (should also complete the whole vaccine series)
Newborn HBIG*	At birth or in first 12 hours of life
Maternal Tenofovir Prophylaxis**	Week 28 of pregnancy until birth
Prevention in Children/Adults	
HBV Vaccination	All children and adults should receive complete vaccine series

*If HBIG is unavailable, at-birth vaccination significantly decreases HBV transmission.
**Indicated when maternal DNA VL ≥200,000 IU *or* HBeAg+ (when VL testing unavailable).

References

1. Howell J, Pedrana A, Schroeder SE, et al. A global investment framework for the elimination of hepatitis B. *J Hepatol.* 2021;74(3):535-549. doi:10.1016/j.jhep.2020.09.013.
2. World Health Organization. *Hepatitis B Fact Sheet.* Accessed February 2, 2022. Available at: https://www.who.int/news-room/fact-sheets/detail/hepatitis-b.
3. Asrani SK, Devarbhavi H, Eaton J, Kamath PS. Burden of liver diseases in the world. *J Hepatol.* 2019;70(1):151-171. doi:10.1016/j.jhep.2018.09.014.
4. Veronese P, Dodi I, Esposito S, Indolfi G. Prevention of vertical transmission of hepatitis B virus infection. *World J Gastroenterol.* 2021;27(26):4182-4193. doi:10.3748/wjg.v27.i26.4182.
5. Cheemerla S, Balakrishnan M. Global epidemiology of chronic liver disease. *Clin Liver Dis (Hoboken).* 2021;17(5):365-370. doi:10.1002/cld.1061.
6. El-Serag HB. Epidemiology of viral hepatitis and hepatocellular carcinoma. *Gastroenterology.* 2012;142(6):1264-1273.e1. doi:10.1053/j.gastro.2011.12.061.
7. Mokdad AA, Lopez AD, Shahraz S, et al. Liver cirrhosis mortality in 187 countries between 1980 and 2010: a systematic analysis. *BMC Med.* 2014;12:145. doi:10.1186/s12916-014-0145-y.
8. Global Hepatitis Report 2017. Geneva: World Health Organization; 2017. Licence: CC BY-NC-SA 3.0 IGO.
9. Liang TJ. Hepatitis B: the virus and disease. *Hepatology.* 2009;49(suppl 5):S13-S21. doi:10.1002/hep.22881.
10. Terrault NA, Lok ASF, McMahon BJ, et al. Update on prevention, diagnosis, and treatment of chronic hepatitis B: AASLD 2018 hepatitis B guidance. *Hepatology.* 2018;67(4):1560-1599. doi:10.1002/hep.29800.
11. Tian Y, Kuo CF, Akbari O, Ou JH. Maternal-derived hepatitis B virus e antigen alters macrophage function in offspring to drive viral persistence after vertical transmission. *Immunity.* 2016;44(5):1204-1214. doi:10.1016/j.immuni.2016.04.008.
12. Buti M, Riveiro-Barciela M, Rodríguez-Frías F, Tabernero D, Esteban R. Role of biomarkers in guiding cure of viral hepatitis B. *Semin Liver Dis.* 2020;40(1):49-60. doi:10.1055/s-0039-3401031.
13. Hou J, Brouwer WP, Kreefft K, et al. Unique intrahepatic transcriptomics profiles discriminate the clinical phases of a chronic HBV infection. *PLoS One.* 2017;12(6):e0179920. doi:10.1371/journal.pone.0179920.
14. Rico Montanari N, Ramirez R, Van Buuren N, et al. Transcriptomic analysis of livers of inactive carriers of hepatitis B virus with distinct expression of hepatitis B surface antigen. *J Infect Dis.* 2022;225(6):1081-1090. doi:10.1093/infdis/jiab381.
15. Montanari NR, Ramírez R, Aggarwal A, et al. Multi-parametric analysis of human livers reveals variation in intrahepatic inflammation across phases of chronic hepatitis B infection. *J Hepatol.* 2022;77(2):332-343. doi:10.1016/j.jhep.2022.02.016.
16. Mavilia MG, Wu GY. Mechanisms and prevention of vertical transmission in chronic viral hepatitis. *J Clin Transl Hepatol.* 2017;5(2):119-129. doi:10.14218/jcth.2016.00067.
17. Fattovich G, Bortolotti F, Donato F. Natural history of chronic hepatitis B: special emphasis on disease progression and prognostic factors. *J Hepatol.* 2008;48(2):335-352. doi:10.1016/j.jhep.2007.11.011.
18. Seto WK, Lo YR, Pawlotsky JM, Yuen MF. Chronic hepatitis B virus infection. *Lancet.* 2018;392(10161):2313-2324. doi:10.1016/S0140-6736(18)31865-8.
19. Salomone F, Micek A, Godos J. Simple scores of fibrosis and mortality in patients with NAFLD: a systematic review with meta-analysis. *J Clin Med.* 2018;7(8):219. doi:10.3390/jcm7080219.
20. Leathers JS, Pisano MB, Re V, et al. Evaluation of rapid diagnostic tests for assessment of hepatitis B in resource-limited settings. *Ann Glob Health.* 2019;85(1):98. doi:10.5334/aogh.2562.
21. Terrault NA, Bzowej NH, Chang KM, Hwang JP, Jonas MM, Murad MH. AASLD guidelines for treatment of chronic hepatitis B. *Hepatology.* 2016;63(1):261-283. doi:10.1002/hep.28156.
22. Yuen MF, Chen DS, Dusheiko GM, et al. Hepatitis B virus infection. *Nat Rev Dis Primers.* 2018;4:18035. doi:10.1038/nrdp.2018.35.
23. Chang TT, Gish RG, de Man R, et al. A comparison of entecavir and lamivudine for HBeAg-positive chronic hepatitis B. *N Engl J Med.* 2006;354(10):1001-1010. doi:10.1056/NEJMoa051285.
24. *Guidelines for the Prevention, Care and Treatment of Persons With Chronic Hepatitis B Infection.* Geneva: World Health Organization (WHO); March 2015.

25. Marcellin P, Heathcote EJ, Buti M, et al. Tenofovir disoproxil fumarate versus adefovir dipivoxil for chronic hepatitis B. *N Engl J Med.* 2008;359(23):2442-2455. doi:10.1056/NEJMoa0802878.
26. Warner N, Locarnini S. Mechanisms of hepatitis B virus resistance development. *Intervirology.* 2014;57(3-4):218-224. doi:10.1159/000360940.
27. Udompap P, Kim WR. Development of hepatocellular carcinoma in patients with suppressed viral replication: changes in risk over time. *Clin Liver Dis (Hoboken).* 2020;15(2):85-90. doi:10.1002/cld.904.
28. Maya R, Gershwin ME, Shoenfeld Y. Hepatitis B virus (HBV) and autoimmune disease. *Clin Rev Allergy Immunol.* 2008;34(1):85-102. doi:10.1007/s12016-007-8013-6.
29. Anugwom CM, Allaire M, Akbar SMF, et al. Hepatitis B-related hepatocellular carcinoma: surveillance strategy directed by immune-epidemiology. *Hepatoma Res.* 2021;7:23. doi:10.20517/2394-5079.2021.06.
30. Chen CJ, Iloeje UH, Yang HI. Long-term outcomes in hepatitis B: the REVEAL-HBV study. *Clin Liver Dis.* 2007;11(4):797-816, viii. doi:10.1016/j.cld.2007.08.005.
31. Marrero JA, Kulik LM, Sirlin CB, et al. Diagnosis, staging, and management of hepatocellular carcinoma: 2018 Practice Guidance by the American Association for the Study of Liver Diseases. *Hepatology.* 2018;68(2):723-750. doi:10.1002/hep.29913.
32. Yi D, Wen-Ping W, Lee WJ, et al. Hepatocellular carcinoma in the non-cirrhotic liver. *Clin Hemorheol Microcirc.* 2021;80(4):423-436. doi:10.3233/ch-211309.
33. Schillie S, Vellozzi C, Reingold A, et al. Prevention of hepatitis B virus infection in the United States: recommendations of the Advisory Committee on immunization practices. *MMWR Recomm Rep.* 2018;67(1):1-31. doi:10.15585/mmwr.rr6701a1.
34. Schillie S, Walker T, Veselsky S, et al. Outcomes of infants born to women infected with hepatitis B. *Pediatrics.* 2015;135(5):e1141-e1147. doi:10.1542/peds.2014-3213.
35. Poland GA, Jacobson RM. Clinical practice: prevention of hepatitis B with the hepatitis B vaccine. *N Engl J Med.* 2004;351(27):2832-2838. doi:10.1056/NEJMcp041507.
36. *Hepatitis: Preventing Mother-to-Child Transmission of the Hepatitis B Virus.* World Health Organization (WHO). Accessed February 2, 2022. https://www.who.int/news-room/questions-and-answers/item/hepatitis-preventing-mother-to-child-transmission-of-the-hepatitis-b-virus
37. Hyams KC. Risks of chronicity following acute hepatitis B virus infection: a review. *Clin Infect Dis.* 1995;20(4):992-1000. doi:10.1093/clinids/20.4.992.

CHAPTER 3

Hepatitis C Infection

Amir Sultan Seid ■ Abate Bane Shewaye

KEY POINTS

- Hepatitis C is a common cause of chronic hepatitis associated with a significant global burden
- It is mainly transmitted by percutaneous route with contact from sharp objects and blood products
- Most patients are asymptomatic, and diagnosis is made by serologic tests followed by virologic confirmatory tests
- Extrahepatic manifestations (i.e., cryoglobulinemia, lichen planus, etc.) are more common than in other forms of viral hepatitis
- Treatment involves oral directly acting antiviral agents, with high success rates of cure

Introduction

Hepatitis C virus (HCV) is a hepatotropic viral hepatitis affecting the liver.[1] It results in chronic hepatitis and associated life-threatening complications such as decompensated cirrhosis and hepatocellular carcinoma (HCC). Although not vaccine preventable, it can now be successfully treated with newly discovered oral directly acting antivirals (DAAs).

Virology

HCV is a single-stranded RNA virus belonging to the class of Flaviviridae, with a small structure and a helical viral genome.[2] There is a significant genetic variation of the viral genome, likely related to the high rate of mutations seen during its replication process. Up to a 5% difference in the viral genome is considered quasispecies, and 30% variation is generally regarded as a genotype.[3] Such a degree of genetic content variation has made the development of vaccines difficult so far despite several trials. There are seven major genotypes (1–7) of the virus with varying global distribution and response rates for therapy.[4]

TRANSMISSION

The commonest route of transmission is percutaneous, that is, bloodborne. HCV is mainly transmitted from person to person through shared sharp objects such as unsafe needle injections, reused or inadequately sterilized medical equipment, and traditional healing practices, like scarification. Blood transfusion used to be a significant contributor to HCV transmission prior to mandatory universal screening.[5] Unfortunately, in low-income settings screening before transfusion is sometimes performed via non–WHO-accredited standards, and the threat for HCV transmission via blood transfusion remains present.[6] Historical cohort effects of transmission in relation to vaccination and treatment campaigns (e.g., trypanosomiasis in west Africa[7] and schistosomiasis in Egypt[8]) have been reported as modes of large-scale transmission. Non-percutaneous methods of transmission like sexual transmission, albeit much less common when compared to hepatitis B, also play a role, particularly in the setting of multiple sexual encounters.[9] Additionally, vertical transmission from a mother to a newborn is possible yet rare, especially in the setting of HIV coinfection and lack of proper obstetric care.[10]

EPIDEMIOLOGY

According to WHO data 2021, globally, an estimated 58 million people have chronic hepatitis C virus infection, with about 1.5 million new infections occurring per year.[11] There is a trend toward decreasing prevalence with the provision of curative DAA therapies, as evidenced by the fact that the 2017 WHO global hepatitis report showed that 71 million people were actively infected with the virus.[12] The bulk of the decrement is from the more affluent countries, and efforts are underway to reflect that across other parts of the world.

In Africa an estimated 9 million people are infected with the virus. According to the WHO data, in southeast Asia and Western Pacific region, 10 million people are considered chronically infected, while it is estimated that 5 million people are chronically infected in WHO America regions.[11]

Historically, the highest seroprevalence of HCV was reported in Egypt in 1996, where up to 24% of the population in the Nile delta had a positive antibody result.[13] This is likely due to iatrogenic transmission of the infection during the eradication of schistosomiasis using injectable drugs via reusable needles and syringes in the 1950s.[8] Subsequently, a large-scale national testing and treatment program led to a significant decrease in the prevalence of HCV in the country.[14] A recent study that screened more than 48 million people in the country showed that the prevalence in the country dropped to 4.6%, with that of the Nile delta dropping to 8.4 %.[15] In the Sub-Saharan Africa context relatively higher prevalence of the infection is reported from Benin (3.8%) and Cameroon (4.9%).[16] In Latin America the overall prevalence is low (approximately 1%) with still limited access to therapy.[17]

Clinical Presentation

Acute hepatitis C is asymptomatic in 80% of cases. A small proportion of patients could present with nonspecific symptoms, including fatigue, joint pain, and nausea, up to 8 to 12 weeks after infection. Most symptomatic patients have a limited clinical course, and symptoms resolve with no complications. Nonetheless, the chance of chronic HCV infection is very high, roaming around 55% to 85%.[18]

Chronic hepatitis C infection is also asymptomatic in most patients, while some might exhibit nonspecific symptoms like fatigue, arthralgias, nausea, and lack of concentration. Among patients with chronic HCV infection, up to 50% can develop cirrhosis according to one study[19]; however, the rate might be lower in different groups of patients.[20] If untreated, the possibility of developing HCC is 1% to 3% per year in patients who have developed cirrhosis.[21]

Once patients develop cirrhosis, they can progressively advance to decompensation over a relatively short period, usually ranging from 5 to 15 years.[22] Patients with decompensated cirrhosis might exhibit nonspecific fatigue, decrement in appetite, abdominal swelling from ascites, upper GI bleeding, and features of hepatic encephalopathy.

Some patients present with extrahepatic manifestations.[23] This is secondary to a continuous, yet ineffective, immune response toward the virus. Strong associations have been established with lichen planus, cryoglobulinemia, and porphyria cutanea tarda (Figure 3.1) (Table 3.1). In addition, likely relationships with type 2DM, membranoproliferative glomerulonephritis, sicca

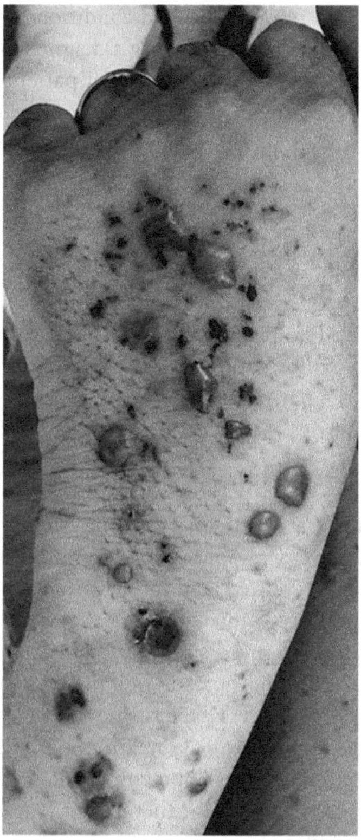

Figure 3.1 Porphyria cutanea tarda (PCT) in an Ethiopian with hepatitis C infection. (Courtesy of Dr. Kassa Tameru, Addis, Ababa, Ethiopia.)

TABLE 3.1 ■ **Extraintestinal Manifestations of Hepatitis C**

Generalized	Fatigue
Renal	Membranoproliferative Glomerulonephritis
Hematologic and Immunologic	Essential Mixed Cryoglobulinemia, Lymphoma, Polyarteritis nodosa, Idiopathic Thrombocytopenic Purpura
Dermatologic	Porphyria Cutanea Tarda, Lichen Planus, Necrolytic Acral Erythema, Sjögren Syndrome
Endocrine	Diabetes Mellitus, Thyroiditis

syndrome, and other uncommon conditions have been reported. It is vital to have a high index of suspicion in patients with HCV diagnosis presenting with vague symptoms.

Diagnosis

As most HCV infections remain asymptomatic, diagnosis is usually made incidentally. Screening for hepatitis C is serologic, using ELISA against the HCVAb. In resource-limited settings the commonest available test is the rapid diagnostic test developed as a point-of-care test. A serologic diagnosis of HCV should be confirmed by RNA tests, which can be of qualitative or quantitative type. However, this might have cost implications as repeated tests are needed to confirm the infection and quantify the virus.[24] In resource-limited conditions conducting a serologic test followed by a quantitative RNA test is justifiable. Making a diagnosis of active hepatitis C infection with no RNA test is inappropriate as up to 15% to 45% of patients might not be viremic. Non-viremic patients are not eligible for treatment since they do not harbor the infection actively (their immune systems effectively controlled and eliminated the virus), and patients should be counseled as such.

Evaluation of livers with hepatitis C infection is usually done using ultrasound, a tool commonly available in resource-limited settings. Ultrasound can aid in making a diagnosis of cirrhosis; however, the sensitivity of doing so is limited as it misses the early stages of cirrhosis.[25] Alternatively, noninvasive markers of liver fibrosis can be utilized in making a diagnosis of significant fibrosis and cirrhosis.[26] AST to platelet ratio index (APRI) and FIB-4 are common tests used in this regard and can provide information about degree of fibrosis with relatively acceptable accuracy. Transient elastography is a newer and very helpful tool to assess liver fibrosis. However, its availability in low-income countries is currently limited.

Management

In the early days hepatitis C infection was treated with interferon therapy. Pegylated interferon and interferon/ribavirin therapy have a response rate of around 50-70%, dependent on HCV genotype.[27] Several side effects were reported, and intolerance was a major issue in management. Moreover, treatment administration was difficult as the drugs were injectable.

The management of patients has improved significantly in the past decade with the advent of oral direct-acting antivirals (DAAs). The goal of therapy is a sustained virological response (SVR), which is defined as a negative HCV RNA 12 weeks after completion of therapy.[28] SVR is considered a cure in the treatment of hepatitis C treatment as it is associated with a decrement in all-cause mortality, liver-related death, development of HCC, and liver failure. Globally, all patients with detectable viral RNA are eligible for therapy, although urgency for treatment might not be similar across all patient profiles.

DAAs are generally classified as protease inhibitors (-previrs) that inhibit the NS3 protein and NS5 inhibitors (-buvirs). Clinical importance of such distinction lies in the fact that protease inhibitors need to be avoided in situations where there is significant liver impairment. The classification and drug types are presented below (Table 3.2).

In resource-limited settings therapy can be considered using pan-genotypic drugs, therefore avoiding the need for further genotype testing, which is costly.[24] Hitherto, the treatment of hepatitis C has been riddled with several nuances of therapy approaches, some of which are very complex. Hence in resource-limited settings the recommended approach to therapy is one with

TABLE 3.2 ■ **General Class of Drugs for HCV Treatment**

NS3/4A (Protease) Inhibitors		Glecaprevir, Grazoprevir, Voxilaprevir, paritaprevir, Simeprevir
NS5A Inhibitors		Velpatasvir, Ledipasvir, Ombitasvir, Daclatasvir, Pibrentasvir, Elbasvir
NS5B Inhibitors	Nucleotide Analogue	Sofosbuvir
	Non-Nucleoside Analogue	Dasabuvir
Pan-Genotypic Drugs		
Sofosbuvir/Velpatasvir		
Glecaprevir/Pibrentasvir		
Sofosbuvir/Velpatasvir/Voxilaprevir		
Sofosbuvir/Daclatasvir		

a simple yet effective approach that is also cost-effective. Assessment of cirrhosis should also be done, and WHO recommends using cheaper non-invasive markers of liver fibrosis like APRI score and sonography.[24]

Currently, there are two widely used pan-genotypic drugs, details of which are outlined in Table 3.2. These are combinations of sofosbuvir/velpatasvir and glecaprevir/pebrintasvir.[29,30] Both regimens achieve a high rate of SVR in treatment-naïve patients with no prior therapy. The combination of sofosbuvir and daclatasvir has been used in Egypt and has shown significantly high rates of SVR.[31] However, the efficacy of this regimen use across the world is inconsistent. These drugs consist of an all-oral regimen, with recommended treatment for 2 to 3 months (depending on specific cases), and are very well tolerated.

Historically during the era of interferon therapy, there were different milestones of therapy where RNA levels were assessed in different weeks of therapy. With DAAs, treatment monitoring of RNA is no longer indicated during therapy, as it is not predictive of SVR rates after completion of treatment.[32] In addition, most patients do not require monitoring of laboratory tests as these drugs are safe and are not associated with organ impairment. For patients with comorbidities or HBV coinfection or those who are taking other drugs, specific function tests monitoring is recommended. In addition, cirrhotic patients taking ribavirin/DAA combination (used sometimes in specific cases with cirrhosis) need to have a serial evaluation of complete blood count (CBC) as ribavirin is associated with anemia. Overall the effectiveness of DAAs in the treatment of HCV is very high even in limited resource setups.[31,33,34]

In patients with failed HCV treatment evaluation should be directed toward ascertaining adherence to treatment regimen and assessing potential drug-drug interaction. Evaluating for resistance might be costly in resource-limited countries, but checking the genotype status of the patient if previously not done can be considered a cheaper option. Treatment can be planned subsequently with alternative DAAs. The pan-genotypic combination of sofosbuvir/velpatasvir/voxilaprevir has been shown to have a superior outcome in patients with prior failure to DAA therapy.[35] Alternatively, for those with prior sofosbuvir-based therapy, glecaprevir/pibrentasvir can be used as second-line therapy. In addition, therapy can be planned with genotype-specific regimens in consultation with an experienced physician in the care of hepatitis C–infected patients. A difficult scenario might be patients with genotype 3 infection with prior treatment failure and cirrhosis, where the choice of therapy might require sofosbuvir/velpatasvir/voxilaprevir and ribavirin.

Special Population of Patients and Public Health Considerations. In patients with hepatitis B and C coinfection there is a possibility of hepatitis B reactivation with the treatment of hepatitis C.[36] In the tropics, where these two conditions are prevalent, the possibility of such a scenario needs to be recognized, and patients need to be assessed for dual infection. In patients with HCV/HIV coinfection the emphasis is on drug-drug interaction, and monitoring is recommended.[24] With other comorbidities, like chronic kidney disease, the safety of sofosbuvir-based treatments needs to be weighed against the potential risk, especially in those with advanced kidney disease.

WHO aims to eliminate hepatitis C infection in the near future, and large-scale HCV treatment programs are being implemented in different countries. In Egypt significant progress has been shown with screening, confirmatory testing, and treating patients at a population level.[15] Globally there are segments of the population identified where elimination might be difficult, including people who inject drugs (PWIDs), people in prison, men who have sex with men, sex workers, and indigenous populations in certain countries. A particular strategy of HCV micro-elimination is being implemented in many affluent countries to address these groups of patients.[37] Regardless, there is a need to scale up treatment for hepatitis C in resource-limited countries, where the proportion of undiagnosed and untreated patients is still high.

References

1. Eorg G, Auer ML, Ruce B, Alker DW. Hepatitis C virus infection. *N Engl J Med.* 2009;345(1):41-52. doi:10.1056/NEJM200107053450107.
2. Roger S, Ducancelle A, Le Guillou-Guillemette H, Gaudy C, Lunel F. HCV virology and diagnosis. *Clin Res Hepatol Gastroenterol.* 2021;45(3):101626. doi:10.1016/J.CLINRE.2021.101626.
3. Tsukiyama-Kohara K, Kohara M. Hepatitis C virus: viral quasispecies and genotypes. *Int J Mol Sci.* 2017;19(1):23. doi:10.3390/IJMS19010023.
4. Smith DB, Bukh J, Kuiken C, et al. Expanded classification of hepatitis C virus into 7 genotypes and 67 subtypes: updated criteria and genotype assignment web resource. *Hepatology.* 2014;59(1):318-327. doi:10.1002/HEP.26744.
5. Alter HJ, Purcell RH, Shih JW, et al. Detection of antibody to hepatitis C virus in prospectively followed transfusion recipients with acute and chronic non-A, non-B hepatitis. *N Engl J Med.* 1989;321(22): 1494-1500. doi:10.1056/NEJM198911303212202.
6. Sonderup MW, Afihene M, Ally R, et al. Hepatitis C in sub-Saharan Africa: the current status and recommendations for achieving elimination by 2030. *Lancet Gastroenterol Hepatol.* 2017;2(12):910-919. doi:10.1016/S2468-1253(17)30249-2.
7. Njouom R, Nerrienet E, Dubois M, et al. The hepatitis C virus epidemic in Cameroon: genetic evidence for rapid transmission between 1920 and 1960. *Infect Genet Evol.* 2007;7(3):361-367. doi:10.1016/J.MEEGID.2006.10.003.
8. Frank C, Mohamed MK, Strickland GT, et al. The role of parenteral antischistosomal therapy in the spread of hepatitis C virus in Egypt. *Lancet.* 2000;355(9207):887-891. doi:10.1016/S0140-6736(99)06527-7.
9. Terrault NA, Dodge JL, Murphy EL, et al. Sexual transmission of hepatitis C virus among monogamous heterosexual couples: the HCV partners study. *Hepatology.* 2013;57(3):881-889. doi:10.1002/HEP.26164.
10. Benova L, Mohamoud YA, Calvert C, Abu-Raddad LJ. Vertical transmission of hepatitis C virus: systematic review and meta-analysis. *Clin Infect Dis.* 2014;59(6):765-773. doi:10.1093/CID/CIU447.
11. WHO. *Hepatitis C.* Avilable at: https://www.who.int/news-room/fact-sheets/detail/hepatitis-c. Accessed December 27, 2021.
12. Web Annex B. *WHO Estimates of the Prevalence and Incidence of Hepatitis C Virus Infection by WHO Region, 2015 Centre for Disease Analysis.* 2018. Available at: http://apps.who.int/bookorders. Accessed December 27, 2021.
13. Abdel-Aziz F, Habib M, Mohamed MK, et al. Hepatitis C virus (HCV) infection in a community in the Nile Delta: population description and HCV prevalence. *Hepatology.* 2000;32(1):111-115. doi:10.1053/JHEP.2000.8438.
14. Abdel-Razek W, Hassany M, El-Sayed MH, et al. Hepatitis C virus in Egypt: interim report from the world's largest national program. *Clin Liver Dis.* 2019;14(6):203-206. doi:10.1002/CLD.868.
15. Waked I, Esmat G, Elsharkawy A, et al. Screening and treatment program to eliminate hepatitis C in Egypt. *N Engl J Med.* 2020;382(12):1166-1174. doi:10.1056/NEJMSR1912628/SUPPL_FILE/NEJMSR1912628_DISCLOSURES.PDF.
16. Riou J, Aït Ahmed M, Blake A, et al. Hepatitis C virus seroprevalence in adults in Africa: a systematic review and meta-analysis. *J Viral Hepat.* 2016;23(4):244-255. doi:10.1111/jvh.12481.
17. Roblero JP, Arab JP, Mezzano G, Mendizabal M. Hepatitis C virus infection: what are we currently doing in Latin America about WHO's proposals for 2030? *Clin Liver Dis.* 2021;18(2):72-75. doi:10.1002/CLD.1084.
18. Grebely J, Page K, Sacks-Davis R, et al. The effects of female sex, viral genotype, and IL28B genotype on spontaneous clearance of acute hepatitis C virus infection. *Hepatology.* 2014;59(1):109-120. doi:10.1002/HEP.26639.
19. Tong MJ, El-Farra NS, Reikes AR, Co RL. Clinical outcomes after transfusion-associated hepatitis C. *N Engl J Med.* 1995;332(22):1463-1466. doi:10.1056/NEJM199506013322202.
20. Thein HH, Yi Q, Dore GJ, Krahn MD. Estimation of stage-specific fibrosis progression rates in chronic hepatitis C virus infection: a meta-analysis and meta-regression. *Hepatology.* 2008;48(2):418-431. doi:10.1002/HEP.22375.
21. Westbrook RH, Dusheiko G. Natural history of hepatitis C. *J Hepatol.* 2014;61(suppl 1):S58-S68. doi:10.1016/J.JHEP.2014.07.012.

22. Fattovich G, Giustina G, Degos F, et al. Morbidity and mortality in compensated cirrhosis type C: a retrospective follow-up study of 384 patients. *Gastroenterology*. 1997;112(2):463-472. doi:10.1053/GAST.1997.V112.PM9024300.
23. El-Serag HB, Hampel H, Yeh C, Rabeneck L. Extrahepatic manifestations of hepatitis C among United States male veterans. *Hepatology*. 2002;36(6):1439-1445. doi:10.1053/JHEP.2002.37191.
24. World Health Organization. *Global Hepatitis Programme. Guidelines for the care and treatment of persons diagnosed with chronic hepatitis C virus infection*. 2018. https://www.who.int/publications/i/item/9789241550345. Accessed March 24, 2023.
25. Šimonovský V. The diagnosis of cirrhosis by high resolution ultrasound of the liver surface. *Br J Radiol*. 1999;72(853):29-34. doi:10.1259/BJR.72.853.10341686.
26. Wai CT, Greenson JK, Fontana RJ, et al. A simple noninvasive index can predict both significant fibrosis and cirrhosis in patients with chronic hepatitis C. *Hepatology*. 2003;38(2):518-526. doi:10.1053/JHEP.2003.50346.
27. McHutchison JG, Gordon SC, Schiff ER, et al. Interferon alfa-2b alone or in combination with ribavirin as initial treatment for chronic hepatitis C. Hepatitis Interventional Therapy Group. *N Engl J Med*. 1998;339(21):1485-1492. doi:10.1056/NEJM199811193392101.
28. Simmons B, Saleem J, Hill A, Riley RD, Cooke GS. Risk of late relapse or reinfection with hepatitis C virus after achieving a sustained virological response: a systematic review and meta-analysis. *Clin Infect Dis*. 2016;62(6):683-694. doi:10.1093/CID/CIV948.
29. Everson GT, Towner WJ, Davis MN, et al. Sofosbuvir with velpatasvir in treatment-naive noncirrhotic patients with genotype 1 to 6 hepatitis C virus infection: a randomized trial. *Ann Intern Med*. 2015;163(11):818-826. doi:10.7326/M15-1000.
30. Forns X, Lee SS, Valdes J, et al. Glecaprevir plus pibrentasvir for chronic hepatitis C virus genotype 1, 2, 4, 5, or 6 infection in adults with compensated cirrhosis (EXPEDITION-1): a single-arm, open-label, multicentre phase 3 trial. *Lancet Infect Dis*. 2017;17(10):1062-1068. doi:10.1016/S1473-3099(17)30496-6.
31. Elsharkawy A, El-Raziky M, El-Akel W, et al. Planning and prioritizing direct-acting antivirals treatment for HCV patients in countries with limited resources: lessons from the Egyptian experience. *J Hepatol*. 2018;68(4):691-698. doi:10.1016/J.JHEP.2017.11.034.
32. Sidharthan S, Kohli A, Sims Z, et al. Utility of hepatitis C viral load monitoring on direct-acting antiviral therapy. *Clin Infect Dis*. 2015;60(12):1743-1751. doi:10.1093/CID/CIV170.
33. Sultan A, Bane A, Braimoh G, Debes JD. Treatment of hepatitis C genotypes 1 to 5 in sub-Saharan Africa using direct-acting antivirals. *Am J Trop Med Hyg*. 2020;103(5):2083-2084. doi:10.4269/ajtmh.20-0367.
34. Lobato CM de O, Codes L, Silva GF, et al. Direct antiviral therapy for treatment of hepatitis C: a real-world study from Brazil. *Ann Hepatol*. 2019;18(6):849-854. doi:10.1016/J.AOHEP.2019.08.001.
35. Bourlière M, Gordon SC, Flamm SL, et al. Sofosbuvir, velpatasvir, and voxilaprevir for previously treated HCV infection. *N Engl J Med*. 2017;376(22):2134-2146. doi:10.1056/NEJMOA1613512.
36. Serper M, Forde KA, Kaplan DE. Rare clinically significant hepatic events and hepatitis B reactivation occur more frequently following rather than during direct-acting antiviral therapy for chronic hepatitis C: data from a national US cohort. *J Viral Hepat*. 2018;25(2):187-197. doi:10.1111/JVH.12784.
37. Lazarus JV, Wiktor S, Colombo M, Thursz M. Micro-elimination—A path to global elimination of hepatitis C. *J Hepatol*. 2017;67(4):665-666. doi:10.1016/J.JHEP.2017.06.033/ATTACHMENT/8DE647F0-FF6E-4158-938C-028636A12F85/DISCLOSURES.PDF.

CHAPTER 4

Hepatitis Delta Virus

Ifeorah M. Ijeoma ■ Yusuf Musa

KEY POINTS

- Hepatitis delta virus (HDV) is a satellite of hepatitis B virus (HBV) and requires the HBV envelope protein for its assembly and transmission.
- Although countries affected by HBV infection in many parts of the world are well identified, data on HDV infection are still scarce.
- HDV is one of the smallest viral agents known to cause human disease, yet it is responsible for the most severe form of viral hepatitis.
- HDV infection may occur concurrently with HBV in a previously healthy subject in a co-infection pattern or may affect persons with chronic HBV as superinfection with an accelerated risk of cirrhosis and hepatocellular carcinoma (HCC) compared to HBV monoinfection.
- HDV surveillance has been suboptimal especially in middle- and low-income countries, thereby masking its actual burden in these settings.
- Prevention of HDV infection is best achieved by prompt implementation of measures aimed at HBV control. Current treatments for HDV are suboptimal.

Introduction

Hepatitis delta virus (HDV), a member of the *Delta virus* genus (Kolmyoviridea family), is a distinct RNA virus associated with severe forms of viral hepatitis. It was discovered over four decades ago by Rizzetto et al.[1] among patients with chronic hepaittis B virus (CHB) infection. Originally assumed to be another antigen of HBV, it was later clarified as a defective virus that required HBV envelop proteins (HBsAg) to establish a successful infection. Due to its dependency on HBV, both viruses share similar routes of transmission. The virion is a small spherical particle of about 36 nm in diameter containing the ribonucleoprotein (RNP) coated with HBsAg. The genome is a circular, single-stranded negative-sense RNA that is about 1700 bp in size.[2] The antigenome encodes the sole protein of the virus (HDAg), which exists in two isoforms, namely small (S-HDAg/p24) and large (L-HDAg/p27) proteins.

HDV Life Cycle

The hepatocytes remain the only natural cells susceptible to HDV infection, although the virus can be grown in vitro using primary human hepatocytes and HepaRG cell lines.[3] Notably, HDV can effectively replicate in any animal cell if the entry restriction placed on it by HBV dependency is bypassed via transfection. HDV life cycle can be summarized as follows[2] (Figure 4.1):

1. Using the HBsAg, HDV attaches to the cell surface receptors.
2. The virus enters the hepatocyte by endocytosis and releases its genome into the cytoplasm. Unlike other human RNA viruses, HDV does not encode an RNA-dependent RNA

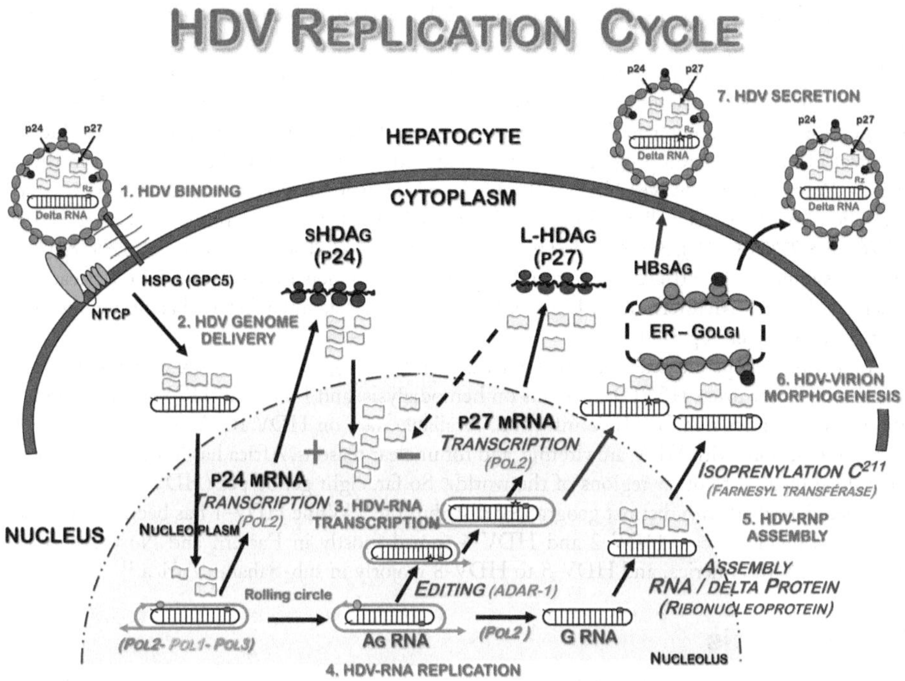

Figure 4.1 HDV replication cycle. (Reproduced with permission from Pr. Emmanuel Gordien.)

polymerase (RdRp) but rather depends on the host polymerases for replication. Thus upon delivery into the cytoplasm, it translocates to the nucleus.

3. Inside the nucleus the genome is transcribed and subsequently translated (in the cytoplasm) into p24, which then moves back into the nucleus to drive viral replication.
4. As replication progresses, another host enzyme, adenosine deaminase acting on RNA 1 (ADAR1), edits the antigenomic RNA to produce transcripts that are translated into p27.
5. p27 enters the nucleus to inhibit further replication and drive the cycle into a packaging phase. The assembled ribonucleoprotein (RNA and Delta proteins) is then exported out of the nucleus.
6. In the endoplasmic reticulum p27 interacts with HBsAg to assemble a new viral particle that is released through Golgi complex.
7. HDV is then secreted out of the infected cell.

Epidemiology

Estimates of the global burden of HDV vary,[4-6] portraying the difficulty in obtaining reliable data to fully understand HDV epidemiology. This may be due to several reasons such as lack of universal screening for HDV-Ab among HBsAg carriers and variations in testing methodology. Globally, of the estimated 257 to 291 million HBsAg carriers, about 4.5% (95% CI 3.6–5.7) have serological evidence of HDV infection.[6] This implies that worldwide between 12 and 13 million individuals are at exacerbated risk of liver cirrhosis and hepatocellular carcinoma (HCC) due to HDV infection. Expectedly, the estimate is higher among patient population drawn from hepatology clinics (16.4%; CI 14.6–18.6). On the other hand, the proportion of children under the age of 5 with CHB is low (<1%).[7] Therefore HDV infection is likely to be uncommon in this population.

Heterogeneity in HDV distribution even within close geographic areas or microepidemiology is typical in HDV.[6,8,9] Broadly, there has been a remarkable reduction in HDV infection in younger generations among indigenous populations in high-income countries, perhaps due to universal HBV vaccination programs that have reduced the pool of HBsAg individuals in these nations. Prevalence is, however, high (>10%) in some countries in western and central Africa and Republic of Moldova as well as Mongolia (Figure 4.2). Pooled HDV seroprevalences of 5.97% (12.26%), 5.91% (3.34%), 3.54% (17.36%), 3.00% (19.48%), 3.20% (4.00%), and 4.09% (8.07%) among asymptomatic HBsAg carriers (and patients from hepatology clinics) in Africa, the Americas, Eastern Mediterranean, Europe, Southeastern Asia, and Western Pacific regions, respectively, have been reported.[6]

Population groups like men having sex with men (MSM), commercial sex workers (CSW), people who inject drugs (PWID), persons on hemodialysis, and HIV- and HCV-positive populations are at higher risk for HDV infection. Available data on HDV RNA suggest that about 7.1 million persons with HDV are viremic, and for unclear reasons, Africa has lower RNA detection rate compared to other regions of the world.[6] So far, eight genotypes (HDV-1 to HDV-8) have been described with distinct geographic distribution.[10] While HDV-1 has been reported to have a worldwide spread, HDV-2 and HDV-4 spread mostly in Eastern and Northern Asia, HDV-3 in South America, and HDV-5 to HDV-8 majorly in sub-Saharan Africa.[11]

Pathogenesis

The mechanism through which HDV causes the most severe forms of viral hepatitis is still not well understood. The virus replicates solely in the hepatocytes, thus limiting the pathology to the liver. Host and viral (HDV and HBV) associated factors have been suggested to play key roles in HDV pathogenesis.[12] Different opinions exist with regard to the relative role played by host immune system versus direct liver injury by the virus in the pathogenesis of HDV infection.[13] Earlier experiments[14-16] suggested a direct cytopathic effect, especially during acute infection, while others implied immune-mediated liver pathology.[17,18]

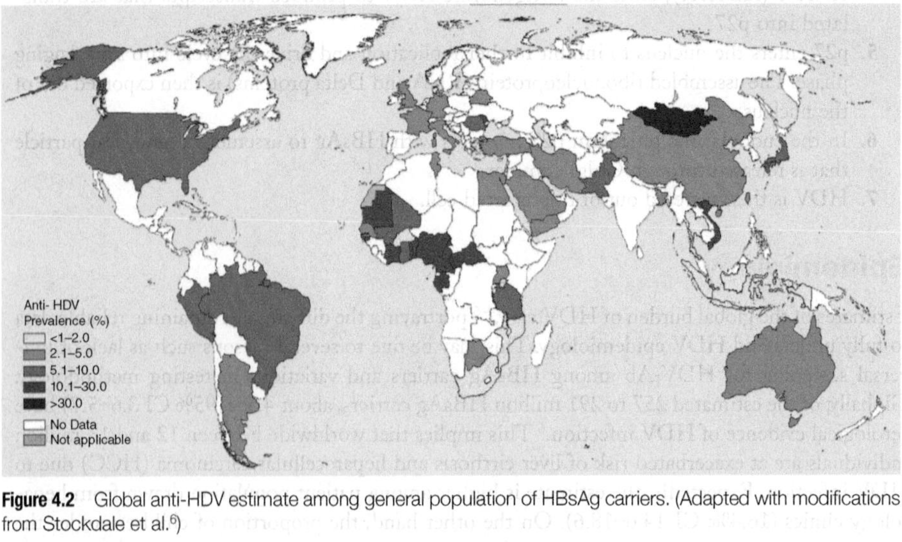

Figure 4.2 Global anti-HDV estimate among general population of HBsAg carriers. (Adapted with modifications from Stockdale et al.[6])

Direct action of p27 on several cell signaling pathways such as those involved in oxidative stress, activation of transcription factors involved in proliferation of inflammation, and apoptosis has been demonstrated.[19] Specifically, p27 is known to promote inflammatory responses by the activation of nuclear factor kappa-light-chain-enhancer of activated B cells (NFκ-B) and signal transducer and activator of transcription (STAT 3) via oxidative stress pathway. Although these responses may help clear HDV-infected cells, they also lead to necro-inflammation and endoplasmic reticulum stress, which may promote HCC development. It is still undefined if HDV possesses intrinsic oncogenic properties. Data showed that HDV replication enhances the expression of clusterin, which is greatly expressed in HCC and plays a role in tumorigenesis.[20] HDV persistence may be through exhaustion of the immune system by chronic inflammation as well as p27 actions against cell signaling pathways.

The specific mechanism by which HDV genotypes influence clinical outcome remains to be elaborated. Indeed, HDV-3 has been associated with a more aggressive form of liver disease,[21-23] whereas HDV-2 presents with milder clinical symptoms.[24] Also HBV replication (although largely suppressed in acute HDV infection) and genotypes may modulate the pathogenesis of HDV.[25-27]

Clinical Features and Course of HDV Infection

Infection with HDV can present as one of the following two patterns: **coinfection or superinfection** depending on the HBsAg state of the individual. Coinfection is assumed when there is simultaneous acute infection of HBV/HDV in a susceptible person. Here the extent of HDV viral expression will depend on that of HBV. Consequently, the clinical symptoms can vary from self-limiting, mild to very severe or fulminant infections, and in about 2% to 4% of the cases it can progress to chronicity.[28] Superinfection pattern occurs when individuals with CHB becomes secondarily infected with HDV. The outcome of this infection pattern may present with severe acute hepatitis with a shorter incubation period or fulminant hepatitis or chronic HDV (CHD) in more than 90% of the cases due to continual presence of HBsAg.[28]

The symptoms of acute HDV infection are indistinguishable from viral hepatitis caused by other viral agents, although hepatitis of HDV origin tends to be more severe. Certain risk factors including older age, male sex, and HIV coinfection have been shown to correlate with worse clinical outcome of HDV infection.[29-31] After an incubation period of about 3 to 7 weeks, clinical symptoms like fatigue, nausea, and lethargy develop with increase in transaminases (ALT and AST) and a reduction in viral load ensues. This is then followed by the appearance of jaundice (icteric phase) with increased bilirubin levels, dark-colored urine, and continued fatigue and nausea. In a self-limiting infection the convalescence phase begins with disappearance of clinical symptoms. In other cases acute infection can lead to a more fulminant course leading to acute liver failure characterized by sudden loss of hepatocytes causing multiple organ failure in an individual with no previous liver disease.

Fulminant hepatitis due to HDV exhibits symptoms like malaise, nausea, jaundice, coagulopathy, and encephalopathy, causing confusion, somnolence, and coma. There is a less dramatic level of serum ALT, AST, and viral load due to marked decrease in viable hepatocytes. The course is usually very rapid (2–10 days), with mortality occurring in about approximately 80% of patients. However, with the advent of orthotropic liver transplantation, the mortality rate has decreased.

In HDV superinfection progression to CHD is a common consequence, and it is typically associated with the most severe form of chronic hepatitis leading to cirrhosis. Establishment of CHD often exacerbates the already existing liver disease caused by HBV. A faster progression to cirrhosis occurs in over 70% of HBV/HDV superinfected population, among which 15% can develop cirrhosis within 1 to 2 years of initial diagnosis.[32]

Diagnosis and Approach

Ideally, HBV positive individuals should be screened for HDV infection, but this is not a common practice in many countries. At the very least, HBV patients with worsening liver disease of unexplainable cause should be tested for HDV. Laboratory investigations may include serological tests, viral RNA detection, and quantification by reverse transcription polymerase chain reaction (qRT-PCR). Typically, diagnosis should be made with detection of HDV antibody as well as RNA.

- **a.** *Serological Tests:* They are mainly qualitative detection of anti-HDV (especially IgG) in the patient's serum either by enzyme-linked immunosorbent assay (ELISA) or radioimmunoassay (RIA). Detection of IgM antibody is not very specific in HDV diagnosis, as it becomes detectable within 14 to 21 days of symptom appearance and clears after 2 months in acute infection[33] but often persists in chronic infection.[34] Limitations to the diagnostic use of serological tests exist especially in early infection when anti-HDV is not yet detectable (making test results falsely negative) or post infection persistence of antibodies despite viral clearance (in which case HDV RNA is negative while HDV-IgG positivity persists). HDV antigen expressed by the liver can be demonstrated using immunohistochemistry methods. However, detection of HDV-Ag in acute infection is not very useful, as it is present only transiently. Quantitative microarray antibody capture (QMAC) assay for anti-HDV IgG has been shown to correlate well with HDV RNA.[35]
- **b.** *Molecular Diagnosis:* Demonstrating HDV RNA in the blood or liver tissue of HDV-infected individual remains the confirmatory test for HDV infection and is useful in treatment monitoring. Individuals with undetectable HDV RNA but positive for HDV-Ab will require follow-up, as late rebounds are often observed. Of note, HDV RNA level does not directly imply active hepatic injury; rather, it is used to monitor response to therapy and viral clearance.
- **c.** *Other Investigations:* Liver biopsy can be employed to assess liver fibrosis or cirrhosis using immune-histochemical technique (although with newer methods of fibrosis detection, this is used less frequently). The use of imaging technologies such as ultrasound, abdominal computed tomographic scans, liver elastography, and magnetic resonance imaging (MRI) of the liver can be a noninvasive alternative to assess the liver in HDV infection. Other supporting investigations including screening for HCV and HIV coinfections, thorough evaluation of HBV markers, liver and renal function test, complete blood count, prothrombin time, and international normalized ratio are critical in HDV evaluation.

Treatment

Although care in acute HBV/HDV coinfection setting is mostly supportive, since over 90% of the cases resolve spontaneously, still close monitoring is required for early detection of progression to fulminant hepatitis. Presently, orthotropic liver transplant remains the ultimate treatment for HDV-induced fulminant hepatitis.[36] In CHD without decompensated liver cirrhosis treatment should be considered as soon as diagnosis is made after a clear discussion of side effects and expectations with the patient. Moreover, we recommend treatment by an experienced provider only.

The primary treatment goal in CHD is sustained virological response (SVR) marked by undetectable HDV RNA for 2 years or more post treatment with resultant normalization of ALT and liver histology.[37] Undetectable HDV-RNA and HBsAg clearance with HBsAb seroconversion is considered complete resolution of the infection but this is rarely achieved even in patients with SVR.

Although multiple agents have been used and others are still under evaluation, at the moment, interferon-based (IFN-based) treatment remains the best option. Variable responses based on dosage and treatment duration have been shown for IFN with overall success of about 20% to 30% after a 1-year regimen.[38,39] Higher IFN dose (9–10 million units three times/week) administered subcutaneously for sufficient duration is more effective.[36] However, side effects represent a major hurdle. Response to IFN treatment in HDV can take up to 10 months; thus a patient is regarded as a non-responder only after 12 months of no response. Pegylated IFN-alpha (PEG-IFNα) has been noted to be better tolerated with more favorable outcome than IFN therapy.[40] Precisely, using 1.5 μg/kg/week of PEG-IFN-α-2b for a duration of 48 weeks.[41] It should be noted then in the majority of large studies for HDV, a decrease in viral load (rather than SVR) has been the main target, and in most studies a significant number of patients rebound to their preivous viral load upon end of treatment. Optimal duration of PEG-IFN treatment has not been defined[37]; therefore decisions on treatment duration should be based on treatment and post-treatment evaluation of each individual. Predictors of IFN treatment response may include higher baseline platelet count and lower HBsAg levels.[37]

Nucleoside/nucleotide analogues have been reported to have no viral suppression effect on HDV.[42] Eighty-two CHD patients (including 23 with cirrhosis and 59 without cirrhosis) receiving a combination of tenofovir disoproxil fumarate (TDF) with PEG-IFN-2α (180 μg/week PEG-IFN-2α and 300 mg/day of TDF) for 96 weeks showed no beneficial difference in comparison with PEG-IFN monotherapy.[43] However, another study[44] showed treatment response in 86.4% and >95% at 24 and 48 weeks, respectively, in 22 subjects with HDV-3 who received 180 μg/week of PEG-IFN-α-2a plus entecavir (0.5 mg/day). They noted SVR among the responders 6 months post treatment. Most studies reported above have had very short follow-up terms, and the long-term effects are still unclear.

Pegylated interferon-lambda (PEG-IFN-λ), RNA interference, HBV/HDV entry inhibitors, prenylation inhibitors, and nucleic acid–based polymers (NAPs) are examples of other promising investigational anti-HDV agents that will hopefully change the narrative in HDV management.[45] Entry inhibitor (bulevirtide/Myrcludex B) monotherapy or in combination with IFN or entecavir has shown promising results in phase II clinical trials.[46-48] Due to its orphan diseases status and limited treatment option as well as the encouraging results from the trials, the European Medical Agency gave a conditional approval for the use of bulevirtide in HDV treatment. Phase III studies are still ongoing, but presently in the European Union patients with detectable HDV RNA and compensated liver disease can be given bulevirtide 2 mg/day subcutaneously as a monotherapy. Although treatment duration is yet to be defined as data on prolonged treatment is scarce, continued treatment as long as it is beneficial to the patient is currently recommended.[49]

References

1. Rizzetto M, Canese MG, Arico S, et al. Immunofluorescence detection of new antigen-antibody system (δ/anti-δ) associated to hepatitis B virus in liver and in serum of HBsAg carriers. *Gut.* 1977;18(12): 997-1003. doi:10.1136/gut.18.12.997.
2. Taylor JM. Structure and replication of hepatitis delta virus RNA. *Curr Top Microbiol Immunol.* 2006;307:1-23. doi:10.1007/3-540-29802-9_1.
3. Sureau C. The use of hepatocytes to investigate HDV infection: the HDV/HepaRG model. *Methods Mol Biol.* 2010;640:463-473. doi:10.1007/978-1-60761-688-7_25.
4. Chen HY, Shen DT, Ji DZ, et al. Prevalence and burden of hepatitis D virus infection in the global population: a systematic review and meta-analysis. *Gut.* 2019;68(3):512-521. doi:10.1136/GUTJNL-2018-316601.
5. Miao Z, Zhang S, Ou X, et al. Estimating the global prevalence, disease progression, and clinical outcome of hepatitis delta virus infection. *J Infect Dis.* 2020;221(10):1677-1687. doi:10.1093/INFDIS/JIZ633.
6. Stockdale AJ, Kreuels B, Henrion MYR, De C, Hutin Y, Geretti AM. The global prevalence of hepatitis D virus infection: systematic review and meta-analysis. *J Hepatol.* 2020;73(3):523-532. doi:10.1016/j.jhep.2020.04.008.

7. World Hepatitis Day: Fast-Tracking the Elimination of Hepatitis B Among Mothers and Children. Accessed February 16, 2022. Available at: https://www.who.int/news/item/27-07-2020-world-hepatitis-day-fast-tracking-the-elimination-of-hepatitis-b-among-mothers-and-children.
8. Aberra H, Gordien E, Desalegn H, et al. Hepatitis delta virus infection in a large cohort of chronic hepatitis B patients in Ethiopia. *Liver Int.* 2018;38(6):1000-1009. doi:10.1111/liv.13607.
9. Winter A, Letang E, Vedastus Kalinjuma A, et al. Absence of hepatitis delta infection in a large rural HIV cohort in Tanzania. *Int J Infect Dis.* 2016;46:8-10. doi:10.1016/j.ijid.2016.03.011.
10. Botelho-Souza LF, Vasconcelos MPA, Dos Santos AO, Salcedo JMV, Vieira DS. Hepatitis delta: virological and clinical aspects. *Virol J.* 2017;14(1):177. doi:10.1186/s12985-017-0845-y.
11. Le Gal F, Brichler S, Drugan T, et al. Genetic diversity and worldwide distribution of the deltavirus genus: a study of 2,152 clinical strains. *Hepatology.* 2017;66(6):1826-1841. doi:10.1002/hep.29574.
12. Tseligka ED, Clément S, Negro F. HDV pathogenesis: unravelling ariadne's thread. *Viruses.* 2021;13(5): 778. doi:10.1002/hep.29574.
13. Chang J, Gudima SO, Tarn C, Nie X, Taylor JM. Development of a novel system to study hepatitis delta virus genome replication. *J Virol.* 2005;79(13):8182-8188. doi:10.1128/JVI.79.13.8182-8188.2005.
14. Cole SM, Gowans EJ, Macnaughton TB, Hall PDLM, Burrell CJ. Direct evidence for cytotoxicity associated with expression of hepatitis delta virus antigen. *Hepatology.* 1991;13(5):845-851. doi:10.1002/HEP.1840130508.
15. Lefkowitch JH, Goldstein H, Yatto R, Gerber MA. Cytopathic liver injury in acute delta virus hepatitis. *Gastroenterology.* 1987;92(5 Pt 1):1262-1266. doi:10.1016/S0016-5085(87)91086-9.
16. Govindarajan S, Fields HA, Humphrey CD, Margolis HS. Pathologic and ultrastructural changes of acute and chronic delta hepatitis in an experimentally infected chimpanzee. *Am J Pathol.* 1986;122(2):315-322.
17. Braga WSM, de Oliveira CMC, de Araújo JR, et al. Chronic HDV/HBV co-infection: Predictors of disease stage: a case series of HDV-3 patients. *J Hepatol.* 2014;61(6):1205-1211. doi:10.1016/J.JHEP.2014.05.041.
18. Negro F, Baldi M, Bonino F, et al. Chronic HDV (hepatitis delta virus) hepatitis: Intrahepatic expression of delta antigen, histologic activity and outcome of liver disease. *J Hepatol.* 1988;6(1):8-14. doi:10.1016/S0168-8278(88)80457-4.
19. Williams V, Brichler S, Khan E, et al. Large hepatitis delta antigen activates STAT-3 and NF-κB via oxidative stress. *J Viral Hepat.* 2012;19(10):744-753. doi:10.1111/j.1365-2893.2012.01597.x.
20. Liao FT, Lee YJ, Ko JL, Tsai CC, Tseng CJ, Sheu GT. Hepatitis delta virus epigenetically enhances clusterin expression via histone acetylation in human hepatocellular carcinoma cells. *J Gen Virol.* 2009;90(Pt 5):1124-1134. doi:10.1099/VIR.0.007211-0.
21. Hadler SC, de Monzon MA, Rivero D, Perez M, Bracho A, Fields H. Epidemiology and Long-Term Consequences of Hepatitis Delta Virus Infection in the Yucpa Indians of Venezuela. *Am J Epidemiol.* 1992;136(12):1507–1516. doi:10.1093/oxfordjournals.aje.a116472.
22. Bensabath G, Hadler SC, Soares MCP, et al. Hepatitis delta virus infection and Labrea hepatitis: prevalence and role in fulminant hepatitis in the Amazon Basin. *JAMA.* 1987;258(4):479-483. doi:10.1001/JAMA.1987.03400040077025.
23. Casey JL, Niro GA, Engle RE, et al. Hepatitis B virus (HBV)/hepatitis D virus (HDV) coinfection in outbreaks of acute hepatitis in the Peruvian Amazon Basin: the roles of HDV genotype III and HBV genotype F. *J Infect Dis.* 1996. Accessed February 16, 2022. Available at: https://academic.oup.com/jid/article/174/5/920/806006.
24. Su CW, Huang YH, Huo TI, et al. Genotypes and viremia of hepatitis B and D viruses are associated with outcomes of chronic hepatitis D patients. *Gastroenterology.* 2006;130(6):1625-1635. doi:10.1053/j.gastro.2006.01.035.
25. Smedile A, Rosina F, Chiaberge E, et al. Presence and significance of hepatitis B virus replication in chronic type D hepatitis. *Prog Clin Biol Res.* 1991;364:185-195.
26. Smedile A, Rosina F, Saracco G, et al. Hepatitis B virus replication modulates pathogenesis of hepatitis D virus in chronic hepatitis D. *Hepatology.* 1991;13(3):413-416.
27. Madejón A, Romero M, Hernández Á, et al. Hepatitis B and D viruses replication interference: influence of hepatitis B genotype. *World J Gastroenterol.* 2016;22(11):3165-3174. doi:10.3748/wjg.v22.i11.3165.
28. Botelho-souza LF, Vasconcelos MPA, Dos Santos AO, Salcedo JMV, Vieira DS. Hepatitis delta: virological and clinical aspects. *Virol J.* 2017;14(1):177. doi:10.1186/s12985-017-0845-y.

29. Soriano V, Grint D, d'Arminio Monfort A, et al. Hepatitis delta in HIV-infected individuals in Europe. *AIDS*. 2011;25(16):1987-1992. doi:10.1097/QAD.0B013E32834BABB3.
30. Gilman C, Heller T, Koh C. Chronic hepatitis delta: A state-of-the-art review and new therapies. *World J Gastroenterol.* 2019;25(32):4580. doi:10.3748/WJG.V25.I32.4580.
31. Serrano BC, Großhennig A, Homs M, et al. Development and evaluation of a baseline-event-anticipation score for hepatitis delta. *J Viral Hepat.* 2014;21(11):e154. doi:10.1111/JVH.12251.
32. Pascarella S, Negro F. Hepatitis D virus: an update. *Liver Int.* 2011;31(1):7-21. doi:10.1111/j.1478-3231.2010.02320.x.
33. Koh C, Heller T, Glenn JS. Pathogenesis of and new therapies for hepatitis D. *Gastroenterology.* 2019;156(2):461-476.e1. doi:10.1053/J.GASTRO.2018.09.058.
34. Wranke A, Heidrich B, Ernst S, et al. Anti-HDV IgM as a marker of disease activity in hepatitis delta. *PLoS One.* 2014;9(7):e101002. doi:10.1371/JOURNAL.PONE.0101002.
35. Chen X, Oidovsambuu O, Liu P, et al. A novel quantitative microarray antibody capture (Q-MAC) assay identifies an extremely high HDV prevalence amongst HBV infected Mongolians. *Hepatology.* 2017;66(6):1739. doi:10.1002/HEP.28957.
36. Niro GA, Rosina F, Rizzetto M. Treatment of hepatitis D. *J Viral Hepat.* 2005;12(1):2-9. doi:10.1111/J.1365-2893.2005.00601.X.
37. Yurdaydin C, Keskin O, Kalkan Ç, et al. Interferon treatment duration in patients with chronic delta hepatitis and its effect on the natural course of the disease. *J Infect Dis.* 2018;217(8):1184-1192. doi:10.1093/INFDIS/JIX656.
38. Hsieh TH, Liu CJ, Chen DS, Chen PJ. Natural course and treatment of hepatitis D virus infection. *J Formos Med Assoc.* 2006;105(11):869-881. doi:10.1016/S0929-6646(09)60172-8.
39. Sagnelli C, Sagnelli E, Russo A, Pisaturo M, Occhiello L, Coppola N. HBV/HDV co-infection: epidemiological and clinical changes, recent knowledge and future challenges. *Life (Basel, Switzerland).* 2021;11(2):1-17. doi:10.3390/life11020169.
40. Niro GA, Ciancio A, Gaeta GB, et al. Pegylated interferon alpha-2b as monotherapy or in combination with ribavirin in chronic hepatitis delta. *Hepatology.* 2006;44(3):713-720. doi:10.1002/HEP.21296.
41. Castelnau C, Le Gal F, Ripault MP, et al. Efficacy of peginterferon alpha-2b in chronic hepatitis delta: relevance of quantitative RT-PCR for follow-up. *Hepatology.* 2006;44(3):728-735. doi:10.1002/HEP.21325.
42. Wedemeyer H, Manns MP. Epidemiology, pathogenesis and management of hepatitis D: update and challenges ahead. *Nat Rev Gastroenterol Hepatol.* 2010;7(1):31-40. doi:10.1038/NRGASTRO.2009.205.
43. Wedemeyer H, Yurdaydin C, Hardtke S, et al. Peginterferon alfa-2a plus tenofovir disoproxil fumarate for hepatitis D (HIDIT-II): a randomised, placebo controlled, phase 2 trial. *Lancet Infect Dis.* 2019;19(3):275-286. doi:10.1016/S1473-3099(18)30663-7.
44. Borzacov LMP, de Figueiredo Nicolete LD, Souza LFB, dos Santos AO, Vieira DS, Salcedo JMV. Treatment of hepatitis delta virus genotype 3 infection with peg-interferon and entecavir. *Int J Infect Dis.* 2016;46:82-88. doi:10.1016/J.IJID.2016.03.017.
45. Sandmann L, Cornberg M. Experimental drugs for the treatment of hepatitis D. *J Exp Pharmacol.* 2021;13:461-468. doi:10.2147/JEP.S235550.
46. Wedemeyer H, Schöneweis K, Bogomolov PO, et al. GS-13-Final results of a multicenter, open-label phase 2 clinical trial (MYR203) to assess safety and efficacy of myrcludex B in cwith PEG-interferon Alpha 2a in patients with chronic HBV/HDV co-infection. *J Hepatol.* 2019;70(1):e81. doi:10.1016/S0618-8278(19)30141-0.
47. Wedemeyer H, Bogomolov P, Blank A, et al. Final results of a multicenter, open-label phase 2b clinical trial to assess safety and efficacy of Myrcludex B in combination with Tenofovir in patients with chronic HBV/HDV co-infection. *J Hepatol.* 2018;68:S3. doi:10.1016/s0168-8278(18)30224-1.
48. Wedemeyer H, Schöneweis K, Bogomolov PO, et al. 48 weeks of high dose (10 mg) bulevirtide as monotherapy or with peginterferon alfa-2a in patients with chronic HBV/HDV co-infection. *J Hepatol.* 2020;73:S52-S53. doi:10.1016/S0168-8278(20)30651-6.
49. European Medicines Agency. Hepcludex. Accessed February 17, 2022. Available at: https://www.ema.europa.eu/en/medicines/human/EPAR/hepcludex.

CHAPTER 5

Hepatitis E Virus

Mandip KC ■ Ananta Shrestha

KEY POINTS

- Most common HEV route is fecal-oral transmission
- Manifests as sporadic cases, epidemic, or focal outbreaks in confined institutions
- Genotypes 1 and 2 are mostly responsible for epidemics or focal outbreaks in resource-limited countries
- Clinical features include asymptomatic disease (majority), icteric hepatitis, anicteric hepatitis, or acute liver failure
- Majority of the cases are self-limiting and managed with supportive care
- Pregnant women are at high risk for severe hepatitis and acute liver failure
- There are no indications for antivirals during acute hepatitis in HEV genotype 1 and 2
- Chronic hepatitis caused by HEV genotype 3 is treated with ribavirin
- Extrahepatic manifestations are rare but should be recognized and may provide clues to the diagnosis of HEV
- Focus should be on prevention of disease especially during outbreaks, with assurance of clean and properly treated drinking water

Introduction

Hepatitis E virus (HEV) is one of the youngest viruses in the hepatitis family of viruses and accounts for the majority of sporadic cases and epidemics of infective hepatitis in Asia and Africa.[1,2] Hepatitis caused by HEV is clinically distinct, as it mainly affects young adults and has high risk of progression into acute liver failure (ALF) among pregnant women, leading to substantial fetal and maternal morbidity and mortality. Until a decade ago, HEV was assumed to be limited to tropics and resource-limited countries, but recently it has been observed that HEV is endemic in industrialized countries, albeit with different clinical, epidemiological, and virological characteristics. HEV in tropical regions manifests as acute hepatitis caused by HEV genotypes 1 and 2. They are transmitted through contaminated drinking water (fecal-oral route) and are limited to humans. HEV genotypes 3 and 4 were originally limited to non-human species but crossed species barrier likely due to consumption of raw meat and raw unprocessed food. Genotypes 3 and 4 are more common in industrialized regions and manifests as a less severe form of acute hepatitis. Nonetheless, these genotypes can establish a chronic infection among immunosuppressed individuals. This chapter intends to focus on HEV genotypes 1 and 2 in the tropics and will briefly discuss HEV genotypes 3 and 4.

Virology

HEV belongs to the family Hepeviridae with genus *Orthohepevirus*. It is a non-enveloped positive single-stranded RNA virus with genome of 7.2 kb with three open reading frames (ORF1,

ORF2, and ORF3). ORF1 contributes to replication of the virus by encoding enzymes like methyltransferase (Met), helicase (Hel), and RNA-dependent RNA polymerase (RdRP). ORF2 contributes to structural capsid proteins and is the major determinant of antigenicity. The function of ORF3 is yet to be clearly understood.[3]

EPIDEMIOLOGY

There have been several large outbreaks of acute hepatitis due to HEV worldwide. The first documented large outbreak was in New Delhi, India, in 1955–1956. Subsequently, several outbreaks were reported in other countries in Southeast Asia. In 1983, Mikhail Balayan, a Russian virologist, was able to demonstrate transmission of the virus to himself and acquire the disease after voluntarily consuming pooled stool extracts from subjects of acute hepatitis outbreak in Soviet military camp in Afghanistan. During that time, the only known hepatitis viruses were hepatitis A and hepatitis B (HAV and HBV). However, serological studies in most of these outbreaks were negative for both HAV and HBV. Furthermore, these outbreaks had distinct characteristics, which included compressed curve, that is, peak within a few months, affected young adults, and high rate of acute liver failure and mortality among pregnant women especially during their third trimester. Based on these characteristics, a new virus, "Non-A Non-B" (NANB), was proposed, which was later sequenced by Reyes et al. in 1990 and was named hepatitis E virus.[4,5]

Acute HEV infection in the community manifests in three forms: (1) sporadic, (2) epidemic, and (3) focal outbreaks in closed, confined institutions. The sporadic form occurs in endemic areas every year, with a peak during rainy seasons. The number of cases in a specific area is fairly comparable every year until an epidemic or a community outbreak where a large population is affected within a short period of time. Contamination of drinking water is often identifiable during large epidemics. These outbreaks tend to recur over a certain interval of time, which is probably due to waning of herd immunity. The third form is "focal outbreaks" in closed, confined institutions like hostels, army camps, and prisons.

Epidemics or large community outbreaks have been reported in many Asian countries like India, Pakistan, Nepal, Bangladesh, and Afghanistan, mainly due to HEV genotype 1. Fecal contamination of local water sources such as ponds or contamination of water pipelines running in proximity to sewer lines has been identified in many cases. Multiple large outbreaks have been reported in Africa including Egypt, Kenya, Sudan, Central African Republic, Uganda, Chad, Namibia, Algeria, Morocco, Somalia, and Ethiopia. Similarly, outbreaks in North, Central, and South America have been reported, including Cuba and Mexico. Most of the African epidemics have been linked to HEV genotype 1 and some to HEV genotype 2. These outbreaks were also linked to contamination of drinking water sources comparable to the ones in Asian countries. In contrast, outbreaks in Japan have been related to HEV genotype 4 and linked to consumption of uncooked or raw meat.[6] The geographic distribution of HEV genotypes is shown in Figure 5.1.

CLINICAL FEATURES OF HEPATITIS E VIRAL INFECTION

The most common presentation of HEV is an acute, self-limiting hepatitis. The incubation period is about 2 to 10 weeks following the exposure of HEV; on average, it is about 5 to 6 weeks. The majority of the patients are asymptomatic or mildly symptomatic. Typical timeline of HEV infection is shown in Figure 5.2.

In patients who are symptomatic, the typical symptoms are similar to other hepatitis viruses. It is important to know that the manifestation of HEV infection is highly variable and has a wide range. Patients develop low-grade fevers, malaise, and anorexia in the early days of infection.

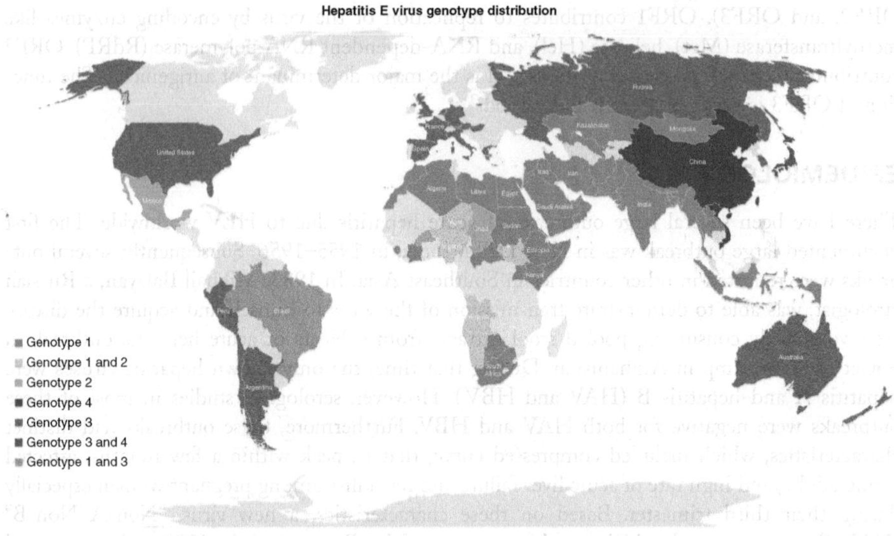

Figure 5.1 Geographic distribution of various genotypes of HEV.

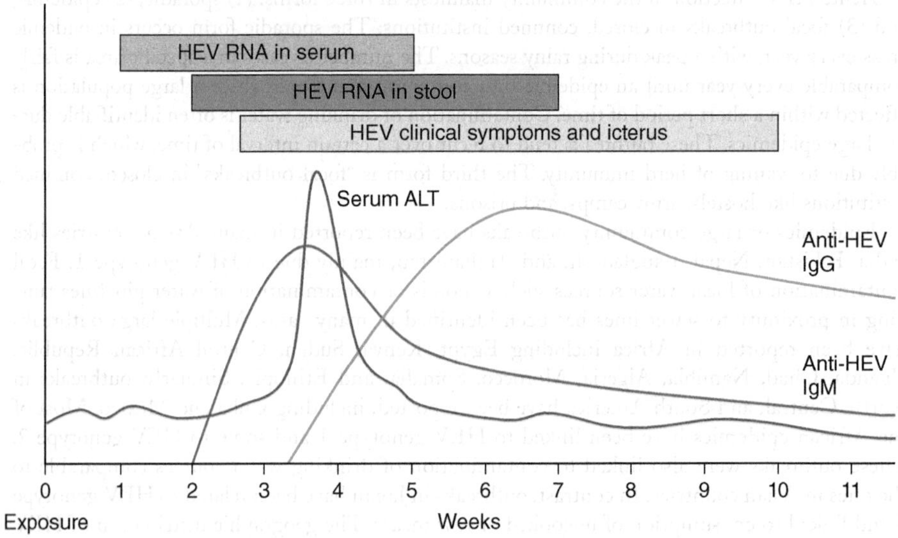

Figure 5.2 Typical timeline of HEV infection.

Vomiting, if present, is typically non-bloody. A transient macular rash may also be seen in some patients. In the following weeks jaundice occurs in about 40% of the patients, with the chance of darkened urine and pale stools occurring. On examination, patients may also have mild hepatomegaly with tenderness. Splenomegaly may also be noted. Most of these symptoms are self-limited and may last several days to a few weeks. A fraction of patients may have a protracted course with cholestatic symptoms for several weeks to months; however, most will resolve on their own.

In regions where genotype 3 or 4 is more predominant the disease course may be asymptomatic with modest derangement of LFTs. However, in patients who are immunosuppressed including transplant recipients, it may cause persistent viremia leading to chronic infection, eventually leading to advanced fibrosis and cirrhosis.

Extrahepatic Manifestation of HEV

On occasions, HEV manifests with extrahepatic symptoms. These manifestations are uncommon and are generally limited to case reports or series. HEV has been associated with a wide array of neurological symptoms, hematologic disorders, renal diseases, pancreatic manifestations including pancreatitis, myocarditis, autoimmune thyroiditis, and musculoskeletal disorders such as myositis. The pathophysiology of the extrahepatic manifestations is unclear. It has been hypothesized that these are typically body's inflammatory response toward the viral infection, or an autoimmune response from the viral antibodies that are generated. The most common of these are neurological symptoms (Guillain-Barre syndrome, neuralgic amyotrophy, transverse myelitis, acute meningoencephalitis, Bell's palsy), and studies have reported up to 16.5% of neurological symptoms associated with HEV in some regions of the world where genotype 3 is most prevalent (France).[7] Other studies have shown rates as low as 0.68%, where genotype 4 was more predominant (China).[8] The neurological symptoms resolve after resolution of the HEV hepatitis. Similarly, renal manifestations such as glomerulonephritis and mixed cryoglobulinemia have also been reported. Early presentation of renal dysfunction is proteinuria, which can be a useful tool for detection of renal involvement. The majority of renal cases have been seen in immunosuppressed patients or in patients with history of renal transplants after infection with HEV genotype 3.[9] One other important manifestation is acute pancreatitis seen in HEV genotype 1 infection, which can itself lead to significant morbidity and therefore should be recognized and managed accordingly.[10] The list of extrahepatic manifestations is enlisted in Table 5.1.

Acute Liver Failure

ALF is characterized by development of coagulopathy and encephalopathy after the onset of jaundice and prodrome. The disease can be explosive in nature, with median time of 4 to 5 days between presentation and outcome, which could be death, transplant, or recovery. Less than 1% of healthy subjects who acquire HEV develop ALF. The mortality without transplant among those who develop ALF is approximately 50%. Cerebral edema and herniation are the leading

TABLE 5.1 ■ **Extrahepatic Manifestations of Hepatitis E**

Organ System	Manifestation Type
Neurological	Guillain-Barre Syndrome Neuralgic Amyotrophy Transverse Myelitis Acute Meningoencephalitis Bell's Palsy
Hematologic	Hemolytic Anemia Aplastic Anemia Thrombocytopenia
Renal	Glomerulonephritis Mixed Cryoglobulinemia
Pancreatic	Acute Pancreatitis
Endocrine	Autoimmune Thyroiditis
Cardiac	Myocarditis
Other	Autoimmune Thyroiditis Henoch-Schonlein Purpura

causes of death in ALF. The clinical feature of ALF is discussed in detail in a chapter elsewhere in this book.

Hepatitis E in Special Populations

PREGNANCY AND HEV INFECTION

Hepatitis E infection in pregnant women carries a significant risk for morbidity, and mortality since it causes more complications in pregnant women compared to other viral hepatitis. Compared to non-pregnant women, the early clinical course of the HEV infection is similar in pregnant women; however, rapid deterioration and acute liver failure may develop more commonly with mortality up to 25% to 30%. During epidemics and outbreaks of HEV infection, the rate of fulminant hepatic failure may reach up to 22% to 69% in pregnant women.

Death is typically from ALF; however, antepartum hemorrhage, eclampsia, preterm delivery, and fetal death are more common in women who are HEV infected. It should be noted that most severe HEV infections in pregnancy are reported from specific Asian countries such as India and Pakistan.[11]

ACUTE-ON-CHRONIC LIVER FAILURE

Acute-on-chronic liver failure (ACLF) refers to a distinct clinical syndrome where any acute hepatic insult, including HEV, infection leads to rapid decompensation (ascites, encephalopathy, coagulopathy) of underlying preexisting liver disease. These underlying chronic liver diseases may be diagnosed or undiagnosed and may range from non-alcoholic steatohepatitis with variable degrees of fibrosis to compensated liver cirrhosis. In the Asia Pacific region nearly 21% of all ACLF cases are due to HEV, with a median mortality of 34% (0–67%).[12] HEV-related ACLF typically starts with jaundice and coagulopathy, which worsens with development of ascites and/or encephalopathy and subsequent multiorgan failure. Early recognition of this syndrome and aggressive intensive care management may help to improve survival in these patients.

IMMUNOSUPPRESSED INDIVIDUALS

Chronic hepatitis can be seen with genotype-3 HEV in patients who are immunosuppressed. This is characterized by persistent viremia and fecal excretion beyond three months of initial infection. This is attributed to immunosuppression from solid organ transplantation mainly[13] but also reported in chemotherapy/immunotherapy, or in HIV-infected patients. Moreover, it seems to be specific to certain areas of the world such as Europe. Patients show persistent elevation in liver enzymes, which can lead to fibrosis and cirrhosis if not treated.

Laboratory Diagnosis

The index of suspicion for HEV infection should be high based on epidemiological as well as clinical scenario. As with any patient presenting with jaundice, initial laboratory workup should include liver panel (to include AST, ALT, alkaline phosphatase [ALP], total bilirubin, conjugated bilirubin, total protein), prothrombin time (PT), complete blood counts, and basic electrolyte panel (Na, K, Cl, CO_2, Ca, PO_4).

The typical laboratory features in HEV infection include marked transaminitis with ALT levels reaching more than 100 to 200 times the upper limit of normal (ULN). Variable degree of hyperbilirubinemia is also noted in about 40% of patients. Rising prothrombin time (PT) is an indicator of failing liver or fulminant course and has to be carefully addressed, as discussed in the chapter.

Confirmation of HEV infection is usually done by means of serological assays and nucleic acid testing.[14] Serological methods include (1) IgM for anti-HEV using ELISA, (2) IgM for anti-HEV using rapid diagnostic tests, or (3) HEV antigen levels using ELISA.

While anti-HEV IgM using ELISA has been widely used around the world, discrepancies in performance have been noted between various ELISA kits based on the manufacturer. Properly validated kits need to be ensured before interpreting their results. Various rapid diagnostic kits are available that are inexpensive, including point-of-care. Anti-HEV IgG is used to assess seroprevalence in community and gives an estimate of exposure to HEV. Though rising titer of anti-HEV IgG is also seen during convalescence period of acute HEV infection, it is less frequently used in clinical practice. HEV antigen detection by ELISA is also shown to be very sensitive at least in early viremic period and correlates well with HEV viremia. HEV antigen is more sensitive than anti-HEV IgM in detecting asymptomatic HEV viremic subjects. However, this test has not been widely used and still needs validation before it can be used in routine clinical practice.

Nucleic acid testing (NAT) by PCR is the confirmatory test for active infection. It is a surrogate indicator of viremia and can be detected in stool and blood. It is rarely required for diagnosis of acute viral hepatitis E but is mandatory in diagnosis of chronic HEV infection where persistent chronic viremia needs to be established. Further, HEV RNA PCR is essential for molecular epidemiological studies and genotyping and for research purposes.

Management of Hepatitis E

The management of HEV infection depends on the acuity of viral infection as well as the immune status of the infected patient.

In immunocompetent patients, acute HEV infection is mild and self-limited in majority of the cases; therefore management is primarily supportive. Icteric hepatitis will resolve within a few weeks, and long-term sequelae (such as cirrhosis or renal failure) are extremely rare. In these populations there is no role for any antiviral medications. Any medications that may have hepatotoxicity (such as high-dose acetaminophen, NSAIDs, or herbal medications) should be avoided. Selected patients who develop severe acute hepatitis and those with underlying chronic liver disease who develop ACLF may be cautiously considered for ribavirin therapy based on available limited anecdotal data.

Pregnant patients with HEV genotype 1 or genotype 2 infection should be transferred to higher level of care if possible, preferably to centers with specialists including hepatologist, intensivist, and maternal-fetal medicine experts due to high risk of liver failure and fetal complications. Recognition of early complications is the key. Management is primarily supportive and staying vigilant for features of acute liver failure (ALF), premature delivery, stillbirths, and peripartum bleeding. There is no proven role of specific antiviral agents, and ribavirin is contraindicated in pregnancy. Therapeutic termination of pregnancy or early induction of labor is not recommended as this does not change outcome in the mother. Mode of delivery should be normal vaginal delivery with expectant management. Cesarian section should only be considered if there are standard indications. It is helpful to remain prepared, having blood products and coagulation factors available for potential peripartum blood loss, which is exacerbated by underlying coagulopathy.

The most dreaded complication of acute HEV infection in pregnant women is acute liver failure, which is often life threatening and associated with high mortality rate. Management of ALF is the same as managing ALF of other etiologies. Though there have been efforts to develop better prognostic models in HEV-related ALF, King's College Criteria are still being followed for selecting candidates for liver transplantation in HEV-related ALF. Pregnant women with ALF are managed similarly to nonpregnant patients.

Herbal and traditional medicine have become increasingly popular in many parts of the world.[15] There is a wide variation of the medications based on the location and beliefs. The use of these remedies is often without advice or knowledge of any medical professional. There are no standardized studies to show the efficacy and safety of these regimens in the setting of liver diseases or hepatitis E. Moreover, there is always a risk of superimposed liver injury because of herbal/traditional medicine and hence should be avoided.[16]

Chronic HEV infection in immunosuppressed individuals is associated with progression to chronic liver disease and reduced graft and patient survival. Reduction of immunosuppressive medications, especially tacrolimus and switching to another immunosuppressant, could lead to resolution of viremia and fecal excretion in one-third of the patients. Persistence of viremia beyond 3 months is generally an indication for antiviral therapy. Ribavirin 600 mg-1200 mg a day for 3 months is the recommended first-line therapy; however, this comes from evidence from limited number of cases. Variation of dose based on type of immunosuppression or organ transplantation has also been described.[17,18] If there is relapse of viremia on stopping ribavirin, an additional course of 6 months of ribavirin has been recommended. Second-line therapy with pegylated interferon-alpha could be considered, for those who relapse after retreatment with 6 months of ribavirin therapy, those who are intolerant to ribavirin therapy, or those not achieving virological response to ribavirin therapy. However, this may lead to acute rejection in organ transplant patients.

Prevention of HEV

WATER SANITATION

Assurance of safe drinking water is the key to prevention of HEV at community level. Water disinfection may be done by various methods including boiling and chlorination. Chlorination of water is relatively cheap and widely available. Free residual chlorine (FRC) of >0.5 mg/L at tap stands level has been accepted as adequate to define safe drinking water, which may be raised to 1.0 mg/L during outbreak settings. Boiling of drinking water is more accessible; however, it may be cumbersome and associated with additional cost of fuel/electricity usage. Studies have shown that heating water at 56°C for 15 minutes was sufficient to inactivate 95% of HEV.[19,20]

HEV VACCINES

A recombinant HEV vaccine HEV 239 (Hecolin, Xiamen Innovax Biotech Co., Ltd., Xiamen, China) has completed phase 3 trial and has been approved for use in China.[21] It is safe and shows efficacy of 100% after three doses of vaccine at 1 year and 87% at 4.5 years. It was also seen that single dose of HEV 239 provided 95% protection at the end of 1 year. An accelerated course of vaccination where three doses are given within 21 days has shown to be effective, which could potentially help to curb the cases during outbreaks and humanitarian settings. Though safety of HEV 239 during pregnancy is yet to be established, there were no adverse events noted among 37 inadvertently vaccinated pregnant subjects during its phase 3 trial. HEV 239 has not yet been used to prevent or as a response to an outbreak of HEV infection, so it is not known how these efficacies translate into reduction of mortality in real-world scenarios.

HEV 239 is yet to be approved for use beyond China, and until then, it seems imperative to emphasize proper disinfection and safe drinking water supply in endemic areas in order to prevent HEV-related morbidity and mortality.

References

1. Hoofnagle JH, Nelson KE, Purcell RH. Hepatitis E. *N Engl J Med.* 2012;367:1237-1281. doi:10.1056/NEJMra1204512.
2. Kamar N, Bendall R, Legrand-Abravanel F, et al. Hepatitis E. *Lancet.* 2012;379:2477-2488. doi:10.1016/S0140.

3. Nan Y, Zhang YJ. Molecular biology and infection of hepatitis E virus. *Front Microbiol.* 2016;7:1419. doi:10.3389/FMICB.2016.01419.
4. Reyes GR, Purdy MA, Kim JP, et al. Isolation of a cDNA from the virus responsible for enterically transmitted non-A, non-B hepatitis. *Science.* 1990;247(4948):1335-1339. doi:10.1126/SCIENCE.2107574.
5. Khuroo MS, Khuroo MS, Khuroo NS. Hepatitis E: discovery, global impact, control and cure. *World J Gastroenterol.* 2016;22(31):7030. doi:10.3748/WJG.V22.I31.7030.
6. Hakim MS, Wang W, Bramer WM, et al. The global burden of hepatitis E outbreaks: a systematic review. *Liver Int.* 2017;37(1):19-31. doi:10.1111/LIV.13237.
7. Fousekis FS, Mitselos IV, Christodoulou DK. Extrahepatic manifestations of hepatitis E virus: an overview. *Clin Mol Hepatol.* 2020;26(1):16. doi:10.3350/CMH.2019.0082.
8. Wang Y, Wang S, Wu J, et al. Hepatitis E virus infection in acute non-traumatic neuropathy: a large prospective case-control study in China. *EBioMedicine.* 2018;36:122. doi:10.1016/J.EBIOM.2018.08.053.
9. Kamar N, Abravanel F, Lhomme S, Rostaing L, Izopet J. Hepatitis E virus: chronic infection, extrahepatic manifestations, and treatment. *Clin Res Hepatol Gastroenterol.* 2015;39:20-27. doi:10.1016/j.clinre.2014.07.005.
10. Haffar S, Bazerbachi F, Garg S, Lake JR, Freeman ML. Frequency and prognosis of acute pancreatitis associated with acute hepatitis E: a systematic review. *Pancreatology.* 2015;15(4):321-326. doi:10.1016/J.PAN.2015.05.460.
11. Patra S, Kumar A, Trivedi SS, Puri M, Sarin SK. Maternal and fetal outcomes in pregnant women with acute hepatitis E virus infection. *Ann Intern Med.* 2007;147(1):28-33. doi:10.7326/0003-4819-147-1-200707030-00005.
12. Kumar A, Saraswat VA. Hepatitis E and acute-on-chronic liver failure. *J Clin Exp Hepatol.* 2013;3(3):225-230. doi:10.1016/J.JCEH.2013.08.013.
13. Kamar N, Garrouste C, Haagsma EB, et al. Factors associated with chronic hepatitis in patients with hepatitis E virus infection who have received solid organ transplants. *Gastroenterology.* 2011;140(5):1481-1489. doi:10.1053/J.GASTRO.2011.02.050.
14. Khudyakov Y, Kamili S. Serological diagnostics of hepatitis E virus infection. *Virus Res.* 2011;161:84-92. doi:10.1016/j.virusres.2011.06.006.
15. Nsibirwa S, Anguzu G, Kamukama S, Ocama P, Nankya-Mutyoba J. Herbal medicine use among patients with viral and non-viral Hepatitis in Uganda: prevalence, patterns and related factors. *BMC Complement Med Ther.* 2020;20(1):169. doi:10.1186/S12906-020-02959-8.
16. Bernuau JR, Durand F. Herbal medicines in acute viral hepatitis: a ticket for more trouble. *Eur J Gastroenterol Hepatol.* 2008;20(3):161-163. doi:10.1097/MEG.0B013E3282F2BBF7.
17. Kamar N, Izopet J, Tripon S, et al. Ribavirin for chronic hepatitis E virus infection in transplant recipients. *N Engl J Med.* 2014;12(20):1111-1131. doi:10.1056/NEJMoa1215246.
18. De Winter BCM, Hesselink DA, Kamar N. Dosing ribavirin in hepatitis E-infected solid organ transplant recipients. *Pharmacol Res.* 2018;130:308-315. doi:10.1016/J.PHRS.2018.02.030.
19. Guerrero-Latorre L, Gonzales-Gustavson E, Hundesa A, Sommer R, Rosina G. UV disinfection and flocculation-chlorination sachets to reduce hepatitis E virus in drinking water. *Int J Hyg Environ Health.* 2016;219(4-5):405-411. doi:10.1016/j.ijheh.2016.04.002.
20. Spina A, Beversluis D, Irwin A, et al. Learning from water treatment and hygiene interventions in response to a hepatitis E outbreak in an open setting in Chad. *J Water Health.* 2018;16(2):223-232. doi:10.2166/WH.2018.258.
21. Zhu FC, Zhang J, Zhang XF, et al. Efficacy and safety of a recombinant hepatitis E vaccine in healthy adults: a large-scale, randomised, double-blind placebo-controlled, phase 3 trial. *Lancet.* 2010;376(9744):895-902. doi:10.1016/S0140-6736(10)61030-6.

SECTION II

Liver Masses

CHAPTER 6

Hepatocellular Carcinoma

Manaswita Tappata ■ Jose D. Debes

KEY POINTS

- Hepatocellular carcinoma (HCC) is among the most common causes of cancer-related death worldwide
- Hepatitis B virus (HBV) is the most common cause of HCC worldwide, followed by hepatitis C and fatty liver disease (alcoholic and nonalcoholic)
- The majority of HCCs occur in the setting of cirrhosis; therefore screening for HCC in cirrhotic patients is critical
- HCC can occur without cirrhosis in patients with hepatitis B (and to a lesser extent those with nonalcoholic fatty liver disease (NAFLD)
- Screening for HCC is performed with ultrasound with or without a serum marker called alpha-fetoprotein (AFP)
- HCC treatment is different from that of other tumors as it does not respond to conventional chemotherapy
- Locoregional therapies like radiofrequency ablation (RFA), percutaneous ethanol injection (PEI), and surgery, as well as liver transplantation with curative intent can be used if the tumor is detected early

Introduction

Hepatocellular carcinoma (HCC) is the third leading cause of cancer-related death worldwide.[1,2] HCC mostly occurs in a background of chronic liver disease with advanced liver fibrosis known as cirrhosis. Therefore, the frequency and pathogenesis of underlying liver disease in each region has a major impact on the incidence and progression of HCC. In this chapter, we review the epidemiology, symptoms, screening, diagnosis, and treatment of HCC in the context of tropical settings.

Epidemiology

The highest incidence of HCC is in Asia and Africa, with approximately 75% of liver cancers in the world occurring in these regions (Figure 6.1).[3] In these high-incidence areas the most common cause of HCC is chronic hepatitis B virus (HBV) infection, which, combined with aflatoxin B1 exposure (AFB1), dramatically affects younger people.[4] In the Americas, Europe, and Japan the most common causes of HCC are hepatitis C virus (HCV) infection alcohol consumption, and obesity/metabolic syndrome leading to nonalcoholic fatty liver disease (NAFLD).[3,5,6] Alcohol consumption is thought to play a major role in the development of HCC and related mortality in Eastern Europe and Russia.[7] HCC has high mortality mainly due to the advanced stage at

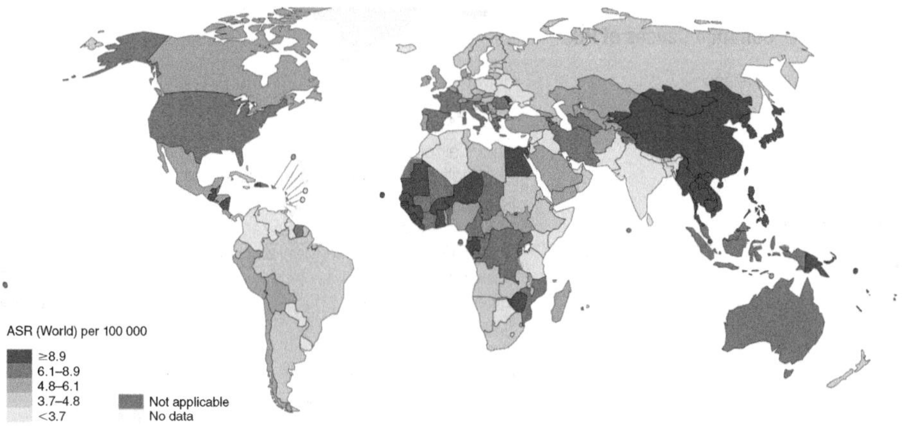

Figure 6.1 Incidence of liver cancer across the world in both sexes. (Data graph from GLOBOCAN 2018: https://gco.iarc.fr/today/data/factsheets/cancers/11-Liver-fact-sheet.pdf.)

presentation as patients are often asymptomatic. This is a particular issue in resource-limited settings due to lack of surveillance programs and treatment options.

The underlying etiology of HCC does impact the clinical progression of the tumor. Indeed, age of onset of HCC is lower in sub-Saharan Africa when compared with Asia and other areas of the world.[8-10] This is thought to be due to the higher incidence of hepatitis B associated with HCC due to early infection with the virus, as well as the synergistic effect of dietary aflatoxins and the virus, which can induce TP53 mutations.[4,11] Aflatoxins are mycotoxins produced by molds of the *Aspergillus* species, found in maize, groundnuts, and tree nuts in humid environments, and are known to be a hepatic carcinogen. Since hepatitis B vaccination has been implemented worldwide, it has decreased the incidence of HCC in resource-limited and rich settings. Many resource-limited regions have lower frequencies of vaccination, and vaccination does not occur until 6 weeks of age, thus decreasing its efficacy.[11]

In regions of higher HBV incidence in Latin America, HBV-associated HCC has shown onset at a younger age, though reasons for this have not yet been elucidated.[12] In Asia aristolochic acid (AA) is found in plants known as *Aristolochia*/*Asarum* (Chinese wild ginger), which have been used in traditional Chinese herbal medicines for centuries. AA has been shown to be mutagenic, and a subset of HCCs from east Asia have been found to have the mutational signature of AA exposure.[13,14]

In western regions HCV is the more common underlying liver disease causing HCC.[3] In some countries such as Egypt, which used intravenous anti-schistosomal therapies with suboptimal needle assessment in the early 20th century, the association of HCV and HCC has been out of proportion compared to other countries with a significant HCV population.[3,15] With the advent of curative therapy for HCV, it is expected that rates of HCC related to HCV infection will become less common, and NAFLD, which has been increasing due to increasing rates of obesity, will become a more common cause of HCC (Table 6.1).

Symptoms

HCC at early stages is often asymptomatic in most patients.[16] Those who are symptomatic, often at the later stages, commonly report right upper quadrant pain and early satiety and can have signs of hepatic decompensation such as jaundice and hepatic encephalopathy. If the tumor invades

TABLE 6.1 ■ **Common Causes of HCC**

Resource-limited areas	Hepatitis B Aflatoxin exposure Aristolochic acid exposure Heavy alcohol intake Coinfection with HIV, hepatitis delta virus
Resource-rich areas	Hepatitis C Aflatoxin exposure (in certain regions) Metabolic liver disease (non-alcoholic fatty liver disease) Heavy alcohol intake Excess body weight Tobacco smoking Hemochromatosis Alpha-1 antitrypsin deficiency

portal structures, sequelae of portal hypertension such as ascites and variceal bleeding can develop. Rarely, patients can have tumor rupture, cutaneous manifestations, and diarrhea.[16-18]

Screening

Surveillance for HCC is aimed at reducing disease-related mortality by identifying a tumor at an early stage where it is small enough to be amenable to curative treatment.[19] Current guidelines vary based on continent and professional association; however, most recommend twice-yearly screening with ultrasound with or without serum alpha-fetoprotein (AFP) in patients with cirrhosis. This level of screening is also recommended for those with chronic hepatitis B even without cirrhosis at certain ages depending on their region of origin.[20-22]

Ultrasound is the preferred method of surveillance since it is well tolerated, inexpensive, and noninvasive. However, it has a sensitivity of 60% to 80% at best.[19,23] Moreover, sensitivity for lesions smaller than 2 cm (early tumors) is even poorer.[24] Challenges include variability of sensitivity based on operator expertise, need for fasting prior to the study, and patient time commitment, all of which lead to poor adherence. In areas with less resources, including rural regions of Latin America and Africa, access to imaging is limited, training of operators is at times unreliable, and work permits for medical exams are scarce, which leads to further lack of screening and contributes to HCC-related mortality.[25] The appearance of HCC is affected by size and background liver disease, and identification can be compromised in nodular livers.[26] HCCs less than 3 cm can appear hypoechoic to adjacent liver, whereas larger lesions and lesions containing fat can appear more heterogeneous.

When combined with serum AFP, ultrasound detection rates are increased, but the rates of false positives are also increased as AFP levels can be elevated in viral hepatitis, pregnancy, and more rarely tumors of gonadal origin and gastric malignancies.[27-31] AFP by itself is not sensitive or specific enough to be used alone as surveillance for HCC, although it is sometimes used in regions with no ultrasound expertise available. International societies recommend the optional use of AFP (Asia Pacific Association for the Study of the Liver [APASL], American Association for the Study of Liver Diseases [AASLD]), and one concluded that no recommendation can be made due to insufficient evidence (European Association for the Study of the Liver [EASL]).[20-22]

Diagnosis

Diagnosis of HCC can be made by imaging alone without the need for biopsy, with triple-phase contrast-enhanced CT or MRI in the setting of liver cirrhosis, or by biopsy of the lesion when

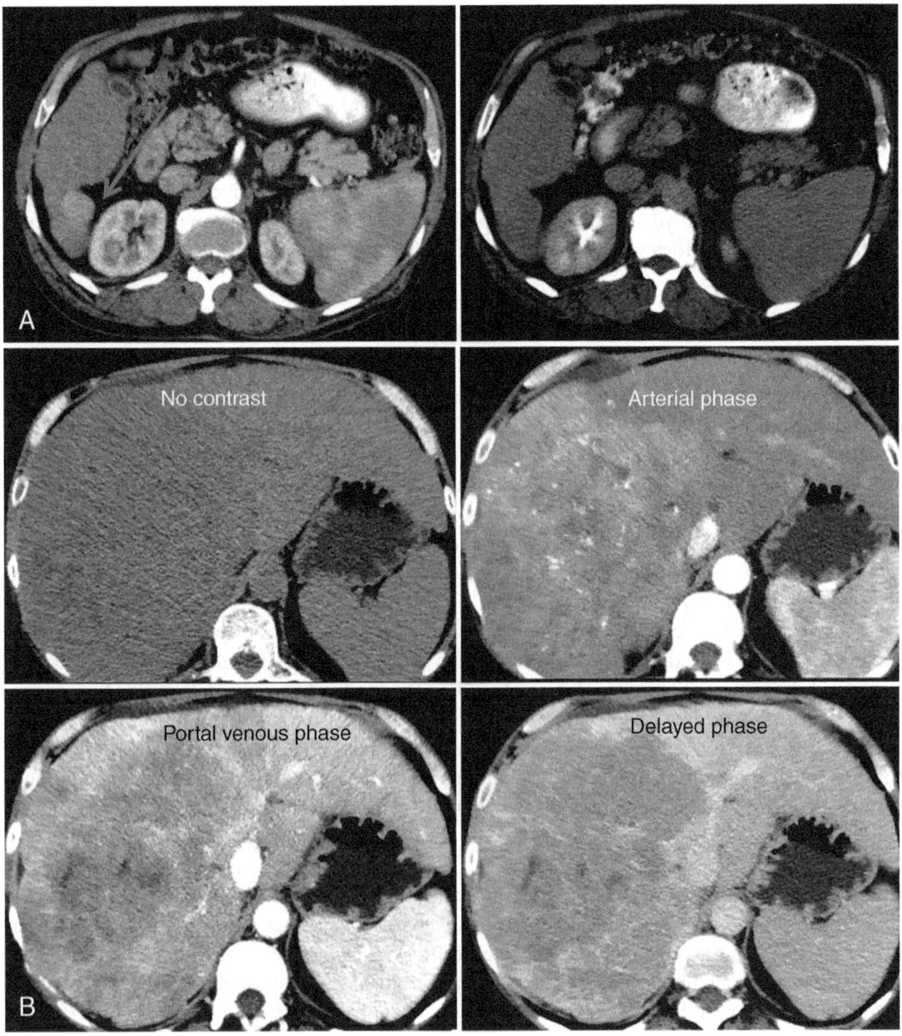

Figure 6.2 **A,** CT scan showing arterial enhancement (image on left) with venous washout (image on right) diagnostic of hepatocellular carcinoma (red arrow indicates lesion). **B,** CT scan showing diagnostic appearance of diffuse hepatocellular carcinoma in various phases. (Courtesy of Dr. Gopal Punjabi.)

the imaging is equivocal.[32,33] Pretest probability plays an important role in the diagnosis of HCC, with any liver mass in a cirrhotic patient considered to be HCC until proven otherwise, but a mass in a non-cirrhotic patient is unlikely to be HCC. The ultrasound appearance of HCC is variable, and the pattern seen on CT/MRI imaging is intense contrast uptake during the arterial phase followed by contrast washout in the portal venous phase in lesions greater than 1 cm (Figure 6.2).[34] Diagnosis depends on the size of the lesion on imaging since nodules less than 1 cm are less likely to be diagnosed as HCC, can be difficult to biopsy, and may not have developed the hypervascular pattern on imaging at this stage. Therefore nondiagnostic nodules are followed by serial imaging for surveillance.[34-37]

Specificity of imaging for HCC is characterized by the Liver Imaging Reporting and Data System (LI-RADS), a widely used methodology of classification to better define HCC, with LR-5 lesions being definite HCC without need for biopsy.[33,38] If the lesions do not have the classic pattern of contrast enhancement and washout, then biopsy could be performed or follow up imaging can be done at a specific interval (3–6 months depending on the clinical situation). At this point in time, contrast-enhanced ultrasound (another imaging alternative) is not recommended as the sole method of evaluation.[39]

Diagnostic biopsy is an alternate method of diagnosis; however, it can have lower yield if the size of the lesion is small and has an associated risk of procedural complications.[40] Significantly elevated AFP ≥400 ng/mL in a high-risk patient can be nearly diagnostic for HCC with a specificity of ≥90%.[41] However, less than 10% of HCCs are associated with such a high AFP.[42,43]

Treatment

Several treatment modalities are available for HCC and these can be stratified into curative and non-curative, or systemic and locoregional therapies. The availability of these therapies varies widely based on resources in the region. The major curative modalities include surgical resection of the lesion, liver transplantation, and percutaneous ablation. Percutaneous ablation modalities include radiofrequency ablation (RFA) or microwave ablation, cryoablation, or percutaneous ethanol injection (PEI), all of which are reasonable treatments but should be performed by experienced providers.[44] Noncurative percutaneous treatments include transarterial chemo-embolization or radio-embolization (TACE or TARE), although these approaches are sometimes used with curative intent as well.

Systemic chemotherapy in HCC is complex, as the tumor does not respond to typical chemo-therapeutic agents. Indeed, there was no systematic therapy for HCC until 2008, with the arrival of sorafenib, an oral multi-kinase inhibitor. For 10 years, sorafenib was the only available systemic therapy, with most studies performed in resource-rich settings, and very few in resource-limited ones.[45-47] Over the last few years, systemic therapy for HCC has expanded dramatically with multiple oral and parenteral treatments, including multi-kinase inhibitors, targeted therapy, and immune therapy.[48,49] These treatments, however, are not currently available in many resource-limited regions.

In resource-limited settings PEI of small HCC lesions (≤3–5 cm) is a reasonable option in the appropriate setting and with appropriate expertise (Figure 6.3).[44] It is low cost, requires minimal equipment, and has clinical benefit relatively similar to that of radiofrequency ablation (although RFA is still preferred and more efficient when possible).[50,51] In addition, systemic therapy, that is, sorafenib, is oral and well tolerated and has been described to have benefit in survival in patients with HBV in Africa.[52] However, an appropriate discussion should be had with

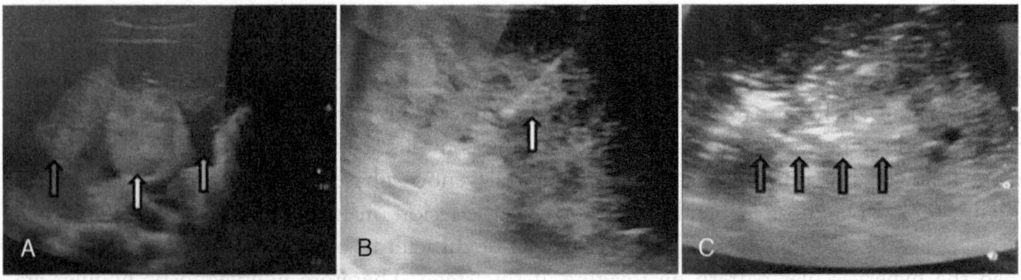

Figure 6.3 Injection of pure ethanol into a liver cancer mass – **A**: Liver mass (yellow arrow) with heterogenous echotexture, with increased echogenicity compared to the non-tumoral liver (red arrow). Hypoechoic ascites (green arrow) is noted surrounding the liver; **B**: Visible needle (white arrow) infecting ethanol in the tumor; **C**: Increased echogenicity in the area (grey arrows), post ethanol injection. (Figure courtesy of J. Debes)

TABLE 6.2 ■ **HCC Treatments**

Curative	Liver transplantation Surgical resection Percutaneous ethanol injection Radiofrequency ablation Microwave ablation Cryoablation
Non-curative	Transarterial chemo-embolization (TACE) Transarterial radio-embolization (TARE) Systemic therapy (multi-kinase inhibitors, antibodies, immune therapy)

patients about the real benefits and risks of using sorafenib. Ultimately, application of a curative treatment at an early stage is the ideal goal to reduce mortality related to HCC. In this regard, identification of individuals at risk for proper surveillance and early tumor identification is critical (Table 6.2).

HBV-Related HCC

As discussed earlier, HBV-related HCC accounts for the majority of HCC in Africa and Asia.[53] Due to significant efforts in implementation of vaccination programs against HBV in high-incidence areas such as east Asia and West and sub-Saharan Africa, HBV incidence has been declining but still represents a major problem worldwide. Notably, in this population, HCC can occur in the absence of cirrhosis, unlike other etiologies of HCC. Moreover, age of occurrence is much earlier in these patients, particularly in Africa.[10] Prevention has been focused on surveillance programs, which have had variable success due to limited resources such as ultrasound operators and barriers to adherence.[53,54] Other aspects that apply to HBV-HCC include treatment of viral hepatitis in those with HCC. Although specific data is lacking, it is overall advisable to treat these patients with HCC and HBV for HBV as it could lead to a slight improvement in survival (since the virus is estimated to be the driver of the tumor).

HIV-Related HCC

A large number of individuals with HIV are also coinfected with HBV or HCV, both of which can lead to development of HCC, usually at a younger age.[55] The mechanism underlying the younger age of HCC in those with HIV infection remains unclear. It has been hypothesized that impairment of the immune system plays a role. HIV is more common in Africa, and screening for HIV-related HCC is challenging due to lower detection of HCC via ultrasound in HIV-infected individuals and lack of large studies to evaluate the role of ultrasound in this population.[56,57] Patients with HIV and HCC should be evaluated by experts with experience in the field as this combination exposes unique complexities.

References

1. McGlynn KA, Petrick JL, El-Serag HB. Epidemiology of hepatocellular carcinoma. *Hepatology.* 2021;73(suppl 1):4-13. doi:10.1002/hep.31288.
2. Sung H, Ferlay J, Siegel RL, et al. Global Cancer Statistics 2020: GLOBOCAN estimates of incidence and mortality worldwide for 36 cancers in 185 countries. *CA Cancer J Clin.* 2021;71(3):209-249. doi:10.3322/caac.21660.

3. McGlynn KA, Petrick JL, London WT. Global epidemiology of hepatocellular carcinoma: an emphasis on demographic and regional variability. *Clin Liver Dis.* 2015;19(2):223-238. doi:10.1016/j.cld.2015.01.001.
4. Kirk GD, Lesi OA, Mendy M, et al. 249ser TP53 mutation in plasma DNA, hepatitis B viral infection, and risk of hepatocellular carcinoma. *Oncogene.* 2005;24(38):5858-5867. doi:10.1038/sj.onc.1208732.
5. Park JW, Chen M, Colombo M, et al. Global patterns of hepatocellular carcinoma management from diagnosis to death: the BRIDGE Study. *Liver Int.* 2015;35(9):2155-2166. doi:10.1111/liv.12818.
6. Debes JD, Chan AJ, Balderramo D, et al. Hepatocellular carcinoma in South America: evaluation of risk factors, demographics and therapy. *Liver Int.* 2018;38(1):136-143. doi:10.1111/liv.13502.
7. Singal AG, El-Serag HB. Hepatocellular carcinoma from epidemiology to prevention: translating knowledge into practice. *Clin Gastroenterol Hepatol.* 2015;13(12):2140-2151. doi:10.1016/j.cgh.2015.08.014.
8. Yang JD, Mohamed EA, Aziz AOA, et al. Characteristics, management, and outcomes of patients with hepatocellular carcinoma in Africa: a multicountry observational study from the Africa Liver Cancer Consortium. *Lancet Gastroenterol Hepatol.* 2017;2(2):103-111. doi:10.1016/S2468-1253(16)30161-3.
9. Okeke E, Davwar PM, Roberts L, et al. Epidemiology of liver cancer in Africa: current and future trends. *Semin Liver Dis.* 2020;40(2):111-123. doi:10.1055/s-0039-3399566.
10. Yang JD, Gyedu A, Afihene MY, et al. Hepatocellular carcinoma occurs at an earlier age in Africans, particularly in association with chronic hepatitis B. *Am J Gastroenterol.* 2015;110(11):1629-1631. doi:10.1038/ajg.2015.289.
11. Anugwom CM, Allaire M, Akbar SMF, et al. Hepatitis b-related hepatocellular carcinoma: surveillance strategy directed by immune-epidemiology. *Hepatoma Res.* 2021;7:23. doi:10.20517/2394-5079.2021.06.
12. Debes JD, Chan AJ, Balderramo D, et al. Hepatocellular carcinoma in South America: evaluation of risk factors, demographics and therapy. *Liv Int.* 2018;38(1):136-143. doi:10.1111/liv.13502.
13. Yang JD, Hainaut P, Gores GJ, Amadou A, Plymoth A, Roberts LR. A global view of hepatocellular carcinoma: trends, risk, prevention and management. *Nat Rev Gastroenterol Hepatol.* 2019;16(10):589-604. doi:10.1038/s41575-019-0186-y.
14. Arlt VM, Stiborova M, Schmeiser HH. Aristolochic acid as a probable human cancer hazard in herbal remedies: a review. *Mutagenesis.* 2002;17(4):265-277.
15. Davis GL, Alter MJ, El-Serag H, Poynard T, Jennings LW. Aging of hepatitis C virus (HCV)-infected persons in the United States: a multiple cohort model of HCV prevalence and disease progression. *Gastroenterology.* 2010;138(2):513-521. doi:10.1053/j.gastro.2009.09.067.
16. Bialecki ES, di Bisceglie AM. Diagnosis of hepatocellular carcinoma. *HPB.* 2005;7(1):26-34. doi:10.1080/13651820410024049.
17. Dogra S, Jindal R. Cutaneous manifestations of common liver diseases. *J Clin Exp Hepatol.* 2011;1(3):177-184. doi:10.1016/S0973-6883(11)60235-1.
18. Xia F, Ndhlovu E, Zhang M, Chen X, Zhang B, Zhu P. Ruptured hepatocellular carcinoma: current status of research. *Front Oncol.* 2022;12:848903. doi:10.3389/fonc.2022.848903.
19. Forner A, Llovet JM, Bruix J, Forner A, Llovet JM. Hepatocellular carcinoma. *Lancet.* 2012;379:1245-1255. doi:10.1016/S0140.
20. Galle PR, Forner A, Llovet JM, et al. EASL clinical practice guidelines: management of hepatocellular carcinoma. *J Hepatol.* 2018;69(1):182-236. doi:10.1016/j.jhep.2018.03.019.
21. Marrero JA, Kulik LM, Sirlin CB, et al. Diagnosis, staging, and management of hepatocellular carcinoma: 2018 Practice Guidance by the American Association for the study of liver diseases. *Hepatology.* 2018;68(2):723-750. doi:10.1002/hep.29913.
22. Omata M, Cheng AL, Kokudo N, et al. Asia-Pacific clinical practice guidelines on the management of hepatocellular carcinoma: a 2017 update. *Hepatol Int.* 2017;11(4):317-370. doi:10.1007/s12072-017-9799-9.
23. Tzartzeva K, Obi J, Rich NE, et al. Surveillance imaging and alpha fetoprotein for early detection of hepatocellular carcinoma in patients with cirrhosis: a meta-analysis. *Gastroenterology.* 2018;154(6):1706-1718.e1. doi:10.1053/j.gastro.2018.01.064.
24. Lim J, Singal AG. Surveillance and diagnosis of hepatocellular carcinoma. *Clin Liver Dis.* 2019;13(1):2-5. doi:10.1002/cld.761.
25. Debes JD, Carrera E, Mattos AZ, Prieto JE, Boonstra A. Hepatocellular carcinoma, a unique tumor with a lack of biomarkers. *Ann Hepatol.* 2019;18(6):786-787. doi:10.1016/j.aohep.2019.07.009.

26. Nowicki TK, Markiet K, Szurowska E. Diagnostic imaging of hepatocellular carcinoma: a pictorial essay. *Curr Med Imaging Rev.* 2017;13(2):140-153. doi:10.2174/1573405612666160720123748.
27. Kew M. Alpha-fetoprotein in primary liver cancer and other diseases. *Gut.* 1974;15(10):814-821. doi:10.1136/gut.15.10.814.
28. Turshudzhyan A, Wu GY. Persistently rising alpha-fetoprotein in the diagnosis of hepatocellular carcinoma: a review. *J Clin Transl Hepatol.* 2022;10(1):159-163. doi:10.14218/JCTH.2021.00176.
29. Hanif H, Ali MJ, Khan IW, et al. Update on the applications and limitations of alpha-fetoprotein for hepatocellular carcinoma. *World J Gastroenterol.* 2022;28(2):216-229. doi:10.3748/wjg.v28.i2.216.
30. Søreide JA. Therapeutic approaches to gastric hepatoid adenocarcinoma: current perspectives. *Ther Clin Risk Manag.* 2019;15:1469-1477. doi:10.2147/TCRM.S204303.
31. Chun H, Kwon SJ. Clinicopathological characteristics of alpha-fetoprotein-producing gastric cancer. *J Gastric Cancer.* 2011;11(1):23-30. doi:10.5230/jgc.2011.11.1.23.
32. Choi JY, Lee JM, Sirlin CB. CT and MR imaging diagnosis and staging of hepatocellular carcinoma: Part I. Development, growth, and spread: key pathologic and imaging aspects. *Radiology.* 2014;272(3): 635-654. doi:10.1148/radiol.14132361.
33. Moura Cunha G, Chernyak V, Fowler KJ, Sirlin CB. Up-to-date role of CT/MRI LI-RADS in hepatocellular carcinoma. *J Hepatocell Carcinoma.* 2021;8:513-527. doi:10.2147/jhc.s268288.
34. Ayuso C, Rimola J, Vilana R, et al. Diagnosis and staging of hepatocellular carcinoma (HCC): current guidelines. *Eur J Radiol.* 2018;101:72-81. doi:10.1016/j.ejrad.2018.01.025.
35. Khalili K, Kyoung Kim T, Jang HJ, Kochak Yazdi L, Guindi M, Sherman M. Indeterminate 1-2-cm nodules found on hepatocellular carcinoma surveillance: biopsy for all, some, or none? *Hepatology.* 2011;54(6):2048-2054. doi:10.1002/hep.24638.
36. Forner A, Vilana R, Ayuso C, et al. Diagnosis of hepatic nodules 20 mm or smaller in cirrhosis: prospective validation of the noninvasive diagnostic criteria for hepatocellular carcinoma. *Hepatology.* 2008; 47(1):97-104. doi:10.1002/hep.21966.
37. Leoni S, Piscaglia F, Golfieri R, et al. The impact of vascular and nonvascular findings on the noninvasive diagnosis of small hepatocellular carcinoma based on the EASL and AASLD criteria. *Am J Gastroenterol.* 2010;105(3):599-609. doi:10.1038/ajg.2009.654.
38. Elmohr M, M. Elsayes K, Chernyak V. LI-RADS: review and updates. *Clin Liver Dis.* 2021;17(3): 108-112. doi:10.1002/cld.991.
39. D'Onofrio M, Faccioli N, Zamboni G, et al. Focal liver lesions in cirrhosis: value of contrast-enhanced ultrasonography compared with Doppler ultrasound and α-fetoprotein levels. *Radiol Med.* 2008;113(7): 978-991. doi:10.1007/s11547-008-0316-z.
40. Forner A, Vilana R, Ayuso C, et al. Diagnosis of hepatic nodules 20 mm or smaller in cirrhosis: prospective validation of the noninvasive diagnostic criteria for hepatocellular carcinoma. *Hepatology.* 2008;47(1):97-104. doi:10.1002/hep.21966.
41. Marrero JA, Feng Z, Wang Y, et al. α-Fetoprotein, des-γ carboxyprothrombin, and lectin-bound α-fetoprotein in early hepatocellular carcinoma. *Gastroenterology.* 2009;137(1):110-118. doi:10.1053/j.gastro.2009.04.005.
42. Chan SL, Mo F, Johnson PJ, et al. Performance of serum α-fetoprotein levels in the diagnosis of hepatocellular carcinoma in patients with a hepatic mass. *HPB.* 2014;16(4):366-372. doi:10.1111/hpb.12146.
43. Kanwal F, Singal AG. Surveillance for hepatocellular carcinoma: current best practice and future direction. *Gastroenterology.* 2019;157(1):54-64. doi:10.1053/j.gastro.2019.02.049.
44. Nault JC, Sutter O, Nahon P, Ganne-Carrié N, Séror O. Percutaneous treatment of hepatocellular carcinoma: state of the art and innovations. *J Hepatol.* 2018;68(4):783-797. doi:10.1016/j.jhep.2017.10.004.
45. Sultan A, Anugwom CM, Wondifraw Z, Braimoh GA, Bane A, Debes JD. Single center analysis of therapy and outcomes of hepatocellular carcinoma in Sub-Saharan Africa. *Expert Rev Gastroenterol Hepatol.* 2020;14(10):1007-1011. doi:10.1080/17474124.2020.1802246.
46. Bruix J, Cheng AL, Meinhardt G, Nakajima K, de Sanctis Y, Llovet J. Prognostic factors and predictors of sorafenib benefit in patients with hepatocellular carcinoma: analysis of two phase III studies. *J Hepatol.* 2017;67(5):999-1008. doi:10.1016/j.jhep.2017.06.026.
47. Leathers JS, Balderramo D, Prieto J, et al. Sorafenib for treatment of hepatocellular carcinoma: a survival analysis from the South American Liver Research Network. *J Clin Gastroenterol.* 2019;53(6):464-469. doi:10.1097/MCG.0000000000001085.

48. Greten TF, Lai CW, Li G, Staveley-O'Carroll KF. Targeted and immune-based therapies for hepatocellular carcinoma. *Gastroenterology.* 2019;156(2):510-524. doi:10.1053/j.gastro.2018.09.051.
49. Bruix J, Chan SL, Galle PR, Rimassa L, Sangro B. Systemic treatment of hepatocellular carcinoma: an EASL position paper. *J Hepatol.* 2021;75(4):960-974. doi:10.1016/j.jhep.2021.07.004.
50. Meloni F, Lazzaroni S, Livraghi T. Percutaneous ethanol injection: single session treatment. *Eur J Ultrasound.* 2001;13(2):107-115. doi:10.1016/S0929-8266(01)00124-0.
51. Bouza C, López-Cuadrado T, Alcázar R, Saz-Parkinson Z, Amate JM. Meta-analysis of percutaneous radiofrequency ablation versus ethanol injection in hepatocellular carcinoma. *BMC Gastroenterology.* 2009;9(1):31. doi:10.1186/1471-230X-9-31.
52. Sultan A, Anugwom CM, Wondifraw Z, Braimoh GA, Bane A, Debes JD. Single center analysis of therapy and outcomes of hepatocellular carcinoma in Sub-Saharan Africa. *Expert Rev Gastroenterol Hepatol.* 2020;14(10):1007-1011. doi:10.1080/17474124.2020.1802246.
53. Anugwom CM, Allaire M, Akbar SMF, et al. Hepatitis b-related hepatocellular carcinoma: surveillance strategy directed by immune-epidemiology. *Hepatoma Res.* 2021;7:23. doi:10.20517/2394-5079.2021.06.
54. Singal AG, Lampertico P, Nahon P. Epidemiology and surveillance for hepatocellular carcinoma: new trends. *J Hepatol.* 2020;72(2):250-261. doi:10.1016/j.jhep.2019.08.025.
55. Bräu N, Fox RK, Xiao P, et al. Presentation and outcome of hepatocellular carcinoma in HIV-infected patients: a U.S.-Canadian multicenter study. *J Hepatol.* 2007;47(4):527-537. doi:10.1016/j.jhep.2007.06.010.
56. Merchante N, Merino E, Rodríguez-Arrondo F, et al. HIV/hepatitis C virus-coinfected patients who achieved sustained virological response are still at risk of developing hepatocellular carcinoma. *AIDS.* 2014;28(1):41-47. doi:10.1097/QAD.0000000000000005.
57. Sahasrabuddhe VV, Shiels MS, McGlynn KA, Engels EA. The risk of hepatocellular carcinoma among individuals with acquired immunodeficiency syndrome in the United States. *Cancer.* 2012;118(24):6226-6233. doi:10.1002/cncr.27694.

CHAPTER 7

Cholangiocarcinoma

Lewis R. Roberts

KEY POINTS

- Cholangiocarcinoma is subclassified into intrahepatic, perihilar, and distal cholangiocarcinoma based on the site of origin of the tumor.
- Intrahepatic cholangiocarcinomas can grow to a large size in the liver, as they remain asymptomatic until they distend the liver capsule or cause mass effect on surrounding organs.
- Perihilar or distal cholangiocarcinomas, together referred to as extrahepatic cholangiocarcinomas, are likely to obstruct the central or distal bile ducts, leading to presentation with painless jaundice, dark urine, and light-colored stools.
- Endoscopic retrograde cholangiopancreatography with brushings and biopsies, percutaneous transhepatic cholangiography, or percutaneous biopsies are required for histologic confirmation of the diagnosis of cholangiocarcinoma.
- Surgical resection is the primary treatment for cholangiocarcinoma, but cholangiocarcinomas have a high rate of recurrence even after apparently curative resection.
- Cholangiocarcinomas frequently have targetable mutations for which specific drugs are available, including FGFR inhibitors, IDH1 inhibitors, immune checkpoint inhibitors for microsatellite high tumors, and TRK inhibitors. Appropriate application of these therapies requires genomic characterization of tissue biopsies or plasma circulating tumor DNA, all of which are difficult to perform in resource-limited settings.

Introduction

Cholangiocarcinomas (CCAs) are malignant neoplasms of the bile ducts. CCA are classified by anatomical location into intrahepatic cholangiocarcinomas (iCCAs), which arise from the most peripheral bile ducts to the second-order bifurcation of the right and left hepatic ducts; perihilar cholangiocarcinomas (pCCAs), which arise from the second-order bifurcation to the junction of the cystic duct with the common hepatic duct to form the common bile duct; and distal cholangiocarcinomas (dCCAs), which arise from the common bile duct extending to the ampulla of Vater (Figure 7.1). pCCA and dCCA are grouped together as extrahepatic CCA, as the right and left bile ducts exit the liver and join to form the common hepatic duct, which traverses the peritoneal cavity outside the liver and merges with the cystic duct to form the common bile duct that then courses through the pancreas to the second portion of the duodenum.

Epidemiology

CCA is associated with a wide variety of risk factors, which also vary by geographical location or region and by the location of the tumor within the biliary tree, with iCCA, pCCA, and dCCA all having distinct but somewhat related etiologic factors[1] (Figure 7.2).

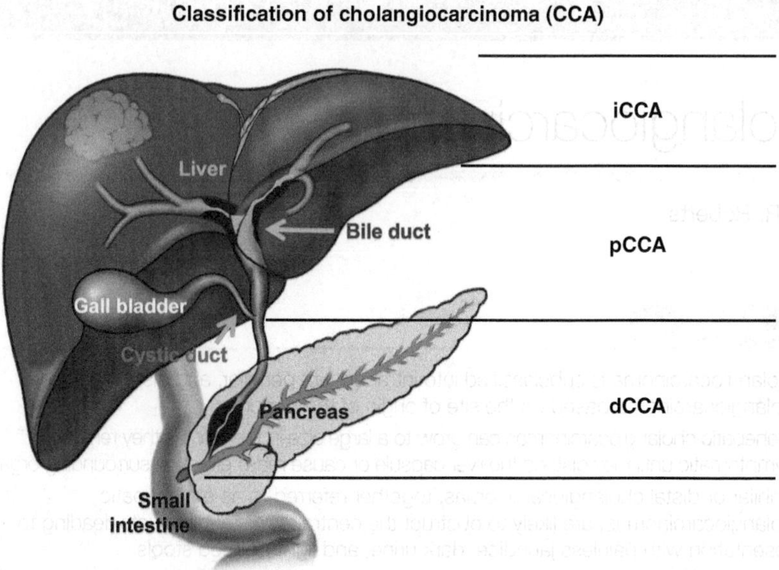

Figure 7.1 Classification of cholangiocarcinoma into intrahepatic (iCCA), perihilar (pCCA), and distal cholangiocarcinoma (dCCA).

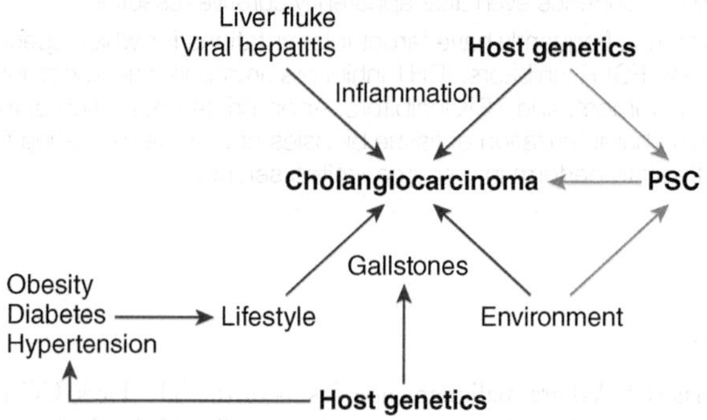

Figure 7.2 Factors associated with risk of cholangiocarcinoma.

The most common characteristic associated with risk of CCA is chronic inflammation affecting the biliary tract or the liver generally. Local bile duct inflammation may be due to biliary obstruction from stones, chronic bacterial or parasitic infestation of the biliary tract—classically occurring in parts of Asia—due to infestation of the bile ducts by the liver flukes *Clonorchis sinensis* or *Opisthorchis viverrini*, congenital cystic disease of the bile ducts including choledochal cysts, or immune-related biliary inflammation and strictures in primary sclerosing cholangitis (PSC). These local biliary inflammatory factors predominantly affect the hilar and distal extrahepatic bile ducts, causing malignant transformation in the medium and larger bile ducts.[1,2]

Chronic inflammation involving the entire liver, due most commonly to chronic viral hepatitis B or C, alcoholic liver disease, or nonalcoholic fatty liver disease (NAFLD) and less commonly to metabolic disorders such as hereditary hemochromatosis or immune-related diseases such as autoimmune hepatitis or primary biliary cirrhosis, is associated with increased risk of iCCA, arising from the smaller bile ducts. These factors, particularly NAFLD, are increasing in many industrial countries, leading to increasing rates of iCCA over the past 30 years. They are also increasing in low-resource countries, in part due to the adoption of high-carbohydrate, high-fat Western diets and more sedentary lifestyles.[1,3]

In addition to specific inflammatory diseases, conditions and factors associated with increased systemic inflammation such as diabetes and obesity are also associated with increased risk of CCA.

One of the key functions of the liver is detoxification of drugs and noxious chemicals. Exposure of the biliary tract to high concentrations of certain chemical toxins has been associated with an increased risk of CCA. Perhaps most notable is the evidence that defects in exhaust systems leading to increased exposure to solvents used in the offset color printing industry, notably 1,2-dichloropropane and dichloromethane, are associated with increased risk of CCA.[3]

Early-stage studies also suggest that there are host genetic variants that contribute to the risk of CCA.

Clinical Presentation

iCCA is initially limited to either the right or left lobe of the liver. iCCA can grow to a large size without obstructing bile flow from both sides of the liver and are therefore usually diagnosed in patients who do not have jaundice. Further, there are no pain fibers within the substance of the liver, only in the liver capsule. Thus iCCA are typically asymptomatic until they grow large enough to exert mass effect on the stomach, causing early satiety; to stretch the liver capsule and cause abdominal pain or diaphragmatic irritation with referred pain to the shoulder, particularly with deep inspiration; or to invade the hilum of the liver and produce obstruction of both the left and right bile duct systems, causing hyperbilirubinemia manifesting as jaundice. Occasionally, the first manifestation of iCCA is when the patient notes a protruding mass in the upper abdomen from the expanding liver.

pCCA typically arise from either the right or left extrahepatic bile duct between the first and second bifurcation of the bile ducts, at the site of the bile duct bifurcation, or in the common hepatic duct between the site of bile duct bifurcation and the junction of the cystic duct with the common hepatic duct. pCCA arising from the right or left hepatic ducts can form a malignant stricture obstructing bile flow from either the right or left lobe of the liver. While bile from the contralateral side of the liver is still able to flow into the duodenum, jaundice does not develop, and the patient remains asymptomatic. However, the obstruction of bile flow leads to hyperbilirubinemia on the affected side, often compounded by portal vein compression or thrombosis on the same side. This results in atrophy of the affected lobe, with compensatory hypertrophy of the other lobe, a classic radiologic feature referred to as the "atrophy-hypertrophy complex" (Figure 7.3). As they progress and expand, many pCCA will eventually occlude the bile duct confluence and the opposite hepatic duct, resulting in complete biliary occlusion and the development of jaundice. pCCA arising from within the common hepatic duct will typically cause complete biliary obstruction early on in tumor progression.

dCCA arise from within the common bile duct beyond the junction of the cystic duct with the common hepatic duct. Like common hepatic duct pCCA, dCCA are prone to causing total biliary obstruction with resulting jaundice relatively early in the course of the disease.

Unfortunately, CCA is one of the more biologically aggressive, invasive, and metastatic tumors. CCA would have frequently already metastasized to regional lymph nodes, the liver, the peritoneal cavity, or the lungs by the time they are clinically apparent. Coupled with their relative resistance to standard chemotherapy, the propensity of CCA to invasive and metastatic spread results in relatively poor survival, even for tumors apparently diagnosed with early-stage, surgically resectable disease, as there is a high rate of recurrence and progression due to micrometastatic tumors that are unrecognized at the time of diagnosis.

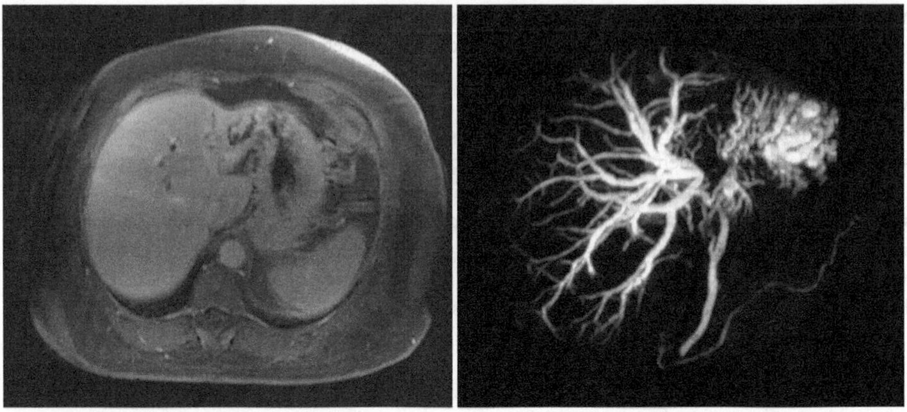

Atrophy-hypertrophy complex MR Cholangiopancreatogram

Figure 7.3 MRI (left) and MRCP (right) images showing the atrophy-hypertrophy complex induced by a cholangiocarcinoma arising in the left biliary system.

In addition to the classical sudden onset of painless jaundice with associated pruritus and pale acholic stools found in patients who develop extrahepatic biliary obstruction, systemic symptoms of CCA include unintended weight loss, unaccustomed fatigue, night sweats, and frailty. Patients with biliary strictures may develop secondary bacterial infections with acute and chronic cholangitis and associated fever, chills, rigors, and neutrophilia, potentially progressing to sepsis syndrome if unrecognized.

Diagnosis

The diagnosis of CCA requires a high degree of suspicion, both in persons with known predisposing conditions or factors and in the majority of patients with CCA who have no known risk factors.

For patients with PSC, approximately a third of the 15% to 20% who will develop CCA during their lifetime will be diagnosed with CCA within 2 to 3 years of the initial diagnosis of PSC. This suggests that changes associated with malignant transformation are the initial triggers for the diagnosis of PSC in some patients. Consequently, it is important to carefully assess and follow patients with newly diagnosed PSC. Current expert recommendations are for surveillance of PSC patients with annual multiphasic magnetic resonance imaging (MRI) with magnetic resonance cholangiopancreatography (MRCP) and serum carbohydrate antigen 19-9 (CA 19-9) biomarker measurements, reflexing to endoscopic retrograde cholangiopancreatography (ERCP) with brushings for cytology and pancreatobiliary fluorescence in situ hybridization (FISH) testing if patients have any suspicious changes in clinical status, including episodes of ascending cholangitis.[4,5]

For patients without known risk factors, symptomatic presentation with painless jaundice, acholic stools, and weight loss, or epigastric or right upper quadrant abdominal pain, early satiety, and an upper abdominal mass should prompt diagnostic imaging initially by ultrasound. Evidence for biliary tract obstruction or a mass should trigger multiphasic cross-sectional imaging by CT or MRI/MRCP. Biliary tract obstruction with a suspicious-looking stricture or periductal mass should prompt the performance of an ERCP, or if this option is not available or warranted, a percutaneous transhepatic cholangiogram performed by an interventional radiologist to dilate the stricture, obtain cytology brushings and biopsies for CCA diagnosis, and perform temporary presurgical or permanent palliative biliary stenting to relieve obstruction and reduce the likelihood of acute bacterial cholangitis. These critical investigations are often unavailable in low-resource settings, making efficient and accurate diagnosis of CCA particularly challenging. Imaging features of iCCA show tumors with a lobular border with progressively increasing enhancement during progression from the arterial through the portal venous and delayed phases; this is different from the early arterial phase enhancement and portal and late venous washout that are typical for HCC. There may be capsular retraction adjacent to the mass and evidence of portal vein occlusion or thrombosis.

For pCCA and dCCA, the most typical imaging appearance is of the previously described "atrophy-hypertrophy complex." There may be evidence of biliary dilatation due to occlusion of the left and/or right or more distal points in the bile duct system. In patients who are potential candidates for surgical resection, careful attention should be paid to assess for involvement of the hepatic artery supplying the uninvolved liver lobe, which is not uncommon and often precludes resection in persons who are otherwise surgical candidates.

Almost all CCA have a propensity to metastases, with intrahepatic, peritoneal, and lymph node metastases being more common and lung and skeletal metastases being somewhat less common.

A key consideration in the differential diagnosis of pCCA and dCCA is IgG4-associated cholangitis. This immune-related inflammatory condition of the bile ducts can mimic obstructive malignant biliary strictures and affects other intraabdominal and systemic organs, being characterized by elevated serum and tissue IgG4 levels.[6] Because some CCA can also be associated with high serum IgG4 levels, it can be challenging to distinguish IgG4-associated cholangitis from CCA.[7] IgG4-associated cholangitis is associated with thickening of the bile and pancreatic ducts and inflammation in other retroperitoneal organs. The tissues are infiltrated with plasma cells and the inflammatory response is very sensitive to treatment with corticosteroids, which can cause remarkably rapid resolution of the inflammation and biliary obstruction. In steroid-refractory cases the anti-B cell monoclonal antibody rituximab is frequently effective.[6]

In addition to the imaging features of CCA, the serum biomarker CA 19-9, or monosialylated Lewis, is a sialyl-Lewis^A blood group antigen (Le^a) that is frequently increased in patients with CCA and has prognostic utility, being higher in persons with more progressive or metastatic disease and also frequently elevated in persons with pancreatic cancer. Acute bacterial cholangitis can lead to spurious elevations of the CA 19-9 into the thousands; thus cholangitis should be excluded or treated before reliance on the CA 19-9 as a marker for CCA. The CA 19-9 has a low positive predictive value in asymptomatic persons and is not a useful test in this setting. Approximately 10% of persons are unable to synthesize CA 19-9 and are referred to as Lewis negative, resulting in false-negative CA 19-9 tests.[8]

Management

Surgical resection is the preferred treatment for CCA developing in patients with no underlying liver disease or with compensated cirrhosis with adequate liver function and without clinically significant portal hypertension. Patients with iCCA often have underlying chronic liver disease and should be evaluated carefully for adequacy of hepatic reserve in order to prevent hepatic decompensation after surgery. Patients with underlying PSC often have significant fibrosis or established cirrhosis by the time of development of CCA, which is most frequently perihilar or distal. In these PSC patients surgical resection is discouraged due to the risk of postoperative hepatic decompensation. Overall, surgical resection with uninvolved margins is associated with a 30% to 40% 5-year survival, reflecting the high rate of postoperative recurrence. There is increasing exploration of the use of neo-adjuvant chemotherapy prior to surgical resection as this has proven to be quite effective in the treatment of early-stage pancreatic cancer and other cancer types and is thought to be beneficial in CCA.

A protocol of preoperative chemoradiation followed by staging laparoscopy to confirm a lack of extrahepatic involvement prior to liver transplantation has been refined at the Mayo Clinic and used successfully in patients with early-stage perihilar and distal cholangiocarcinoma who are not candidates for surgical resection. The protocol is particularly effective in patients with PSC who have been under regular surveillance for CCA and have early tumor detection but are ineligible for surgical resection due to their underlying cirrhosis. The Mayo Clinic protocol is limited to tumors with a radial diameter of no more than 3 cm perpendicular to the bile duct axis, although the linear diameter along the axis of the bile duct can be greater than 3 cm. CCA have a high propensity for intraperitoneal seeding, and during the pre-transplant evaluation, endoscopic ultrasound is often performed to assess for perihilar lymph node involvement. Fine needle aspiration of any suspicious nodes is performed to exclude metastatic disease. In these pre-transplant patients it is important not to traverse the bile duct from the peritoneal surface to confirm the histologic diagnosis of CCA, as this substantially increases the risk of peritoneal seeding and renders the patient ineligible for liver transplantation. In this highly selected population, at high-volume centers, the protocol achieves a 5-year survival of 74% in PSC patients and 58% in those with *de novo* pCCA.[9]

There have also been early attempts to implement protocols of liver transplantation for patients with limited-stage iCCA. These protocols have built on the observation that patients with early-stage iCCA that are mistaken for hepatocellular carcinoma (HCC) and enrolled in liver transplant protocols for HCC appeared to have acceptable long-term outcomes.[10]

Notwithstanding these advances in the treatment of CCA by liver transplantation, this treatment modality is not available in most low- and middle-income settings, due to the sophisticated healthcare infrastructure and technical expertise required for successful implementation. There is also evidence that the outcomes from the Mayo Clinic transplant protocol are poorer in low-volume centers.

Patients with pCCA or dCCA who are not candidates for surgical resection and who have biliary obstruction from tumor invasion or compression of the bile ducts typically require restoration of biliary drainage by stenting, either performed endoscopically at ERCP or through percutaneous transhepatic cholangiography (PTC). Palliative biliary drainage is critical because hyperbilirubinemia is toxic to the liver and also because many chemotherapy agents are metabolized and detoxified by the liver and excreted through the bile. Patients with biliary obstruction are therefore not eligible for most chemotherapy regimens.

Genomic analyses of CCA over the past several years have revealed that there is a gradient of genomic alterations extending from cancers arising in the smallest bile ducts in the periphery of the liver through the perihilar region to distal bile duct cancers. In general, there is an increasing frequency of KRAS gene mutations as one proceeds from the proximal to the distal bile ducts. Proximally, significant proportions of iCCA have mutations in the isocitrate dehydrogenase 1 (*IDH1*) or 2 (*IDH2*) genes or alterations in the fibroblast growth factor receptor 2 (*FGFR2*) gene. The *IDH1* and *IDH2* mutations result in the production of the oncometabolite 2-hydroxyglutarate, which has a distinctive effect on the epigenome, mediating oncogenesis. The most common *FGFR2* alterations seen in iCCA are fusions between the *FGFR2* gene and other partner genes. A proportion of iCCA also have mutations in chromatin remodeling genes, including *ARID1A*, *ARID2*, and *PBRM1*. *BAP1* gene mutations and mutations in cell cycle regulating and receptor kinase pathway genes such as *TP53* and *PIK3CA* are also seen at appreciable frequencies. A small proportion of iCCA also have mismatch repair deficiency or Lynch syndrome.[11,12] A substantial proportion of iCCA developing in persons with chronic hepatitis B virus infection have been shown to have integrations of the HBV DNA into the host genome, with the telomerase reverse transcriptase (*TERT*) gene being the most common site of recurrent HBV integration in iCCA.[13]

CCA have traditionally been treated with chemotherapy, to which most exhibit substantial resistance, with the most effective agents thus far being the combination of the antimetabolite gemcitabine with the alkylating agent cisplatin. Recent studies suggest that the addition of nanoparticle albumin-bound (nab)-paclitaxel or immune checkpoint inhibition with durvalumab provides additional antitumor activity.[14-16] Over the past few years, the recognition of the relatively high proportion of CCA with targetable gene alterations has led to considerable therapeutic development activity.

Targeted Therapies for CCA

Patients with mismatch repair deficiency (dMMR), also referred to as microsatellite instability-high (MSI-H), have a hypermutated state in which they create many tumor neo-antigens. These tumors are highly susceptible to treatment with immune checkpoint inhibitors, regardless of the tissue site of the tumor. The prevalence of dMMR ranges from 2% to 5% of CCA.

BRAF alterations occur in 3% to 5% of CCA and the *BRAF* V600E mutations are targetable with combined BRAF and MEK inhibition. Currently, treatment of non-V600E class II and III *BRAF* alterations is under investigation with novel targeting strategies.

Homologous recombination deficiency, found in tumors bearing mutations in *ARID1A*, *BAP1*, *ATM*, *BRCA2*, *CHEK2*, or *PALB2*, occurs in 5% to 15% of CCA. These tumors are more likely to be platinum sensitive. There are also ongoing trials evaluating the use of poly(adenosine diphosphate ribose) polymerase (PARP) inhibitors in patients harboring germline variants of these genes.

For iCCA, *FGFR2* gene fusions, amplification, or activating mutations, seen in 10% to 20% of iCCA, or *IDH1* and *IDH2* mutations, seen in 15% to 20% of iCCA, are particularly prevalent, resulting in the approvals of the reversible FGFR inhibitors pemigatinib and infigratinib, and the granting of FDA priority review status to the irreversible inhibitor futibatinib for patients with *FGFR2*-altered iCCA, as well as the approval of the IDH1 inhibitor ivosidenib for patients with *IDH1*-mutated iCCA.[17-20]

Other CCA for which FDA-approved tissue agnostic therapies are available include those with neurotrophic tyrosine receptor kinase (NTRK) gene fusions of the C-terminal of the tropomyosin receptor tyrosine kinase (TRK) with an N-terminal fusion partner, leading to ligand-independent phosphorylation and activation. NTRK gene fusions occur in less than 1% of CCA, but the TRK inhibitors entrectinib and larotrectinib show meaningful responses in these tumors.

KRAS mutations occur in 30% to 45% of eCCA and are the most common oncogenic driver in these tumors. *KRAS*-mutated cancers show aggressive tumor growth and are associated with poor survival. While novel therapies have recently been successfully developed that target the *KRAS* G12C mutation, this mutation is only observed in 6% of CCA patients, and the most common *KRAS* mutations in CCA are G12D and G12V mutations, which are yet undruggable.[21]

Based on the rich repertoire of targeted agents now available for treatment of CCA, particularly iCCA, genomic characterization of CCA tumors performed on biopsies obtained at the time of diagnosis has now become a routine standard of practice in high-resource settings. Unfortunately, this level of sophistication is not currently available in most low-resource settings, where relatively rudimentary immunohistochemical and genomic characterization of common cancers, such as breast cancer, remain elusive.

Positive efforts such as the recent announcement by Pfizer management of their intent to provide all their products on a nonprofit basis to low-income countries in Africa and the example of Gilead Sciences, which has provided manufacturing licenses for HIV and viral hepatitis medicines at no cost to manufacturers in low-income countries provide hope for improvement in access to life-saving systemic anti-cancer therapies for CCA in low-income settings such as Africa.

Key needs for improving access to specialist care for patients with CCA include promoting training and expertise in interventional endoscopy/advanced endoscopy, diagnostic and interventional radiology, stereotactic body radiation therapy, and hepatobiliary surgery. There is also a need to provide infrastructure and training to allow improved access to genomic characterization of tumors in low-resource settings.

References

1. Banales JM, Marin JJG, Lamarca A, et al. Cholangiocarcinoma 2020: the next horizon in mechanisms and management. *Nat Rev Gastroenterol Hepatol.* 2020;17(9):557-588.
2. Brindley PJ, Bachini M, Ilyas SI, et al. Cholangiocarcinoma. *Nat Rev Dis Primers.* 2021;7(1):65.
3. Kumagai S, Kurumatani N, Arimoto A, Ichihara G. Cholangiocarcinoma among offset colour proof-printing workers exposed to 1,2-dichloropropane and/or dichloromethane. *Occup Environ Med.* 2013; 70(7):508-510.
4. Rizvi S, Eaton JE, Gores GJ. Primary sclerosing cholangitis as a premalignant biliary tract disease: surveillance and management. *Clin Gastroenterol Hepatol.* 2015;13(12):2152-2165.
5. Barr Fritcher EG, Voss JS, Brankley SM, et al. An optimized set of fluorescence in situ hybridization probes for detection of pancreatobiliary tract cancer in cytology brush samples. *Gastroenterology.* 2015;149(7):1813-1824.e1.
6. Miyabe K, Zen Y, Cornell LD, et al. Gastrointestinal and extra-intestinal manifestations of IgG4-related disease. *Gastroenterology.* 2018;155(4):990-1003.e1.
7. Oseini AM, Chaiteerakij R, Shire AM, et al. Utility of serum immunoglobulin G4 in distinguishing immunoglobulin G4-associated cholangitis from cholangiocarcinoma. *Hepatology.* 2011;54(3):940-948.
8. Parra-Robert M, Santos VM, Canis SM, Pla XF, Fradera JMA, Porto RM. Relationship between CA 19.9 and the Lewis phenotype: options to improve diagnostic efficiency. *Anticancer Res.* 2018;38(10): 5883-5888.
9. Azad AI, Rosen CB, Taner T, Heimbach JK, Gores GJ. Selected patients with unresectable perihilar cholangiocarcinoma (pCCA) derive long-term benefit from liver transplantation. *Cancers (Basel).* 2020;12(11):3157. doi:10.3390/cancers12113157.
10. Sapisochin G, Ivanics T, Heimbach J. Liver transplantation for intrahepatic cholangiocarcinoma: ready for prime time? *Hepatology.* 2022;75(2):455-472.
11. Farshidfar F, Zheng S, Gingras MC, et al. Integrative genomic analysis of cholangiocarcinoma identifies distinct IDH-mutant molecular profiles. *Cell Rep.* 2017;18(11):2780-2794.
12. Simbolo M, Bersani S, Vicentini C, et al. Molecular characterization of extrahepatic cholangiocarcinoma: perihilar and distal tumors display divergent genomic and transcriptomic profiles. *Expert Opin Ther Targets.* 2021;25(12):1095-1105.
13. An J, Kim D, Oh B, et al. Comprehensive characterization of viral integrations and genomic aberrations in HBV-infected intrahepatic cholangiocarcinomas. *Hepatology.* 2022;75(4):997-1011.
14. Shroff RT, Javle MM, Xiao L, et al. Gemcitabine, cisplatin, and nab-paclitaxel for the treatment of advanced biliary tract cancers: a phase 2 clinical trial. *JAMA Oncol.* 2019;5(6):824-830.
15. Cheon J, Lee CK, Sang YB, et al. Real-world efficacy and safety of nab-paclitaxel plus gemcitabine-cisplatin in patients with advanced biliary tract cancers: a multicenter retrospective analysis. *Ther Adv Med Oncol.* 2021;13:17588359211035983.
16. Kang S, El-Rayes BF, Akce M. Evolving role of immunotherapy in advanced biliary tract cancers. *Cancers (Basel).* 2022;14(7):1748. doi:10.3390/cancers14071748.
17. Abou-Alfa GK, Sahai V, Hollebecque A, et al. Pemigatinib for previously treated, locally advanced or metastatic cholangiocarcinoma: a multicentre, open-label, phase 2 study. *Lancet Oncol.* 2020;21(5): 671-684.
18. Javle M, Roychowdhury S, Kelley RK, et al. Infigratinib (BGJ398) in previously treated patients with advanced or metastatic cholangiocarcinoma with FGFR2 fusions or rearrangements: mature results from a multicentre, open-label, single-arm, phase 2 study. *Lancet Gastroenterol Hepatol.* 2021;6(10):803-815.

19. Zhu AX, Macarulla T, Javle MM, et al. Final overall survival efficacy results of ivosidenib for patients with advanced cholangiocarcinoma with IDH1 mutation: the phase 3 randomized clinical ClarIDHy Trial. *JAMA Oncol.* 2021;7(11):1669-1677.
20. Israel MA, Danziger N, McGregor KA, et al. Comparative genomic analysis of intrahepatic cholangiocarcinoma: biopsy type, ancestry, and testing patterns. *Oncologist.* 2021;26(9):787-796.
21. Wang S, Li Q, Ma P, et al. KRAS mutation in rare tumors: a landscape analysis of 3453 Chinese patients. *Front Mol Biosci.* 2022;9:831382.

CHAPTER 8

Hepatic Hemangioma

Joerg Boecker ■ Karl J. Oldhafer

KEY POINTS

- Sufficient imaging should be obtained in order to confirm the diagnosis of hemangioma. Under US they show as homogeneous hyperechoic lesions with sharp margin, posterior enhancement and absence of halo sign
- Regardless of the size, conservative management is appropriate for typical cases, and intervention should be considered for symptomatic lesions, which affect quality of life.
- Clinical surveillance is not required for typical hemangiomas.
- Intake of contraceptives or pregnancy is not contraindicated.

Introduction

Hemangiomas represent benign liver tumors that consist of vascular spaces lined by endothelial cells that are supplied by the hepatic artery. More recently, studies and the International Society for the Study of Vascular Anomalies 2018 classification have recognized that the histology of these lesions in adults is more representative of venous malformations when compared to lesions identified in children,[1] although they are most often called "cavernous hemangiomas" on imaging studies. This particular discussion requires more depth than this brief chapter to discuss the appropriate imaging terminology and histopathology, and we will focus on the "typical" hemangioma. Hemangiomas can be solitary, multiple, or, rarely, diffuse and are typically characterized by benign behavior. They are usually found incidentally on ultrasound studies as well-circumscribed, homogeneous, markedly hyperechogenic lesions. Lesion heterogeneity, cystic change, calcifications, capsular retraction, and avascularity are far less commonly seen and may be associated with larger lesions, vascular shunting, and fibrosis.[2] Several guidelines exist that propose therapeutic options and alternatives for patients with hepatic hemangioma, as well as strategies for risk stratification.[3-5]

EPIDEMIOLOGY

With an incidence of 0.4% to 7.3% in autopsy series, these liver masses are common and have an approximated prevalence of up to 20% of the population.[6-8] There is no evidence that a hepatic hemangioma has any malignant potential. According to the current edition of the World Health Organization, there are three types of hemangioma[9]: (1) hepatic infantile hemangioma (usually a solitary lesion becoming symptomatic in early childhood at the age of about 2 years); (2) hepatic small vessel neoplasia, usually small, about 2 cm, thin-walled blood vessel lesion; and (3) hepatic cavernous hemangioma—with the latter accounting for the largest proportion by far (Figure 8.1).[10] Men and women are affected, albeit men less commonly than women (female:male ratio = 3:1). They can be found in all age groups, although they are typically discovered in those between the ages of 30 and 50 years.[11,12] In the majority of adult patients hemangiomas are very small and

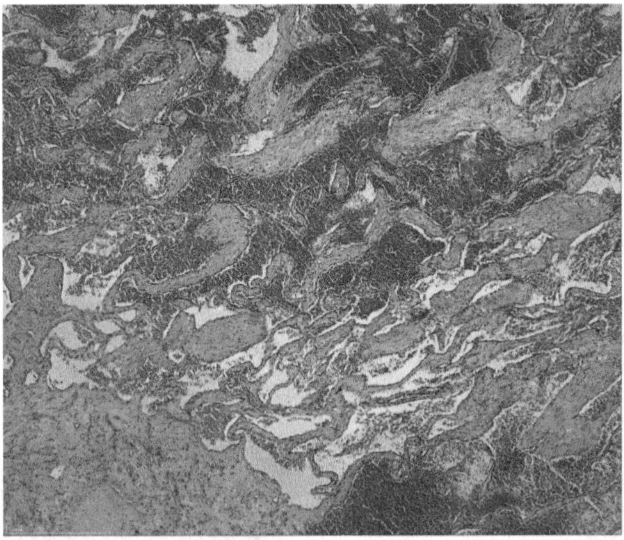

Figure 8.1 Histologic (hematoxylin and eosin staining) section showing thin-walled dilated vascular spaces lined by endothelial cells.

singular masses of less than 3 cm in diameter and are incidentally found on ultrasounds performed for reasons unrelated to the hemangioma. Larger tumors (>10 cm) are categorized as giant hemangiomas and may cause clinical symptoms. Cavernous hemangiomas larger than 40 cm are rarely reported. The etiology of hemangiomas is still not fully understood. A hormonal relationship in the growth of cavernous hemangiomas has been demonstrated. Possible hormonal dependence is suggested to play a role in the enlargement of these lesions, as patients who were exposed to estrogen during pregnancy or who were on hormone replacement therapy showed regression after withdrawal.[8,13] Nevertheless, lesions rarely progress in size enough to cause clinical problems due to pregnancy or estrogen therapy, and growth has been observed even in post-menopausal women.

PRESENTATION

Patients presenting with hepatic hemangioma rarely experience clinical signs or symptoms and typically don't need treatment. Nevertheless, the lesions may be responsible for pain due to Glisson's capsule pressure and partial infarction or may cause compression of adjacent tissue/organs, leading to symptoms such as fullness, nausea, vomiting, and constipation. These symptoms are generic and might be caused by something else. Rarely, hemangiomas may be associated with compression of vessels (Budd-Chari-like syndrome) or bile ducts, leading to cholestasis and/or cholangitis, or abscess formation. Consumptive coagulopathy (Kassabach-Merritt syndrome) and spontaneous rupture are rarely seen.

Diagnostics

IMAGING

With the increasing use of imaging modalities, asymptomatic hemangiomas are detected more frequently, mostly during imaging studies undertaken for other unrelated pathologies.[14] Conventional B-mode and color duplex ultrasound (US) is usually the initial imaging method for the primary assessment of symptoms of the upper abdomen symptoms/pathologies. US displaying a lesion with typical signs such as homogeneous hyperechoic, sharp margin, posterior enhancement, and absence of halo sign can be a very accurate tool to make a diagnosis of hemangioma (Figure 8.2) without the need for further investigation.[15]

For questionable lesions—hepatic hemangiomas disclose a typical contrast behavior so that they can be reliably diagnosed with contrast-enhanced imaging such as contrast-enhanced ultrasound (CEUS) as well as computed tomographic (CT) and magnetic resonance imaging (MRI) Examinations (Figure 8.3). The diagnosis is based on a typical vascular profile, characterized by peripheral and globular enhancement on arterial phase followed by a central enhancement on delayed phases—centripetal contrast uptake. MRI provides additional results such as lesion signal on T1-weighted, T2-weighted sequences, and diffusion-weighted imaging. These characteristics are of importance in differentiating hemangiomas from metastases of primary tumors from other sites.[16,17]

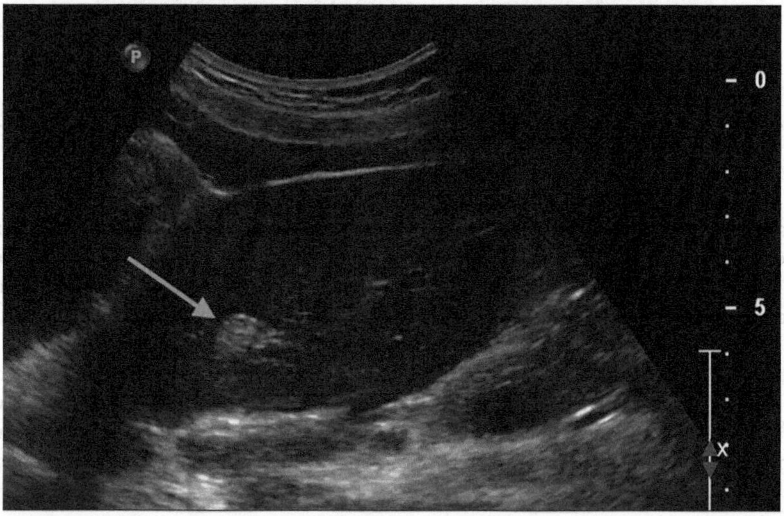

Figure 8.2 A 52-year-old female with rheumatoid arthritis and no cancer diagnosis underwent screening ultrasound to assess for gallstones. Grayscale ultrasound image shows a well-circumscribed, hyperechoic lesion (arrow). MRI later confirmed hemangioma.

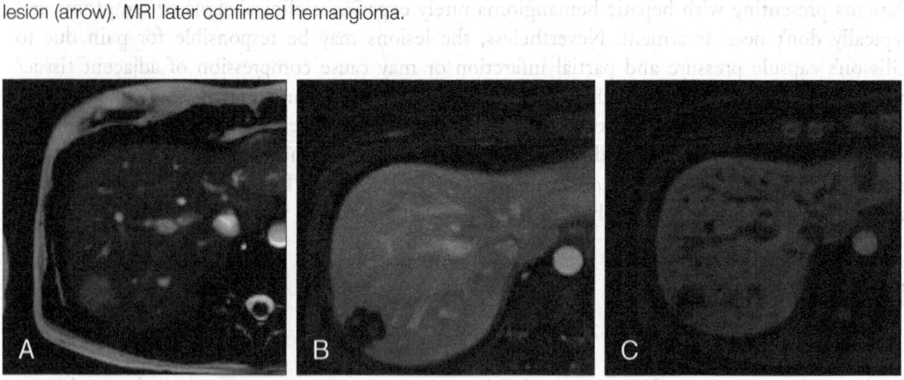

Figure 8.3 Hemangioma in Segment VII: axial T2-weighted (a), arterial phase (b), and late phase (c), after IV injection of contrast agent. Hyperintense signal in the T2 images, peripheral enhancement in the arterial phase, and increasing isointense presentation in the late phase.

BIOPSY

According to existing guidelines, percutaneous needle biopsy can be considered in questionable cases that cannot be clarified by other methods or imaging. Nevertheless, there is a strong discouragement not to do so, due to a high risk of bleeding.[4,5]

Management

There is a general agreement that small asymptomatic hemangiomas should be managed conservatively. Surgical excision for cavernous hemangioma is necessary only for large, symptomatic tumors. Especially in very voluminous cavernous hemangiomas, surgical removal can be considered in individual cases, depending on the degree of affliction. Patients with progressive abdominal discomfort or tumor enlargement can be considered for surgical resection, which is the treatment of choice (Figure 8.4). The risk of potential complications should be carefully weighed against operative risks, and surgery should be considered only after open discussion with the patient. The surgical procedure itself remains the choice of the treating surgeon—the commonest being enucleation and resection, if possible by minimally invasive fashion. However, reports suggest that symptoms can persist in up to 25% of patients following resection of hemangiomas, and therefore clear communication with the patients is essential.[18]

In addition to classic surgical measures, there are other interventional therapy options: sclerotherapy, laser vaporization, transarterial chemoembolization (TACE), medical therapy with corticosteroids or vincristine, or even liver transplantation.[3,4,19] Ultimately, surgery/resection remains the most commonly used treatment for symptomatic hemangiomas.

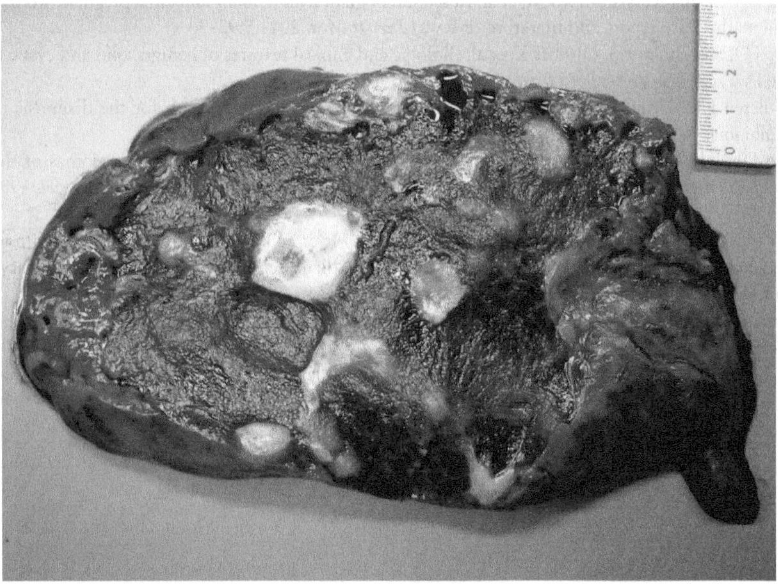

Figure 8.4 Large resected cavernous hemangioma with a red cut surface and many fibrous areas indicating tumor regression.

References

1. Kulungowski AM, Alomari AI, Chawla A, et al. Lessons from a liver hemangioma registry: subtype classification. *J Pediatr Surg.* 2012;47:165-170.
2. Vilgrain V, Boulos L, Vullierme MP, et al. Imaging of atypical hemangiomas of the liver with pathologic correlation. *Radiographics.* 2000;20:379-397.
3. European Association for the Study of the Liver. EASL Clinical Practice Guidelines on the management of benign liver tumours. *J Hepatol.* 2016;65:386-398.
4. Marrero JA, Ahn J, Rajender Reddy K, et al. ACG clinical guideline: the diagnosis and management of focal liver lesions. *Am J Gastroenterol.* 2014;109:1328-1347; quiz 1348.
5. Strauss E, Ferreira Ade S, Franca AV, et al. Diagnosis and treatment of benign liver nodules: Brazilian Society of Hepatology (SBH) recommendations. *Arq Gastroenterol.* 2015;(52 suppl 1):47-54.
6. Ishak KG, Rabin L. Benign tumors of the liver. *Med Clin North Am.* 1975;59:995-1013.
7. Karhunen PJ. Benign hepatic tumours and tumour like conditions in men. *J Clin Pathol.* 1986;39:183-188.
8. Duxbury MS, Garden OJ. Giant haemangioma of the liver: observation or resection? *Dig Surg.* 2010;27:7-11.
9. Nagtegaal ID, Odze RD, Klimstra D, et al. The 2019 WHO classification of tumours of the digestive system. *Histopathology.* 2020;76:182-188.
10. Wakasugi M, Ueshima S, Tei M, et al. Multiple hepatic sclerosing hemangioma mimicking metastatic liver tumor successfully treated by laparoscopic surgery: report of a case. *Int J Surg Case Rep.* 2015;8C:137-140.
11. Sewell JH, Weiss K. Spontaneous rupture of hemangioma of the liver: a review of the literature and presentation of illustrative case. *Arch Surg.* 1961;83:729-733.
12. Reddy KR, Kligerman S, Levi J, et al. Benign and solid tumors of the liver: relationship to sex, age, size of tumors, and outcome. *Am Surg.* 2001;67:173-178.
13. Ebina Y, Hazama R, Nishimoto M, et al. Resection of giant liver hemangioma in a pregnant woman with coagulopathy: case report and literature review. *J Prenat Med.* 2011;5:93-96.
14. Shaked O, Siegelman ES, Olthoff K, et al. Biologic and clinical features of benign solid and cystic lesions of the liver. *Clin Gastroenterol Hepatol.* 2011;9:547-562.e1-4.
15. Sandulescu LD, Urhut CM, Sandulescu SM, et al. One stop shop approach for the diagnosis of liver hemangioma. *World J Hepatol.* 2021;13:1892-1908.
16. Leslie DF, Johnson CD, Johnson CM, et al. Distinction between cavernous hemangiomas of the liver and hepatic metastases on CT: value of contrast enhancement patterns. *AJR Am J Roentgenol.* 1995;164:625-629.
17. Takayama Y, Nishie A, Okamoto D, et al. Differentiating liver hemangioma from metastatic tumor using T2-enhanced spin-echo imaging with a time-reversed gradient-echo sequence in the hepatobiliary phase of gadoxetic acid-enhanced MR imaging. *Magn Reson Med Sci.* 2022;21(3):445-457.
18. Fodor M, Primavesi F, Braunwarth E, et al. Indications for liver surgery in benign tumours. *Eur Surg.* 2018;50:125-131.
19. Li Y, Jia Y, Li S, et al. Transarterial chemoembolization of giant liver haemangioma: a multi-center study with 836 cases. *Cell Biochem Biophys.* 2015;73:469-472.

CHAPTER 9

Other Liver Masses

Siobhan M. Flanagan

KEY POINTS

- Hepatic cyst: Very common liver lesion. US classically shows a simple, anechoic lesion with imperceptible walls and posterior acoustic enhancement.
- FNH: Most common in young women. US appearance is variable, but a central scar is suggestive of FNH. May show mass effect on liver vasculature.
- Hepatic adenoma: More common in women than men and is related to oral contraceptive use, glycogen storage disease, and metabolic syndrome. US appearance is variable, depending on factors such as internal hemorrhage.
- Focal fat deposition: Seen in obesity, alcohol, hyperalimentation, hepatitis. Focal fat deposition is hyperechoic compared to adjacent liver, whereas focal fat sparing shows decreased echogenicity compared to adjacent liver. Both demonstrate sharp geographic borders and impart no mass effect on vasculature.
- Biliary hamartoma: Associated with polycystic kidney disease and polycystic liver disease. Diffuse small lesions give the liver a heterogenous appearance. Small lesions that can be seen are hyperechoic, round, or irregular. Larger lesions are hypoechoic and may show hyperechoic comet tail artifact.
- Liver metastasis: Suspect metastatic lesion in patients with known primary cancer outside the liver. Variable echogenicity depending on site and primary cancer type. A peripheral hypoechoic halo is suggestive of metastatic lesion. Lesions can have mass effect and displace vessels.
- Lymphoma: Risk factors HIV/AIDS, hepatitis C, preexisting or clinical suspicion of lymphoma. Lesions are typically hypoechoic to adjacent liver and can also be differentiated from a cyst by the presence of internal or peripheral vascularity.
- Hydatid cyst: Echinococcal infection. Cysts of various appearances depending on stage of life cycle. Simple cysts, complex cyst containing anechoic daughter cysts, complex mass-like lesions, and calcified lesions can be seen depending on life cycle stage.

Introduction

Liver masses other than HCC, cholangiocarcinoma, or hepatic hemangioma need to be considered in the differential diagnosis of focal liver lesions. These include benign and malignant entities. Benign entities include hepatic cysts (noninfectious), focal nodular hyperplasia, hepatic adenomas, biliary hamartomas, and abscess/infectious (covered elsewhere in the book). Malignant entities include metastases and lymphoma.

A clue to the entity can be the number of lesions (solitary, multiple, or diffuse) and if there is background liver disease. The echogenicity of the lesion can also assist in differential diagnosis; for example, a classic hemangioma is markedly hyperechoic. One must remember that if there is diffuse increased echogenicity of the liver, such as with fatty infiltration, this can give a focal lesion the appearance of decreased echogenicity. Comparing the echogenicity of the liver to adjacent kidney or spleen should help determine if the liver echogenicity is normal. The liver should be of equal or lower echogenicity to normal kidney and normal spleen. Also, fatty liver can hamper ultrasound view by making the deeper areas of the liver more difficult to visualize.[1]

Hepatic Cysts

Hepatic cysts are seen in nearly 5% of individuals. These lesions are anechoic and show through transmission with well-defined borders, an imperceptible wall, and no internal vascularity on Doppler imaging (Figure 9.1). Typical cysts lack internal echoes; therefore internal complexity or thick wall should raise the question of infection such as hydatid cyst or cystic metastatic lesion. Cysts are typically asymptomatic and do not change significantly in size unless there is an underlying entity causing the formation of cysts such as autosomal dominant or recessive polycystic kidney disease. Rarely, large cysts can cause pain or impart mass effect and cause biliary compression, and these lesions can be treated with alcohol sclerosis, surgical fenestration, or resection.[2,3]

Focal Nodular Hyperplasia

Focal nodular hyperplasia is a rare benign neoplasm more common in women (75%) and is composed of hepatocytes, Kupfer cells, and bile ducts.[4] They are not related to exogenous estrogens but can be seen after treatment with oxaliplatin. They are typically found incidentally and are not associated with spontaneous hemorrhage. The appearance on ultrasound can be highly variable, and lesions may be difficult to detect (Figure 9.2). Some lesions are well marginated, whereas others are isoechoic to surrounding liver. When lesions are detectable, a central scar with displacement of peripheral vasculature on Doppler can be seen, although this is only noted in 20% of lesions. Lesions are typically treated conservatively. In a patient with cirrhosis HCC needs to be excluded.

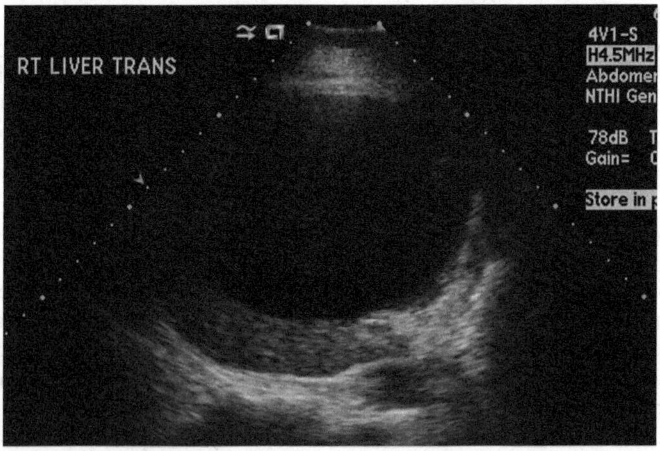

Figure 9.1 Simple hepatic cyst in a 75-year-old male. Note that the lesion is anechoic, is well marginated, and has imperceptible walls. Subtle posterior acoustic enhancement is noted.

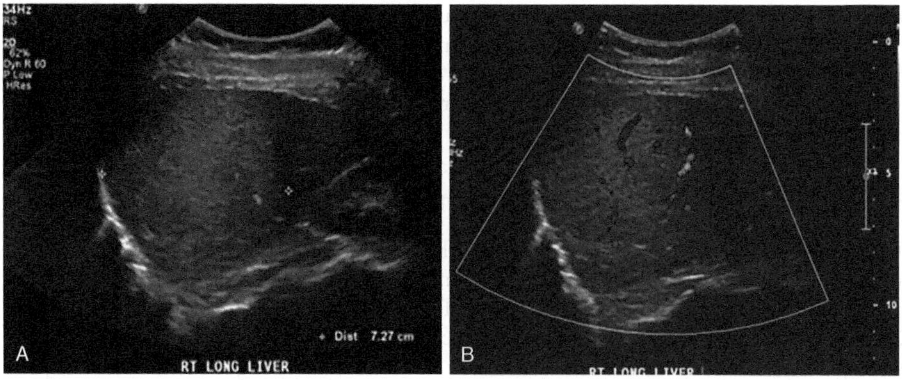

Figure 9.2 A and B: Focal Nodular Hyperplasia. A 36-year-old female with elevated liver enzymes found to have a subtle isoechoic lesion (2a) that was hypervascular on color Doppler (2b).

Hepatic Adenoma

Hepatic adenomas are relatively uncommon and are seen more often in women than men given that the tumors are stimulated by estrogen; however, the prevalence is thought to be increasing as obesity and metabolic syndrome are becoming more common worldwide.[2] Risk factors include oral contraceptive use and glycogen storage disease. Lesions can be solitary or multiple and are usually well demarcated. The echogenicity can be variable depending on size and internal components, including hemorrhage and calcifications.[5] Approximately 20% to 40% of lesions are hypoechoic, and approximately 30% are hyperechoic (Figure 9.3) due to internal fat. Internal hemorrhage can be seen, which contributes to a heterogeneous appearance. Oral contraceptive

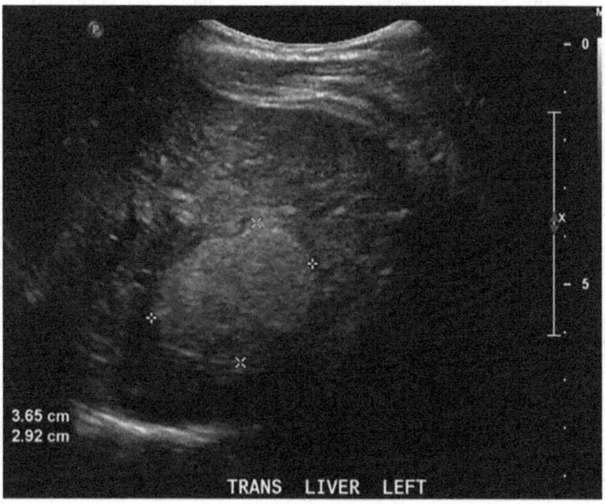

Figure 9.3 A 14-year-old female with history of Kabuki syndrome and fatty liver disease who had a screening ultrasound that showed a mass in the left lobe with increased echogenicity compared to adjacent liver. The lesion increased in size over time and was resected. Pathology showed adenoma.

use is a clue, and lesions should decrease in size after oral contraceptive is discontinued. Biopsy can be considered in a patient with risk factors for malignancy. Lesions larger than 5 cm and those in a subcapsular location can bleed; thus resection or embolization can be considered. Evaluation by a specialist should be performed when women with hepatic adenomas are pregnant, as the lesion has a high risk of growing and bleeding.

Focal Fat Deposition or Sparing

Focal fat deposition or fatty sparing in a liver with diffuse steatosis can mimic lesions. Focal fat deposition is hyperechogenic compared to adjacent liver and demonstrates sharp borders, tends to have nonspherical margins, and has no mass effect on vessels or the biliary tree (Figure 9.4). Distribution tends to be lobar or segmental, and certain areas of the liver are more prone to developing focal fat deposition, such as the liver that abuts the falciform ligament.[6,7] Focal fat sparing in the background of fatty infiltration demonstrates geographic borders and decreased echogenicity compared to adjacent fatty infiltrated liver.[8] Also, it does not impart mass effect on adjacent vessels (Figure 9.5).

Biliary Hamartomas

Multiple biliary hamartomas are rare and benign entities composed of small disorganized clusters of dilated cystic bile ducts lined with a layer of cuboidal cells and surrounded by fibrocollagenous stroma.[1] They are associated with polycystic kidney disease and polycystic liver disease. They do not typically communicate with the biliary tree and are thought to be embryonic bile duct remnants that did not involute. They are small, round, or irregular lesions that range in size from 5 to 30 mm. They are usually hyperechogenic if they are able to be seen. When small and numerous, they give the liver a diffusely heterogenous appearance. When larger and individually seen, they are hypoechoic (Figure 9.6) and may demonstrate a hyperechoic comet tail artifact.[9] Treatment is not typically indicated.

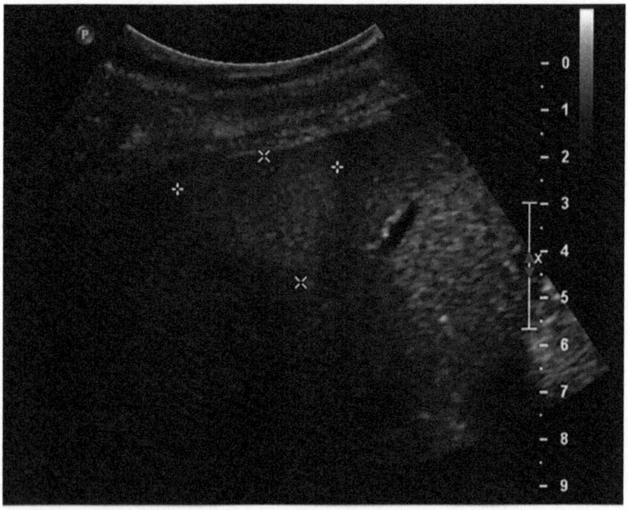

Figure 9.4 Focal fatty deposition in the liver of a 33-year-old male with hyperlipidemia and obesity who underwent screening ultrasound. Gray-scale ultrasound shows hyperechoic lesion with geographic borders abutting a vessel, adjacent to the portal vein.

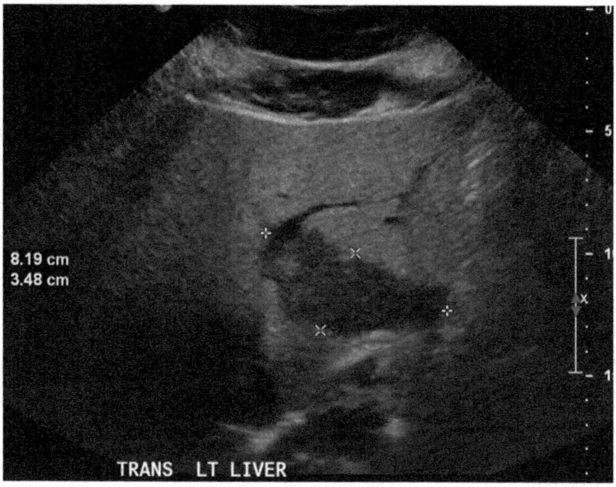

Figure 9.5 Focal fatty sparing in the liver of 34-year-old female with elevated liver enzymes and suspected nonalcoholic fatty liver disease. Ultrasound demonstrates a geographic area of decreased echogenicity with no mass effect on the adjacent vessels consistent with focal fatty sparing.

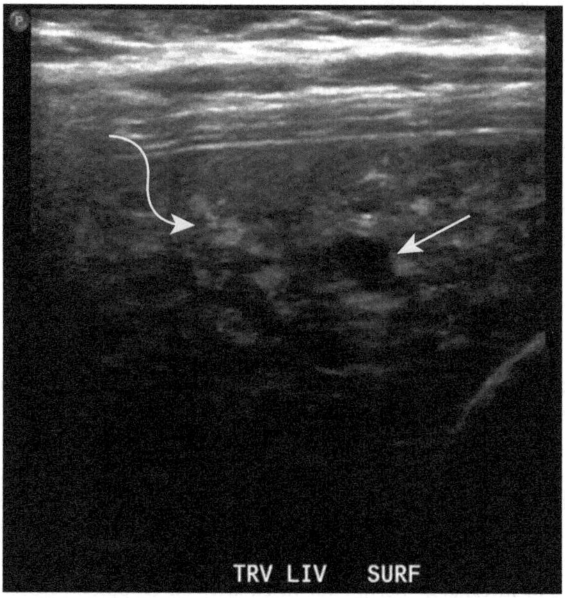

Figure 9.6 Ultrasound in a 46-year-old male shows multiple small hyperechoic (curved arrow) and hypoechoic (straight arrow) lesions.

Liver Metastases

Liver metastases can also have a variable appearance; however, certain characteristics can suggest metastasis versus primary tumor. Metastases are more often (approximately 65% of cases) hypoechoic,[1] the most common being lung, breast, pancreatic cancer, and lymphoma. Hyperechoic metastases include colorectal, renal cell, and neuroendocrine cancers and Kaposi

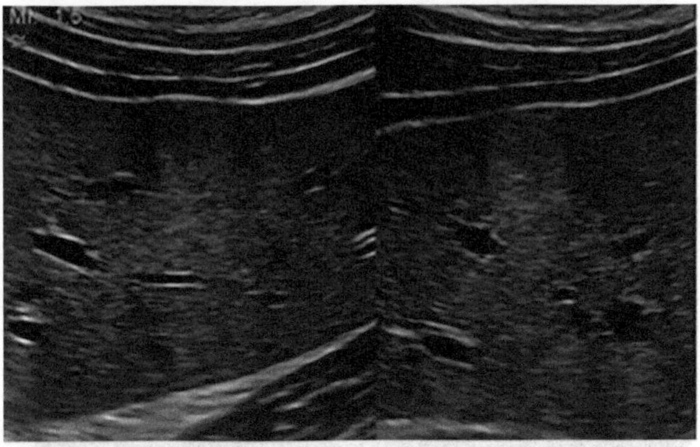

Figure 9.7 A 57-year-old male presented with abdominal pain and weight loss. Gray-scale ultrasound image shows an echogenic liver lesion with hypoechoic halos. Biopsy of the lesion revealed metastatic gastro-esophageal adenocarcinoma.

sarcoma. Of note, a peripheral hypoechoic halo (Figure 9.7) due to compressed and fat-spared liver surrounding the lesion is a feature suggestive of metastasis.[10] In addition, normal liver vasculature is distorted or displaced by the mass effect of the lesion. Mucinous adenocarcinomas can demonstrate internal calcifications, which are hyperechoic and shadowing. Cystic metastases can be seen with ovarian, squamous cell, pancreatic, and colorectal cancers. Infiltrative or poorly defined metastases can be seen with melanoma, breast, and lung cancer. Contrast-enhanced ultrasound, if available, can aid in determining the degree of vascularity of a tumor, which can also be a clue to primary cancer. When a liver lesion is identified in a case of cancer without known primary malignancy, biopsy of the lesion, when possible, is useful in aiding the diagnosis.

Lymphoma

Lymphoma can be seen in the liver as a primary or secondary site of disease. Risk factors for developing hepatic lymphoma include HIV/AIDS and hepatitis C. Primary hepatic lymphoma is very rare but is seen primarily in immunocompromised patients (including those with HIV/AIDS). Secondary involvement of the liver is far more common and tends to be related to non-Hodgkin lymphoma.[11] On ultrasound, lesions tend to be hypoechoic to liver parenchyma, which may be due to the high degree of cellularity without associated stroma (Figure 9.8). Rarely are lesions nearly anechoic and mimic a cyst, but they typically lack the posterior acoustic enhancement seen with cysts. Lymphoma can also be differentiated from a cyst by the presence of internal or peripheral vascularity on Doppler.[12] Vascular channels can be seen coursing through the lesion and this finding has been referred to as the "vessel penetration sign."[13]

Hydatid Cyst

Hydatid disease is caused by the parasitic tapeworm *Echinococcus granulosus*, which is endemic in many parts of the world, including South America, Africa, and the Middle East (further described elsewhere in the book).[14] After the outer shell is digested, the oncosphere passes through the duodenal mucosa and eventually is lodged in a hepatic vasculature. Those trapped in the liver

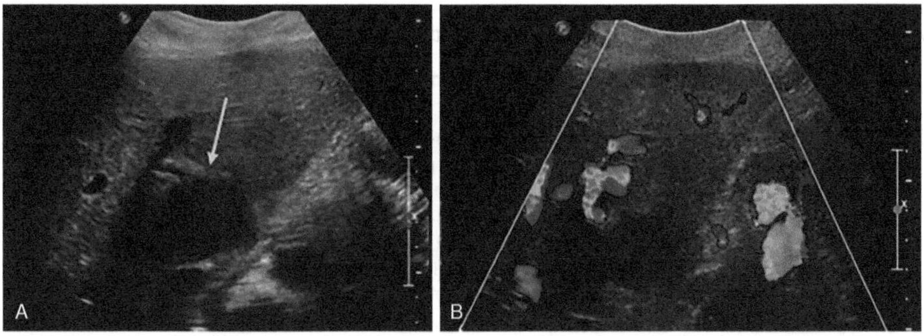

Figure 9.8 A 13-year-old male status post liver transplant presented with elevated transaminases. A: Gray-scale ultrasound image demonstrates a hypoechoic lesion in the caudate lobe (arrow). B: Internal blood flow was not appreciated on Doppler ultrasound. Biopsy revealed post-transplant lymphoma.

may develop into hydatid cysts. Others may enter the hepatic vein drainage and into systemic circulation, where they can lodge elsewhere, such as in lung. Liver cysts can present with abdominal pain and can range in appearance and multiple classification systems exist. Cysts are typically anechoic with well-defined walls. Imaging findings reflect the stage of cyst growth, including whether the cyst is unilocular, contains daughter vesicles, contains daughter cysts, is partially calcified, or is dead/completely calcified. Thus the ultrasound appearance can vary depending on stage and can at times mimic a mass.[15] The Gharbi ultrasound classification consists of five stages. Stage 1 lesions are homogeneously hypoechogenic cystic thin-walled lesions (Figure 9.9a). Stage 2 lesions are septated cysts. Stage 3 lesions demonstrate internal daughter cysts. Stage 4 lesions mimic tumors and stage 5 are inactive cysts that are partially or completely calcified (Figure 9.9b). Cysts causing symptoms can be treated with surgical excision or percutaneous aspiration and sclerotherapy.

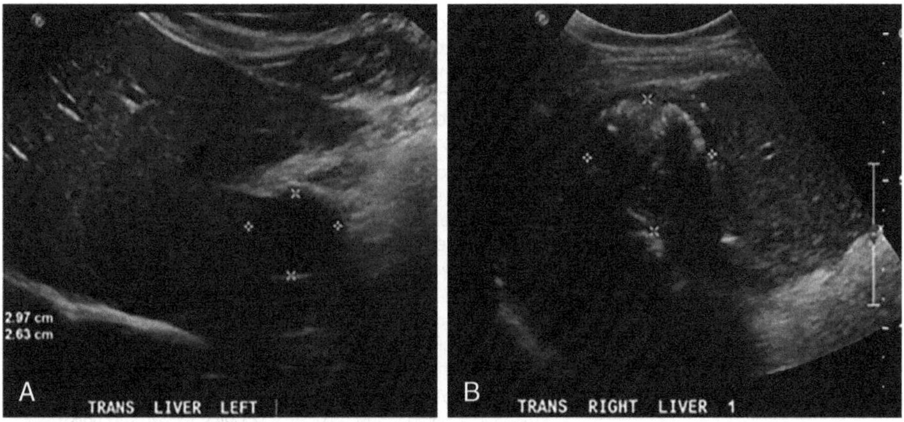

Figure 9.9 A 34-year-old male with abdominal pain. A: Gray-scale ultrasound shows a simple cystic lesion in the left lobe of the liver. B: Gray-scale ultrasound of the right lobe shows a calcified lesion. Subsequent CT scan revealed multiple abdominal cystic lesions of varying complexity. The calcified lesions indicated that the echinococcal infection was chronic.

TABLE 9.1 ■ **Clinical Pearls, Ultrasound Findings, and Management of "Other Liver Lesions"**

Lesion	Clinical Pearls	Ultrasound Findings	Management
Cyst	May be associated with polycystic kidney disease	Anechoic Posterior acoustic enhancement Well-defined borders, imperceptible wall No internal vascularity	Expectant management is typically recommended Surgical management is reserved for symptomatic lesions
FNH	Most common in young women Can be seen after treatment with oxaliplatin	Highly variable US appearance May see central scar May show mass effect on liver vasculature	If no risk of malignancy, can be observed If cirrhosis or other risk for HCC, CT/MRI or biopsy is considered
Adenoma	More common in women than men Related to oral contraceptives and glycogen storage disease	Single or multiple lesions Variable appearance and internal echogenicity depending on size and internal components	Stop oral contraceptives Treatment (surgery or embolization) considered for lesions larger than 5 cm and subcapsular in location
Focal Fat Deposition	Seen in obesity, alcohol, hyperalimentation, hepatitis	Hyperechoic compared to adjacent liver Sharp borders May be non-spherical No mass effect	Treat underlying condition Can follow with ultrasound
Focal Fat Sparing	Seen in obesity, alcohol, hyperalimentation, hepatitis	Decreased echogenicity compared to adjacent liver Geographic borders No mass effect	Treat underlying condition Can follow with ultrasound
Biliary Hamartomas	Associated with polycystic kidney disease and polycystic liver disease	Diffuse small lesions give liver heterogenous appearance Size range 5–30 mm Small lesions that can be seen are hyperechoic, round, or irregular Larger lesions are hypoechoic and may show hyperechoic comet tail artifact	Treatment typically not needed
Metastases	Known primary cancer outside liver	Variable echogenicity depending on size and primary cancer type Peripheral hypoechoic halo Mass effect/vessel displacement	Biopsy if primary unknown Treat primary cancer
Lymphoma	Risk factors HIV/AIDS, hepatitis C, pre-existing or clinical suspicion of lymphoma	Hypoechoic to adjacent liver May mimic cyst Can be differentiated from cyst by presence of internal or peripheral vascularity	Biopsy if diagnosis needed Treat primary lymphoma
Hydatid Cyst	Echinococcal infection causes cysts most commonly in liver. Can be disseminated.	Cysts of various appearances depending on stage of life cycle. Simple cysts, complex cyst containing anechoic daughter cysts, complex mass-like lesions, and calcified lesions can be seen depending on life cycle stage.	Positive Ig ELISA serology aids diagnosis Treatment with anti-helminthic agents is necessary Surgical or percutaneous procedures for symptomatic cysts can be considered

References

1. Middleton WD, Morgan T. *Ultrasound: The Requisites*. Philadelphia, PA: Elsevier Health Sciences; 2015.
2. Venkatesh SK, Chandan V, Roberts LR. Liver masses: a clinical, radiologic, and pathologic perspective. *Clin Gastroenterol Hepatol.* 2014;12(9):1414-1429. doi: 10.1016/j.cgh.2013.09.017.
3. Borhani AA, Wiant A, Heller MT. Cystic hepatic lesions: a review and an algorithmic approach. *AJR Am J Roentgenol.* 2014;203:1192-1204.
4. Cha DI, Yoo SY, Kim JH, Jeon TY, Eo H. Clinical and imaging features of focal nodular hyperplasia in children. *AJR Am J Roentgenol.* 2014;202(5):960-965.
5. Grazioli L, Federle M, Brancatelli G, Ichikawa T, Olivetti L, Blachar A. Hepatic adenomas: imaging and pathologic findings. *RadioGraphics.* 2001;21:877-894.
6. Décarie PO, Lepanto L, Billiard JS, et al. Fatty liver deposition and sparing: a pictorial review. *Insights Imaging.* 2011;2:533-538.
7. Jang JK, Jang HJ, Kim JS, et al. Focal fat deposition in the liver: diagnostic challenges on imaging. *Abdom Radiol (NY).* 2017;42:1667-1678.
8. Décarie PO, Lepanto L, Billiard JS, et al. Fatty liver deposition and sparing: a pictorial review. *Insights Imaging.* 2011;2(5):533-538. doi:10.1007/s13244-011-0112-5.
9. Zheng RQ, Zhang B, Kudo M, Onda H, Inoue T. Imaging findings of biliary hamartomas. *World J Gastroenterol.* 2005;11(40):6354-6359.
10. Shankar A, Varadan B, Kalyanasundaram S, et al. Hypoechoic halo sign: liver metastases. *Abdom Radiol (NY).* 2021;46:2253-2254.
11. Elsayes KM, Menias CO, Willatt JM, Pandya A, Wiggins M. Primary hepatic lymphoma: imaging findings. *J Med Imaging Radiat Oncol.* 2009;53:373-379.
12. Takeuchi N, Naba K. Primary hepatic lymphoma is difficult to discriminate from a liver abscess. *Case Rep Gastrointest Med.* 2014;2014;925307. doi:10.1155/2014/925307.
13. Rajesh S, Bansal K, Sureka B, Patidar Y, Bihari C, Arora A. The imaging conundrum of hepatic lymphoma revisited. *Insights Imaging.* 2015;6(6):679-692. doi:10.1007/s13244-015-0437-6.
14. Turgut AT, Akhan O, Bhatt S, Dogra VS. Sonographic spectrum of hydatid disease. *Ultrasound Q.* 2008;24(1):17-29.
15. Pedrosa I, Saíz A, Arrazola J, Ferreirós J, Pedrosa CS. Hydatid disease: radiologic and pathologic features and complications. *RadioGraphics.* 2000;20:795-817.

SECTION III

Tropical Infectious Liver Disease

CHAPTER 10

Schistosomiasis

Leila M. M. Beltrão Pereira ■ Leila Maria Soares Tojal de Barros Lima ■ Luciano Beltrão Pereira

KEY POINTS

- Schistosomiasis represents a serious public health problem that affects approximately 260 million people worldwide.
- The most important pathogenic event in liver *Schistosomiasis* is hepatic granuloma formation and periportal hepatic fibrosis.
- Hepatosplenic form is the most typical of *Schistosomiasis mansoni*.
- The diagnosis is confirmed by the presence of *Schistosoma mansoni* eggs in stool samples, rectal or liver biopsies, or serological tests.
- Praziquantel is the most widely available drug for the treatment of schistosomiasis.

Introduction

Schistosomiasis represents a serious public health problem that affects approximately 260 million people worldwide, across 78 countries, mainly in South America, the Caribbean, Africa, and the eastern Mediterranean.[1] In Brazil *Schistosoma mansoni* affects >3 million people, and approximately 30 million are exposed to the infection because they reside in endemic areas with a low quality of public sanitation, mainly in the northeast region.[2]

Six species of *Schistosoma* are now known to be mainly responsible for human infection: *S. mansoni* (Figure 10.1A), *S. haematobium* (Figure 10.1B), *S. japonicum* (Figure 10.1C), *S. intercalatum*, *S. mekongi*, and *S. mattheei*. Three other species, namely, *S. bovis*, *S. margrebowiei*, and *S. rodhaini*, infect domestic and wild animals (mainly ungulates and rodents) but affect humans much less frequently.[3] All species require a freshwater snail as an intermediate host, with each inhabiting a particular species of snail, and the geographical distribution of the schistosomes is governed by the range of their molluscan hosts.[4] There is some evidence that rodents and baboons may act as reservoir hosts of *S. mansoni*, but humans, especially children, are the most important definitive hosts of the parasite.[5] Although the morbidity and mortality has decreased in the last 25 years due to use of therapy,[6] the disease still poses a significant risk.[2,7]

Pathogenesis

Infection with *Schistosoma* occurs when infected snails contaminate water and human skin comes in contact with the water allowing the cercariae to penetrate the skin. The most important pathogenic event in schistosomiasis is hepatic granuloma formation and periportal hepatic fibrosis.[8] This fibrosis, initially described by Symmers in 1904, is mediated by several lymphocytic subpopulations, inducing an inflammatory and fibrotic response around the eggs lodged in the liver.

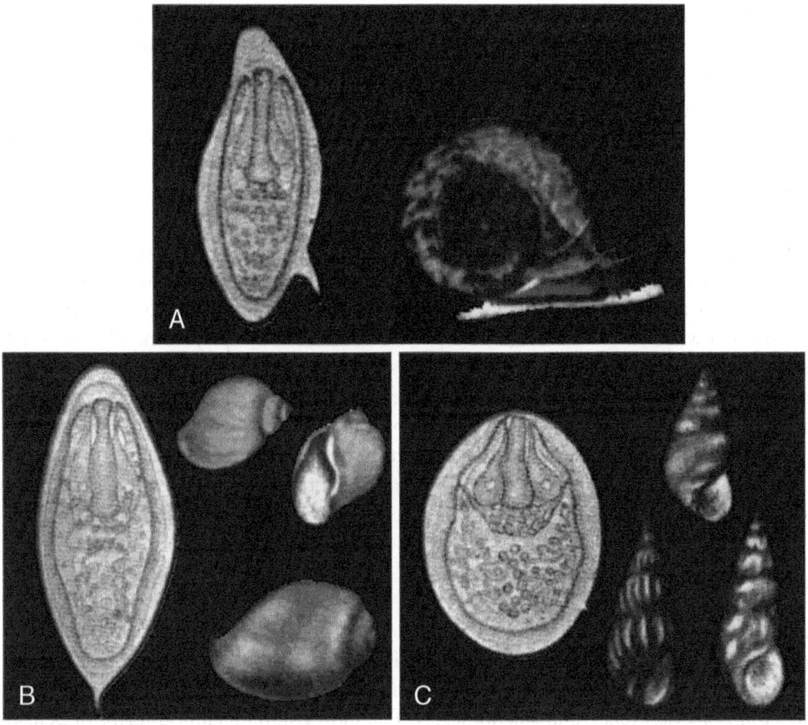

Figure 10.1 *Schistosoma* egg with corresponding snail for (A) *S. mansoni*, (B) *S. haematobium*, (C) *S. japonicum*.

At the time of oviposition, about 60% of the eggs reach the intestinal lumen. Most eggs become "trapped" in the capillaries of the intestinal mucosa. Some eggs remain there, while others are carried by the mesenteric circulation to the liver, where they "strand" in the hepatic sinusoids. The release of soluble antigens from eggs induces the mobilization of macrophages, eosinophils, lymphocytes, and plasmocytes, which is mediated by TNF, CD4 + Th1 and Th2 cells, and CD8 + T lymphocytes. Macrophages put themselves in contact with the egg, forming multinucleated syncytial masses; some of these cells are transformed into fibroblasts, guiding the organization of concentric layers throughout the granuloma's thickness, with extensive collagen production.[9]

In a hepatic granuloma by *Schistosoma*, type III collagen, in the form of procollagen, type I collagen, and fibronectin are usually detected by immunofluorescence.[10] An increase in the mean value of laminin and type IV collagen has also been observed in all clinical forms of schistosomiasis, being more significant in the decompensated hepatosplenic form, suggesting that perisinusoidal fibrosis and sinusoid capillarization may occur early in the disease.[11]

Hypertrophy of the sinusoids and hyperplasia of Kupffer cells and endothelial cells are observed in the schistosomal liver. The perisinusoidal space, which normally contains little collagen, exhibits thin strips of collagen microfibrils in Schistosomiasis mansoni. This space is enlarged, and extracellular elements have been observed in association with strips of collagen or line of granular material.[12]

Periportal fibrosis in its advanced stage may be irreversible, due to the high degree of binding of collagen fibrils. In old granulomas the appearance has been called clay pipe-stem fibrosis (clay pipe-stem cirrhosis or Symmers fibrosis), due to its thickness and whitish color, with greater resistance to collagen degradation and removal.[13]

The study of sinusoids in patients with or without portal hypertension shows a sequence of events, beginning with an increased number of cell nuclei, particularly evident in the centrilobular region. This is followed by the deposition of reticulin fibers along the perisinusoidal space, which is observed posteriorly crossing the lobe.

This perisinusoidal fibrosis probably adds an element of increased intra-sinusoidal pressure to the perisinusoidal hypertension already described. The hepatic sinusoids in *S. mansoni* receive mainly arterial blood.[12,13]

Although egg granuloma formation is probably a cause of tissue damage, the mechanism underlying the variability among patients in the severity of the disease is not well understood. Individual variations in host immune-mediated mechanisms may be important,[14] but it is likely that other factors are also involved. Since hepatitis B virus (HBV) infections are common in patients infected with schistosomiasis,[15] it is possible that this virus plays a major role in the exacerbation of hepatosplenic form of schistosomiasis. Other factors, such as alcoholism or concomitant infection with hepatotropic viruses other than HBV, such as hepatitis C (HCV) or D viruses (HDV), may contribute to the severity of this chronic liver disease.[16] Alternatively, the variability in severity might be due to superimposition of schistosomal infections on an underlying autoimmune liver condition such as autoimmune hepatitis or to parasite-induced autoreactive mechanisms in certain individuals.

Clinical Presentation

The majority of people infected with *Schistosoma mansoni* show limited, intermittent, or unspecific symptoms. The hepatosplenic form of schistosomiasis, the most typical of *Schistosoma mansoni*, usually presents asthenia, anorexia, abdominal pain, diarrhea alternating with constipation, hepatomegaly (left lobe), and splenomegaly. The most common clinical forms of Schistosomiasis mansoni are described in Table 10.1. There are also less frequently occurring infections like schistosomal nephropathy, as well as pseudotumoral, ectopic, and neurological forms.[17]

TABLE 10.1 ■ **Most Common Clinical Forms of *Schistosomiasis mansoni*[17]**

Clinical Form	Characteristics
Acute asymptomatic	Absence of symptoms, positive stool parasitological
Acute symptomatic	Dermatitis cercariae; Katayama fever: lymphadenopathy, malaise, fever, hyporexia, dry cough, sweating, muscle pain, pain in the region of the liver or intestine, diarrhea, headache and prostration, painful hepatomegaly and splenomegaly, tachycardia, and hypotension. Elevated eosinophilia is highly suggestive.
Hepatointestinal form	In general asymptomatic. Positive stool parasitology. Non-specific symptomatology: asthenia, dizziness, headache, diarrheal outbreaks interspersed with constipation, hepatomegaly. The spleen is not palpable. Normal liver function tests.
Hepatic form	Symmers-type periportal fibrosis, without splenomegaly. Symptomatology similar to the hepatointestinal form. Behavior and severity similar to the hepatosplenic form.
Compensated hepatosplenic form	The most typical of *Schistosomiasis mansoni*. Most frequent symptoms: asthenia, anorexia, abdominal pain, alternating diarrhea with constipation. Hepatomegaly (left lobe) with periportal fibrosis, splenomegaly, portal hypertension.
Decompensated hepatosplenic form	Incidence <10% of cases, usually associated with other hepatic pathologies (viral hepatitis B and C, alcoholism, portal vein thrombosis, etc.). Manifest ascites, associated or not with jaundice.

Diagnosis of Schistosoma mansoni

The diagnosis of Schistosomiasis mansoni is based on the history of patients with river bathing in endemic areas, confirmed by the presence of eggs in stool samples (employing at least three samples), rectal or liver biopsies, as well as serological tests,[17,18] described in Table 10.2.

Diagnosis of Periportal Fibrosis

Wedge liver biopsy has always been considered the "gold standard" for the evaluation of schistosomal fibrosis. On the other hand, needle biopsy often neglects periportal fibrosis because it recovers insufficient and fragmented tissue samples, which may lead to significant sampling errors, in addition to being an invasive method and associated with complications.[19]

Since the late 1970s, ultrasonography (US) has been used in *S. mansoni*, proving to be an efficient method in the diagnosis of hepatic fibrosis. It has been demonstrated that the periportal thickening detected by US corresponds to the periportal fibrosis found in histopathological examinations in all cases (Figure 10.2), correlating directly with the clinical conditions and the risks of complications by the disease.[20]

The World Health Organization (WHO) proposed standardization of ultrasound assessment through the Niamey protocol, which allows the grading of schistosomal fibrosis and correlates directly with clinical conditions and the risk of complications from the disease. This has been the most used classification in studies on the disease.[20]

Computed tomography and magnetic resonance imaging were shown to be superior only in the diagnosis of urogenital schistosomiasis and in ectopic lesions such as in the central and pulmonary nervous system compared to US.[21]

Among the direct biomarkers of hepatic fibrosis, there are studies that correlate laminin, collagen IV, and hyaluronic acid with periportal fibrosis and portal hypertension in *S. mansoni*. However, they are not liver specific and may vary according to changes in clearance and excretion.[19] Indirect biomarkers, easily applicable in clinical practice, such as APRI and FIB-4, also showed a correlation with the degree of hepatic fibrosis in *S. mansoni* and *S. japonicum*.[22]

More recently, studies with hepatic transient elastography (TE) have been performed in the assessment of schistosomal fibrosis. Studies with hepatic elastography have been shown to be effective in the diagnosis and grading of fibrosis in Schistosomiasis mansoni, with increased applicability as a noninvasive, easily reproducible method, which may also be correlated with portal

TABLE 10.2 ■ **Diagnostic Methods of *Schistosomiasis mansoni***

Method	Description
Parasitological stool examination	Kato-Katz (egg count) Hoffman (spontaneous sedimentation) Sensitivity 40% single sample (3 samples indicated)
Rectal biopsy	Invasive exam, used if failure of diagnosis repeated, stool exams and high suspicion (sensitivity 80% of cases)
Immunological	Antibody tests:
Circulating antibodies, indirect—do not differentiate between active and past infection, no relation to intensity of infection	Indirect hemagglutination and immunofluorescence (60%–90% sensitivity) ELISA (95% sensitivity)—most used in practice
Circulating antigens—detect active infection, related to the intensity of infection (few commercially available)	Tests with circulating antigens: Circulating cathodic antigen (CCA) Circulating anodic antigen (CAA)

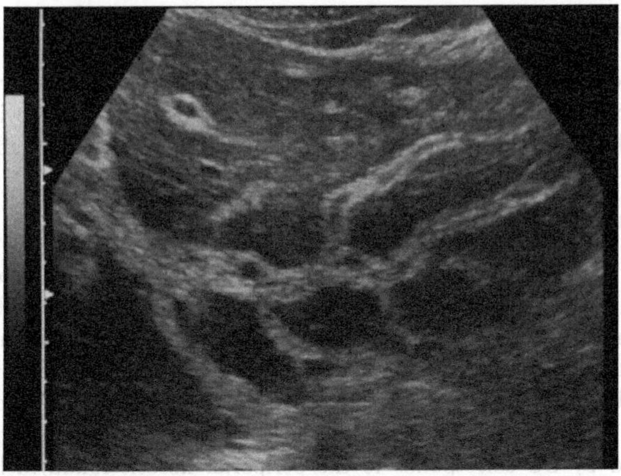

Figure 10.2 Ultrasonography showing periportal fibrosis in schistosomiasis infection. (Da Silva LC, Chieffi PP, Carrilho FJ. Schistosomiasis mansoni: clinical features. *Gastroenterol Hepatol*. 2005;28(1):30-39.)

hypertension in these patients.[22,23] More studies, however, are needed to better define the cutoff points in schistosomal hepatic fibrosis.[24]

Treatment

The treatment of schistosomiasis is aimed at preventing the progression of the disease and limiting existing damage such as hepatosplenomegaly, which is frequent, especially in younger patients.

Praziquantel (PZQ) is the most widely available drug for the treatment of schistosomiasis and remains effective against all schistosomes that infect humans. It is available in 600-mg tablets and administered orally, in a single dose of 50 mg/kg body weight for adults or 60 mg/kg body weight for children, usually administered after a meal. The cure rate is close to 80% for adults and 70% for children. Adverse effects are mild and transient, with no evidence that they cause serious toxic damage to the liver or other organs. Among all the side effects, the following stand out: metallic taste in the mouth, abdominal pain, diarrhea, asthenia, headache, and dizziness.[25]

Although PZQ has been used for over 30 years, the drug's exact mechanism of action remains unknown. A disadvantage is that sexually immature juvenile schistosomes are resistant to its action, and as the drug is usually administered in endemic areas as a single dose, complete efficacy is unlikely, with a reservoir of PZQ-resistant juvenile parasites likely to remain in the host. Therefore, in those patients who remain in areas of high endemicity, therapy should be repeated annually in children and every 2 years for adults.[26]

Oxamniquine is also available in two commercial forms: capsules of 250 mg of active salt and a solution containing 50 mg/mL, for pediatric use. The recommended doses are 20 mg/kg for children and 15 mg/kg for adults, taken as a single dose about 1 hour after a meal. The cure rate is similar to that of PZQ.[25]

Contraindications to the specific treatment of Schistosomiasis mansoni are: severe malnutrition, severe anemia, associated infections, decompensated heart failure, advanced liver disease, and collagen diseases. Although there are no teratogenic effects, most guidelines do not recommend treatment during pregnancy and in children under 2 years of age. However, more than 50 million patients have been treated worldwide and there are no reports of fatal cases associated with the treatment.[25]

In patients with severe acute schistosomiasis treatment should begin with prednisone (1 mg/kg/day). The patient is given schistosomicide (oxamniquine or PZQ) 24 to 48 hours later. The following week, the corticosteroid dose is reduced to 0.5 mg/kg/day and to 0.25 mg/kg/day in the third week.[27]

To evaluate cure, parasitological examinations of stools should be performed in the first, third, and sixth months after treatment. Serology with circulating antigens, which would identify active infection with high sensitivity and specificity, is not yet a reality in clinical practice.[21]

Vaccines Against Schistosomiasis

Three major vaccines against human schistosomiasis (Sh28GST, Sm-14, and Sm-TSP-2) are currently in different stages of clinical development, with a fourth (Sm-P80) to follow shortly.[28]

Despite recent encouraging progress in the development of vaccines against schistosomiasis, the antigens currently used may still not provide the necessary level of protective immunological potency, so it is important to continue the search for new target candidates.

References

1. WHO. *Schistosomiasis Fact Sheet 115*. Geneva: World Health Organization; 2014.
2. Scholte RG, Gosoniu L, Malone JB, Chammartin F, Utzinger J, Vounatsou P. Predictive risk mapping of schistosomiasis in Brazil using Bayesian geostatistical models. *Acta Trop*. 2014;132:57-63.
3. Webbe G, Sturrock RF, James ER, James C. Schistosoma haematobium in the baboon (*Papio anubis*): effect of vaccination with irradiated larvae on the subsequent infection with percutaneously applied cercariae. *Trans R Soc Trop Med Hyg*. 1982;76(3):354-361.
4. Moloney NA, Doenhoff MJ, Webbe G, Hinchcliffe P. Studies on the host-parasite relationship of *Schistosoma japonicum* in normal and immunosuppressed mice. *Parasite Immunol*. 1982;4(6):431-440.
5. Domingues AL, Lima AR, Dias HS, Leao GC, Coutinho A. An ultrasonographic study of liver fibrosis in patients infected with Schistosoma mansoni in northeast Brazil. *Trans R Soc Trop Med Hyg*. 1993; 87(5):555-558.
6. Scholte RG, Gosoniu L, Malone JB, Chammartin F, Utzinger J, Vounatsou P. Predictive risk mapping of schistosomiasis in Brazil using Bayesian geostatistical models. *Acta Trop*. 2014;132:57-63.
7. Pereira LMMB, Domingues ALC, Spinelli V, Mcfarlane IG. Ultrasonography of the liver and spleen in Brazilian patients with hepatosplenic schistosomiasis and cirrhosis. *Trans R Soc Trop Med Hyg*. 1998;92:639-642.
8. Symmers D. Pathogenesis of liver cirrhosis in schistosomiasis. *J Am Med Assoc*. 1951;147(4):304-305.
9. Pearce EJ, MacDonald AS. The immunobiology of schistosomiasis. *Nat Rev Immunol*. 2002;2(7):499-511.
10. Parise ER, Rosa H. Serum laminin in hepatic schistosomiasis. *Trans R Soc Trop Med Hyg*. 1992;86(2): 179-181.
11. Wyszomirska RM, Nishimura NF, Almeida JR, Yamanaka A, Soares EC. High serum laminin and type IV collagen levels in schistosomiasis mansoni. *Arq Gastroenterol*. 2005;42(4):221-225.
12. Grimaud JA, Borojevic R. Chronic human schistosomiasis mansoni. Pathology of the Disse's space. *Lab Invest*. 1977;36(3):268-273.
13. Andrade ZA, Peixoto E, Guerret S, Grimaud JA. Hepatic connective tissue changes in hepatosplenic schistosomiasis. *Hum Pathol*. 1992;23(5):566-573.
14. Ellner JJ, Olds GR, Kamel R, Osman GS, el-Kholy A, Mahmoud AA. Suppression splenic T lymphocytes in human hepatosplenic Schistosomiasis mansoni. *J Immunol*. 1980;125(1):308-312.
15. Pereira LMMB, Melo MCV, Lacerda C, et al. Hepatitis B virus infection in schistosomiasis mansoni. *J Med Virol*. 1994;42:203-206.
16. Pereira LMMB, Melo MCV, Saleh MG, et al. Hepatitis C virus infection in schistosomiasis mansoni in Brazil. *J Med Virol*. 1995;45:423-428.
17. Prata AR, Coura JR. Fases e Formas Clínicas da Esquistossomose Mansoni. Rm: Carvalho OS, Coelho PMZ, Lenzi HL, eds. *Schistosoma mansoni e esquistossomose, uma visão multidisciplinar. 1ª edição*. Rio de Janeiro: Editora Fiocruz; 2008:739-787.

18. Hawkins KR, Cantera JL, Storey HL, Leader BT, de Los Santos T. Diagnostic tests to support late-stage control programs for schistosomiasis and soil-transmitted helminthiases. *PLoS Negl Trop Dis.* 2016; 10(12):e0004985.
19. Castéra L. Invasive and non-invasive methods for the assessment of fibrosis and disease progression in chronic liver disease. *Best Pract Res Clin Gastroenterol.* 2011;25(2):291-303.
20. el Scheich T, Holtfreter MC, Ekamp H, et al. The WHO ultrasonography protocol for assessing hepatic morbidity due to *Schistosoma mansoni:* acceptance and evolution over 12 years. *J Parasitol Res.* 2014; 113(11):3915-3925.
21. Vivek KS, Wang L, Min X, et al. Human schistosomiasis: a diagnostic imaging focused review of a neglected disease. *Radiol Infect Dis.* 2015;2(3):150-157.
22. Wu S, Tseng Y, Xu N, et al. Evaluation of transient elastography in assessing liver fibrosis in patients with advanced schistosomiasis japonica. *Parasitol Int.* 2018;67(3):302-308.
23. Santos JC, Batista AS, Vasconcelos CMM, et al. Liver ultrasound elastography for the evaluation of periportal fibrosis in schistosomiasis mansoni: a cross-sectional study. *PLoS Negl Trop Dis.* 2018; 12(11):e0006868.
24. Lima LMSTB, Lacet CMC, Viana MSVB, Costa BLN, Parise ER. Evaluation of hepatic fibrosis by elastography in patients with schistosomiasis mansoni. *Trans R Soc Trop Med Hyg.* 2020;114(7):531-537.
25. Ministério da Saúde, Secretaria de Vigilância em Saúde, Departamento de Vigilância Epidemiológica. Vigilância da Esquistossomose mansoni: diretrizes técnicas/Ministério da Saúde, Secretaria de Vigilância em Saúde, Departamento de Vigilância das Doenças Transmissíveis. 4th ed. Brasília: Ministério da Saúde; 2014.
26. Sanchez MC, Cupit PM, Bu L, Cunningham C. Transcriptomic analysis of reduced sensitivity to praziquantel in *Schistosoma mansoni. Mol Biochem Parasitol.* 2019;228:6-15.
27. Olveda DU, Inobaya MT, McManus DP, et al. Biennial versus annual treatment for schistosomiasis and its impact on liver morbidity. *Int J Infect Dis.* 2017;54:145-149.
28. McManus DP, Bergquist R, Cai P, Ranasinghe S, Tebeje BM, You H. Schistosomiasis-from immunopathology to vaccines. *Semin Immunopathol.* 2020;42(3):355-371.

CHAPTER 11

Fascioliasis

Roberto Pineda-Reyes ■ Miguel Mauricio Cabada

KEY POINTS

- *Fasciola hepatica* is the most widely distributed foodborne trematode transmitted through contaminated water and water plants.
- *Fasciola* spp. has a complex lifecycle that includes freshwater snails, a tissue migratory phase, and a biliary tree phase.
- The clinical presentation varies from a prolonged febrile illness with abdominal pain and eosinophilia during the migratory phase to symptoms of biliary tree obstruction during the chronic phase.
- The diagnosis of fascioliasis requires a history of exposure in endemic areas. During the migratory phase, serology and imaging can aid in the diagnosis, and during the chronic phase, serology and the examination of at least three stool samples help make the diagnosis.
- Two doses of triclabendazole at 10 mg/kg are recommended for treatment. Treatment failure is not uncommon and patients require a test for cure.

Introduction

The genus *Fasciola* includes two species of parasitic trematodes, *Fasciola hepatica* and *Fasciola gigantica*. These cause liver disease in a wide range of mammals including humans living in sheep- and cattle-rearing areas.[1] *F. hepatica* is the most widely distributed trematode, with cases reported in 81 countries and in ecosystems located at different altitudes in all the continental lands, with the exception of Antarctica.[2,3] The parasite's ability to adapt to various environments and hosts, the development of antiparasitic resistance, and climate change are factors allowing for the emergence of fascioliasis and its global burden.[4,5]

Human fascioliasis is a zoonotic foodborne infection included on the list of neglected tropical diseases by the World Health Organization (WHO).[6] The real global impact of fascioliasis is unknown, but pragmatic estimations suggest there are 2.6 million people infected worldwide and a burden of 35,000 disability-adjusted life years.[3,7] The livestock industry and small-scale farmers, particularly in developing countries, are drastically affected.[8,9] Fascioliasis directly affects income through reductions in meat, milk, and wool production. Indirect effects on small family-owned farms include loss of animal traction power, manure, and food security.[1] Studies in low- and middle-income countries evaluating economic losses due to liver condemnation and loss of carcass weight in abattoirs suggest costs of up to USD 92 million a year.[10-14] The United Nations Food and Agriculture Organization estimated the global economic losses related to fascioliasis at USD 3 billion per year in 1994.[15] However, recent data suggest that the actual costs may be higher.[16] Climate change and resistance to triclabendazole are increasing the total expenditure associated with both human and bovine fascioliasis.[17-21]

Life Cycle

Mature *F. hepatica* parasites inhabit the biliary tract of the definitive hosts, where they can live for up to a decade.[1,2] Adult *Fasciola* parasites produce fertilized, unembryonated eggs that pass through the common bile duct into the intestines and are released into the environment with the feces (Figure 11.1). In freshwater and under appropriate conditions the eggs become embryonated and hatch upon direct sunlight stimulation releasing miracidia.[22] The miracidium seeks a suitable intermediate snail host from the Lymnaeidae family, mainly *Galba truncatula*, to infect.[23,24] The miracidium penetrates the snail tegument and forms a sporocyst.[22] A single sporocyst can asexually produce up to four redial generations and more than 300 cercariae.[25,26] Then, the free-swimming cercariae emerge from the snail and attach to aquatic vegetation, such as watercress, secreting a protective cyst covering called metacercaria, which infects once the vegetation is consumed by humans. Metacercariae can also form in water, and epidemiological data suggest transmission through contaminated water in some endemic regions.[27,28] Metacercariae are the infective stage to mammals, and once ingested by the definitive host, they excyst in the small bowel, penetrate the intestinal wall, and make their way through the peritoneal cavity to the liver.[29] Finally, the juveniles penetrate the Glisson's capsule and migrate across the liver parenchyma into the biliary tree.[2] After this, parasites reach sexual maturity and start egg production.[23,30]

Epidemiology

The complex epidemiology of human fascioliasis is influenced by numerous factors. The geographic distribution of the parasite is associated with the distribution of the snail intermediate host.[4,5,31,32] Weather, seasonality, and climate change are closely related to the lifecycle of the *Fasciola*. Heavy rainfalls and global warming may create new habitats suitable for *Fasciola*

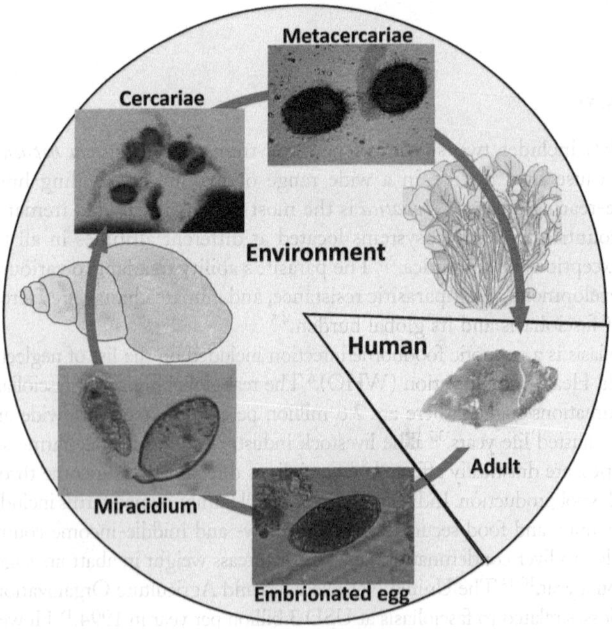

Figure 11.1 *Fasciola hepatica* life cycle. (Images courtesy of Dr. Miguel M. Cabada for the fascioliasis study group laboratory.)

transmission.[20,21,33] Man-made irrigation systems and bodies of water create new ecosystems for the parasite and for the snails to subsist, increasing the risk for outbreaks.[28,34] Migration, globalization, and transportation of livestock help the parasite and snail spread, increasing the distribution and prevalence of fascioliasis and potentially disseminating parasites with decreased drug susceptibility.[1,35]

The parasite-intermediate host interaction is critical in the epidemiology of fascioliasis. *F. gigantica* infects snails of the genus *Radix*, which have shown less capability to adapt to different ecosystems. For that reason, the distribution of *F. gigantica* is limited to tropical and subtropical regions in Africa and Asia.[31,36] In contrast, *F. hepatica* has adapted to different species of snails in the Lymnaeidae family, and its main intermediate host, *G. truncatula*, is highly adaptable to new environments including the high altitudes of the South American Andes.[4,5,31,33] *G. truncatula* from high-altitude environments survive longer and can produce more cercariae than snails from other areas.[32] The characteristic "patchy" geographic distribution of fascioliasis is in direct relationship with the spatial distribution of snails and aquatic vegetation.[37] *F. hepatica* is a cosmopolitan parasite, and human fascioliasis has been reported in all continents. Fascioliasis is a major public health problem in the Andes Mountains in South America (Peru, Bolivia), the Caribbean (Cuba, Puerto Rico), Northern Africa (Egypt), Western Europe (France, Portugal, Spain), Iran, China, and Vietnam.[1,3,7,38] Reports in the United States are mainly related to immigrants, refugees, and returning travelers, although there are autochthonous cases described from Florida, California, Puerto Rico, and Hawaii.[39-42] New endemic regions emerging in South America, Africa, and Asia suggest that our knowledge about fascioliasis burden is incomplete.[43]

Human fascioliasis primarily affects populations living in poverty.[44] Fascioliasis disproportionately affects children living in rural communities. Population-based studies in the Bolivian Altiplano have shown the highest prevalence of *Fasciola* infection among children, reaching 60% to 70% in some communities.[45–47] In the highlands of Peru fascioliasis in children from rural communities was associated with higher-altitude households and poverty.[44,48] School-age children were at higher risk for fascioliasis than preschoolers in studies from Peru, Bolivia, and Vietnam.[44,47,49,50] Adults living with infected children have an increased risk of fascioliasis.[51]

Dietary habits are important determinants of transmission.[52] Consumption of watercress, raw vegetables, and other aquatic plants has been associated with fascioliasis.[31,38,51] In communities without access to clean water and sanitation, drinking untreated water has been associated with infection, suggesting an alternative route of transmission.[27]

Clinical Manifestations

The clinical presentation of fascioliasis depends on the parasite's location in the human body. Two common syndromes have been described, acute or hepatic "migratory" fascioliasis and chronic or "biliary" fascioliasis. During acute fascioliasis, juvenile flukes make their way through the liver parenchyma seeking the biliary ducts. The migration of juvenile parasites and the symptoms associated with it last 3 to 4 months.[29,53] Abdominal pain, especially in the right upper quadrant, and fever associated with asthenia, anorexia, weight loss, and urticaria are reported in acute fascioliasis.[53-55] Less commonly, cough, dyspnea, and pleuritic chest pain with eosinophilic pleural effusions can occur.[56] Marked eosinophilia is observed in most cases and is highly suggestive of the diagnosis.[53,54,57] Anemia and mild elevation of transaminases and alkaline phosphatase may be present. Computed tomography (CT) scan imaging can show hypodense round lesions and tortuous tracts that may persist for months.[56] (Figure 11.2)

After the flukes enter the biliary tract, the symptoms of acute fascioliasis and hypereosinophilia subside. As flukes reach maturity, chronic fascioliasis ensues, and it is thought to last for several years, but natural history studies are limited. Symptoms of chronic infection are associated

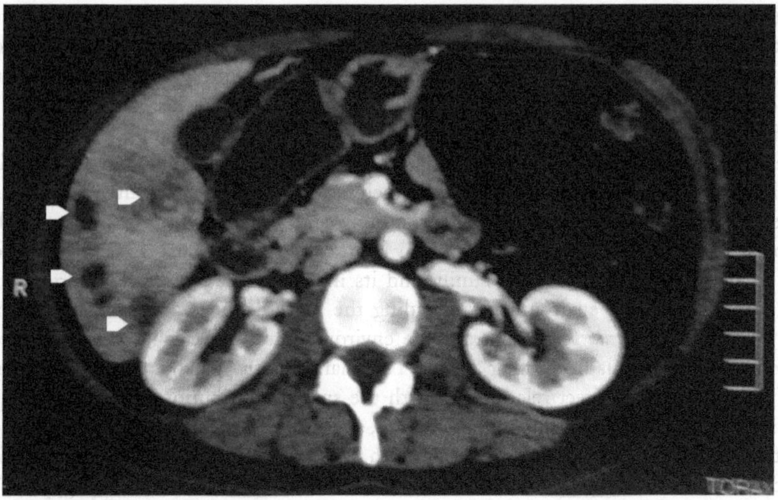

Figure 11.2 Computed tomography scan with intravenous contrast showing hypodense lesion in the liver of a patient with acute fascioliasis. (Image courtesy of Dr. Miguel M. Cabada.)

with obstruction of biliary ducts and include intermittent abdominal pain and jaundice.[58,59] Cholecystitis, extrahepatic biliary obstruction, and pancreatitis have been described.[54,60,61] Importantly, eosinophilia is present only in half of the patients diagnosed with chronic infection and is usually mild.[62,63] Prolonged chronic infections have been associated with liver fibrosis and cirrhosis in children and adults, but strong data are lacking.[64-66]

Atypical presentations or "ectopic fascioliasis" are uncommon and usually caused by aberrant migration of the juvenile parasites. Abdominal skin, subcutaneous tissues, and intestines are the most commonly described ectopic sites.[67] Cases of lung, pancreas, spleen, peritoneum, lymph nodes, ocular, and central nervous system involvement have all been reported.[67-73] Acute fascioliasis in liver transplant recipients from endemic areas is also possible.[74]

Asymptomatic children with anemia and/or stunting with exposure in endemic areas may warrant screening for fascioliasis.

Diagnosis

The diagnosis of fascioliasis can be challenging and requires knowledge of the parasite's life cycle and the assessment of epidemiological, clinical, and laboratory information. It is especially important to gather information on potential exposures to endemic areas and consumption of raw watercress or other vegetables that could have been in contact with contaminated water.

Parasite eggs are not produced during acute fascioliasis. During this phase, the diagnosis relies on clinical presentation, epidemiology, and serologic testing. Antibodies may take 2 to 4 weeks to become detectable after initial infection and should remain detectable for the duration of the disease.[1] Enzyme-linked immunosorbent assays (ELISA) are highly sensitive and specific (>90%). These are based on detection of antibodies against crude excretory/secretory products or purified antigen fractions (e.g., Fas2).[75-78] The Centers for Disease Control and Prevention (CDC) performs an immunoblot assay that detects IgG against the *F. hepatica* recombinant antigen FhSAP2 with a sensitivity of 94% and specificity of 98%.[79]

During chronic fascioliasis, adult flukes produce eggs that may be detectable in stool. Egg production fluctuates in time, causing variability in the sensitivity of tests based on egg detection.

Stool microscopy is the most widely used diagnostic tool for fascioliasis. Examination of multiple stool samples using a combination of techniques increases the diagnostic sensitivity of microscopy. The Kato Katz test is recommended by the WHO for testing patients in highly endemic areas, but it may miss up to a third of cases or more, particularly in low-burden infections or after treatment.[80,81] The Kato Katz test provides a quantitative result expressed in eggs/gram of stool that is useful for epidemiological studies and in certain clinical scenarios. Sedimentation techniques, such as the Lumbreras rapid sedimentation, have a higher sensitivity than Kato Katz and are useful for individual testing.[81] Device-based concentration tests such as mini-FLOTAC and Flukefinder may provide the highest sensitivity but are not widely available for clinical use.[82] Although costs make stool microscopy accessible in endemic countries, these tests are cumbersome and require significant training. Conventional and isothermal molecular tests to detect *Fasciola* DNA in stool are highly sensitive and turn positive before microscopy.[83-86] These tests are promising alternatives for diagnosis but are not widely available outside research laboratories.

Abdominal imaging studies may aid in the diagnosis of acute and chronic fascioliasis. Hypodense and tracks-like lesions in the liver on CT scan and magnetic resonance imaging (MRI) are compatible with acute fascioliasis in the right clinical and epidemiological scenario.[87] These lesions are found in the subcapsular region and may be poorly defined. On rare occasions patients with acute fascioliasis present with subcapsular liver hematomas evident on CT.[88,89] Ultrasound can also demonstrate hypoechoic round lesions and tracks in the liver next to the Glisson's capsule or peribiliary areas.[42,90] In chronic fascioliasis adult parasites may appear as motile hyperechoic objects in the gallbladder and biliary tree.[91] These may be associated with dilatation of the biliary tree or thickening of the gallbladder walls.[91] Liver calcifications can be found on CT of patients with chronic infection or after treatment of acute fascioliasis.[53]

Management and Prevention

Treatment is indicated in all patients with fascioliasis regardless of the presence of symptoms. Effective treatment shortens the duration of symptoms and prevents complications. Triclabendazole is the only medication recommended by the WHO for the treatment of all forms of fascioliasis.[92] The US Food and Drug Administration approved triclabendazole for the treatment of *F. hepatica* infection in patients 6 years of age and older. The recommended treatment consists of two doses of 10 mg/kg separated 12 to 24 hours and administered with food, which increases bioavailability by two- to threefold.[93] In the United States triclabendazole is available upon request from the manufacturer and is no longer provided by the CDC. The mechanism of action of triclabendazole is not fully understood but, as with other benzimidazoles, the drug appears to interfere with the microtubule polymerization and disrupt the tegument and reproductive organs.[94] Triclabendazole is regarded as a safe drug based on limited safety studies. The most common adverse reaction is right upper quadrant abdominal pain that can occur up to 1 week after treatment and is presumably related to migration of dying flukes through the bile ducts. Other reported adverse reactions include headaches, urticaria, and elevation of liver enzymes.[95] Prolongation of the QTc interval in the electrocardiogram has been reported in dogs following administration of high doses of triclabendazole. Caution is advised in humans taking other QTc-prolonging agents.[93] Due to concerns for post-treatment biliary tree obstruction, experts recommend inpatient monitoring of subjects with counts over 300 to 400 eggs/g of stool. However, the limited available data in highly endemic areas fail to support this practice.[96]

Patients treated effectively with triclabendazole experience improvement of their symptoms rapidly. In acute fascioliasis fever and abdominal pain may subside within 1 or 2 weeks. In chronic fascioliasis obstructive symptoms may exacerbate during the first week, with dilatation of the bile ducts on ultrasound, but resolve afterwards.[91] When present, eosinophilia may take months to fully resolve, but significant reductions can be seen within 1 or 2 weeks.[53] Parenchymal liver lesions demonstrated on CT or MRI may also take months to resolve and may turn into calcified lesions. Gallbladder and biliary tree abnormalities found on ultrasound are reversible after successful treatment but may take several weeks to resolve.[91]

Along with clinical improvement, all patients treated for fascioliasis should have a test for cure between 1 and 3 months after treatment. Patients with acute and chronic fascioliasis should be tested by microscopy of multiple stool specimens to ascertain cure. It is important to note that resolution of symptoms and reduction of eosinophilia in patients with acute fascioliasis could represent progression to the biliary phase of the disease, especially after prolonged symptoms. The use of egg concentration techniques for microscopy is recommended, as a lower egg burden is expected after treatment, further decreasing the sensitivity of stool examination. Patients that fail triclabendazole should receive a second treatment course using the same dose schedule and follow-up.

Nitazoxanide, a thiazolide antiparasitic, has been proposed as second-line therapy for acute and chronic fascioliasis.[97] One small clinical trial demonstrated only 40% efficacy in children and 60% in adults with chronic infection.[98] Case series have shown inconsistent results with efficacies of 0% to 100%.[17,99,100] Anthelminthics used to treat other trematodes, such as praziquantel, lack therapeutic benefit in fascioliasis.

Using triclabendazole as a single agent to treat and control fascioliasis represents an important problem for clinicians and public health officials. The widespread use of triclabendazole to avoid economic losses in livestock has caused the appearance of resistance in animals and humans. Reports of triclabendazole resistance and decreased efficacy have emerged from more than 17 countries.[101] Human cases failing multiple doses of triclabendazole have been described in Peru, Chile, Portugal, the Netherlands, Turkey, and Egypt.[17,99,102-105] The WHO encourages control by the implementation of mass chemotherapy in populations living in endemic areas with high burden of infections.[92] In Bolivia a fixed-dose program administering 250 mg triclabendazole to the entire community regardless of weight reduced the prevalence of fascioliasis to <1% from a historical 12% to 27%.[106] Nonetheless, the effects of mass treatment and suboptimal dosing on the emergence of resistant parasites have not been systematically evaluated. Prevention of transmission requires avoiding the ingestion of potentially contaminated water or leafy vegetables in endemic areas. Boling water and cooking vegetables prevents transmission.

References

1. Caravedo MA, Cabada MM. Human fascioliasis: current epidemiological status and strategies for diagnosis, treatment, and control. *Res Rep Trop Med.* 2020;11:149-158.
2. Webb CM, Cabada MM. Recent developments in the epidemiology, diagnosis, and treatment of Fasciola infection. *Curr Opin Infect Dis.* 2018;31(5):409-414.
3. Fürst T, Duthaler U, Sripa B, Utzinger J, Keiser J. Trematode infections: liver and lung flukes. *Infect Dis Clin North Am.* 2012;26(2):399-419.
4. Cwiklinski K, Dalton JP, Dufresne PJ, et al. The *Fasciola hepatica* genome: gene duplication and polymorphism reveals adaptation to the host environment and the capacity for rapid evolution. *Genome Biol.* 2015;16:71.
5. Cwiklinski K, O'Neill SM, Donnelly S, Dalton JP. A prospective view of animal and human Fasciolosis. *Parasite Immunol.* 2016;38(9):558-568.
6. WHO. *Intensified Control of Neglected Diseases: Report of An International Workshop, Berlin, 10–12 December 2003.* Geneva: World Health Organization; 2004. Available at: https://apps.who.int/iris/handle/10665/68529.
7. Mehmood K, Zhang H, Sabir AJ, et al. A review on epidemiology, global prevalence and economical losses of fasciolosis in ruminants. *Microb Pathog.* 2017;109:253-262.
8. Parkinson M, O'Neill SM, Dalton JP. Controlling fasciolosis in the Bolivian Altiplano. *Trends Parasitol.* 2007;23(6):238-239.

9. Carmona C, Tort JF. Fasciolosis in South America: epidemiology and control challenges. *J Helminthol.* 2017;91(2):99-109.
10. Khedri J, Radfar MH, Nikbakht B, et al. Parasitic causes of meat and organs in cattle at four slaughterhouses in Sistan-Baluchestan Province, Southeastern Iran between 2008 and 2016. *Vet Med Sci.* 2021; 7(4):1230-1236.
11. Arias-Pacheco C, Lucas JR, Rodríguez A, Córdoba D, Lux-Hoppe EG. Economic impact of the liver condemnation of cattle infected with *Fasciola hepatica* in the Peruvian Andes. *Trop Anim Health Prod.* 2020;52(4):1927-1932.
12. Nambafu J, Musisi JS, Mwambi B, et al. Prevalence and economic impact of bovine fasciolosis at Kampala City Abattoir, Central Uganda. *Br Microbiol Res J.* 2015;7(3):109-117.
13. Gray GD, Knox MR, Cargill C. Helminth control using local resources in smallholder production systems of Asia. *Trop Biomed.* 2008;25(suppl 1):1-8.
14. Espinoza JR, Terashima A, Herrera-Velit P, Marcos LA. Human and animal fascioliasis in Peru: impact in the economy of endemic zones. *Rev Peru Med Exp Salud Publica.* 2010;27(4):604-612.
15. Animal Production and Health Division. *Diseases of Domestic Animals Caused by Flukes: Epidemiology, Diagnosis and Control of Fasciola, Paramphistome, Dicrocoelium, Eurytrema and Schistosome Infections of Ruminants in Developing Countries.* Rome: FAO; 1994.
16. Gray GD, Copland RS, Copeman DB, eds. *Overcoming liver fluke as a constraint to ruminant production in South-East Asia.* ACIAR Monograph. 2008;133. Available at: https://www.researchgate.net/publication/237664810. Accessed March 28, 2023.
17. Cabada MM, Lopez M, Cruz M, Delgado JR, Hill V, White AC. Treatment failure after multiple courses of triclabendazole among patients with fascioliasis in Cusco, Peru: a case series. *PLoS Negl Trop Dis.* 2016;10(1):e0004361.
18. Morales ML, Tanabe MB, White AC, Lopez M, Bascope R, Cabada MM. Triclabendazole treatment failure for *Fasciola hepatica* infection among preschool and school-age children, Cusco, Peru. *Emerg Infect Dis.* 2021;27(7):1850-1857.
19. Ortiz P, Scarcella S, Cerna C, et al. Resistance of *Fasciola hepatica* against Triclabendazole in cattle in Cajamarca (Peru): a clinical trial and an in vivo efficacy test in sheep. *Vet Parasitol.* 2013;195(1-2):118-121.
20. Haydock LAJ, Pomroy WE, Stevenson MA, Lawrence KE. A growing degree-day model for determination of *Fasciola hepatica* infection risk in New Zealand with future predictions using climate change models. *Vet Parasitol.* 2016;228:52-59.
21. Sabourin E, Alda P, Vázquez A, Hurtrez-Boussès S, Vittecoq M. Impact of human activities on fasciolosis transmission. *Trends Parasitol.* 2018;34(10):891-903.
22. Wilson RA, Draskau T. The stimulation of daughter redia production during the larval development of *Fasciola hepatica. Parasitology.* 1976;72(3):245-257.
23. Kaplan RM. *Epidemiology of Fasciola hepatica in Florida with Emphasis on the Population Dynamics and Infection Prevalence of the Primary Snail Intermediate Host, Fossaria cubensis.* Florida: University of Florida; 1995.
24. Bargues MD, Angles R, Coello J, et al. One Health initiative in the Bolivian Altiplano human fascioliasis hyperendemic area: Lymnaeid biology, population dynamics, microecology and climatic factor influences. *Rev Bras Parasitol Vet.* 2021;30(2):e025620.
25. Rondelaud D, Vignoles P, Dreyfuss G. *Fasciola hepatica*: the developmental patterns of redial generations in naturally infected *Galba truncatula. Parasitol Res.* 2004;94(3):183-187.
26. Rondelaud D, Belfaiza M, Vignoles P, Moncef M, Dreyfuss G. Redial generations of *Fasciola hepatica*: a review. *J Helminthol.* 2009;83(3):245-254.
27. Cabada MM, Goodrich MR, Graham B, et al. Fascioliasis and eosinophilia in the highlands of Cuzco, Peru and their association with water and socioeconomic factors. *Am J Trop Med Hyg.* 2014;91(5): 989-993.
28. Esteban JG, González C, Bargues MD, et al. High fascioliasis infection in children linked to a man-made irrigation zone in Peru. *Trop Med Int Health.* 2002;7(4):339-348.
29. Moazeni M, Ahmadi A. Controversial aspects of the life cycle of *Fasciola hepatica. Exp Parasitol.* 2016;169:81-89.
30. Despommier DD, Griffin D, Gwadz RW, Hotez PJ, Knirsch CA, Karapelou JW. 35. Fasciola hepatica. Parasitic Diseases. New York: Parasites Without Borders, Inc; 2019:413–420. 17th ed.
31. Keiser J, Utzinger J. Food-borne trematodiases. *Clin Microbiol Rev.* 2009;22(3):466-483.

32. Mas-Coma S, Funatsu IR, Bargues MD. *Fasciola hepatica* and lymnaeid snails occurring at very high altitude in South America. *Parasitology.* 2001;123(suppl):S115-S127.
33. Charlier J, Ghebretinsae AH, Levecke B, Ducheyne E, Claerebout E, Vercruysse J. Climate-driven longitudinal trends in pasture-borne helminth infections of dairy cattle. *Int J Parasitol.* 2016;46 (13-14):881-888.
34. Hunter JM, Rey L, Chu KY, Adekolu-John EO, Mott KE, World Health Organization. *Parasitic Diseases in Water Resources Development: The Need for Intersectoral Negotiation.* Geneva: World Health Organization; 1993.
35. Pozio E. How globalization and climate change could affect foodborne parasites. *Exp Parasitol.* 2020;208:107807.
36. Siles-Lucas M, Becerro-Recio D, Serrat J, González-Miguel J. Fascioliasis and fasciolopsiasis: current knowledge and future trends. *Res Vet Sci.* 2021;134:27-35.
37. Owiny MO, Obonyo MO, Gatongi PM, Fèvre EM. Prevalence and spatial distribution of Trematode cercariae in Vector Snails within different Agro-Ecological Zones in Western Kenya, 2016. *Pan Afr Med J.* 2019;32:142.
38. Mas-Coma S, Bargues MD, Valero MA. Fascioliasis and other plant-borne trematode zoonoses. *Int J Parasitol.* 2005;35(11-12):1255-1278.
39. Fried B, Abruzzi A. Food-borne trematode infections of humans in the United States of America. *Parasitol Res.* 2010;106(6):1263-1280.
40. Weisenberg SA, Perlada DE. Domestically acquired fascioliasis in northern California. *Am J Trop Med Hyg.* 2013;89(3):588-591.
41. Bendezú P, Frame A, Hillyer GV. Human fascioliasis in Corozal, Puerto Rico. *J Parasitol.* 1982;68(2): 297-299.
42. Brown JD. Human fascioliasis (liver fluke disease) in Hawai'i: case report and review of human fascioliasis acquired in the United States. *Hawaii J Health Soc Welf.* 2021;80(9):212-217.
43. Cabada MM, Castellanos-Gonzalez A, Lopez M, Caravedo MA, Arque E, White AC. *Fasciola hepatica* infection in an Indigenous Community of the Peruvian Jungle. *Am J Trop Med Hyg.* 2016;94(6): 1309-1312.
44. Cabada MM, Morales ML, Webb CM, et al. Socioeconomic factors associated with *Fasciola hepatica* infection among children from 26 communities of the Cusco region of Peru. *Am J Trop Med Hyg.* 2018;99(5):1180-1185.
45. Bjorland J, Bryan RT, Strauss W, Hillyer GV, McAuley JB. An outbreak of acute fascioliasis among Aymara Indians in the Bolivian Altiplano. *Clin Infect Dis.* 1995;21(5):1228-1233.
46. Parkinson M, O'Neill SM, Dalton JP. Endemic human fasciolosis in the Bolivian Altiplano. *Epidemiol Infect.* 2007;135(4):669-674.
47. Esteban JG, Flores A, Angles R, Mas-Coma S. High endemicity of human fascioliasis between Lake Titicaca and La Paz valley, Bolivia. *Trans R Soc Trop Med Hyg.* 1999;93(2):151-156.
48. Webb CM, Morales ML, Lopez M, et al. Stunting in pre-school and school-age children in the Peruvian highlands and its association with Fasciola infection and demographic factors. *PLoS Negl Trop Dis.* 2021;15(6):e0009519.
49. De NV, Minh PN, Bich NN, Chai JY. Seroprevalence of tissue and luminal helminths among patients in Hanoi Medical University Hospital, Vietnam, 2018. *Korean J Parasitol.* 2020;58(4):387-392.
50. Tanabe MB, Caravedo MA, Morales ML, et al. A comparison of the risk for chronic fascioliasis between children 3 to 5 years and children 6 to 12 years of age in the Cusco Region of Peru. *Am J Trop Med Hyg.* 2021;105(3):684-687.
51. Caravedo MA, Ramirez W, Morales ML, et al. *Fasciola hepatica* infection risk for adult household members living with children with fascioliasis in Cusco, Peru. *Am J Trop Med Hyg.* 2021;104(6):2069-2073.
52. Marcos L, Maco V, Terashima A, Samalvides F, Espinoza JR, Gotuzzo E. Fascioliasis in relatives of patients with *Fasciola hepatica* infection in Peru. *Rev Inst Med Trop Sao Paulo.* 2005;47(4):219-222.
53. Marcos LA, Tagle M, Terashima A, et al. Natural history, clinicoradiologic correlates, and response to triclabendazole in acute massive fascioliasis. *Am J Trop Med Hyg.* 2008;78(2):222-227.
54. Kaya M, Beştaş R, Cetin S. Clinical presentation and management of *Fasciola hepatica* infection: single-center experience. *World J Gastroenterol.* 2011;17(44):4899-4904.
55. Díaz Fernández R, Garcés Martínez M, Millán Alvarez LM, Pérez Lastre J, Millán Marcelo JC. Clinical and therapeutic behaviour of *Fasciola hepatica* in a series of 87 patients. *Rev Cubana Med Trop.* 2011; 63(3):268-274.

56. Pulpeiro JR, Armesto V, Varela J, Corredoira J. Fascioliasis: findings in 15 patients. *Br J Radiol.* 1991;64(765):798-801.
57. Fica A, Dabanch J, Farias C, Castro M, Jercic MI, Weitzel T. Acute fascioliasis—Clinical and epidemiological features of four patients in Chile. *Clin Microbiol Infect.* 2012;18(1):91-96.
58. Rana SS, Bhasin DK, Nanda M, Singh K. Parasitic infestations of the biliary tract. *Curr Gastroenterol Rep.* 2007;9(2):156-164.
59. Umac H, Erkek AB, Ayaşlioğlu E, Erkek E, Ozluk U, Onen N. Pruritus and intermittent jaundice as clinical clues for *Fasciola hepatica* infestation. *Liver Int.* 2006;26(6):752-753.
60. Bulbuloglu E, Yuksel M, Bakaris S, Celik M, Kokoglu OF, Kale IT. Diagnosis of *Fasciola hepatica* cases in an operating room. *Trop Doct.* 2007;37(1):50-52.
61. Kwok J, Buxbaum JL. Liver fluke. *N Engl J Med.* 2019;381(19):e34.
62. Marcos LA, Maco V, Terashima A, Samalvides F, Gotuzzo E. Clinical characteristics of *Fasciola hepatica* chronic infection in children. *Revista de Gastroenterologia del Peru.* 2002;22:228-233.
63. Marcos LA, Terashima A, Gotuzzo E. Update on hepatobiliary flukes: fascioliasis, opisthorchiasis and clonorchiasis. *Curr Opin Infect Dis.* 2008;21(5):523-530.
64. Abou-Basha LM, Salem A, Osman M, el-Hefni S, Zaki A. Hepatic fibrosis due to fascioliasis and/or schistosomiasis in Abis 1 village, Egypt. *East Mediterr Health J.* 2000;6(5-6):870-878.
65. Machicado C, Machicado JD, Maco V, Terashima A, Marcos LA. Association of *Fasciola hepatica* infection with liver fibrosis, cirrhosis, and cancer: a systematic review. *PLoS Negl Trop Dis.* 2016;10(9):e0004962.
66. Marcos LA, Maco V, Castillo M, Terashima A, Gotuzzo E. Report of cases of fascioliasis in the Specialized Children Health Institute in Peru (1988–2003). *Rev Gastroenterol Peru.* 2005;25:198-205.
67. Taghipour A, Zaki L, Rostami A, et al. Highlights of human ectopic fascioliasis: a systematic review. *Infect Dis (Lond).* 2019;51(11-12):785-792.
68. Musa D, Godbole G, Chiodini PL, Phillips R. Unusual case of a lung abscess. *BMJ Case Rep.* 2013;2013: bcr2012008306.
69. Mas-Coma S, Agramunt VH, Valero MA. Direct and indirect affection of the central nervous system by Fasciola infection. *Handb Clin Neurol.* 2013;114:297-310.
70. Dalimi A, Jabarvand M. *Fasciola hepatica* in the human eye. *Trans R Soc Trop Med Hyg.* 2005;99(10): 798-800.
71. Zali MR, Ghaziani T, Shahraz S, Hekmatdoost A, Radmehr A. Liver, spleen, pancreas and kidney involvement by human fascioliasis: imaging findings. *BMC Gastroenterol.* 2004;4:15.
72. Kim AJ, Choi CH, Choi SK, et al. Ectopic human *Fasciola hepatica* infection by an adult worm in the mesocolon. *Korean J Parasitol.* 2015;53(6):725-730.
73. Mohammadi-Ghalehbin B, Chinifroush-Asl MM, Ramzi F. Extra-hepatic fascioliasis with peritoneal malignancy tumor feature. *J Parasit Dis.* 2012;36(1):78-80.
74. Capobianco I, Frank M, Königsrainer A, et al. Liver fluke-infested graft used for living-donor liver transplantation: case report and review of the literature. *Transpl Infect Dis.* 2015;17(6):880-885.
75. Muñoz Zambrano ME, Placencia Medina M, Del Pozo Muñoz JA, Sevilla Andrade C, Huiza Franco A. Serological diagnosis of *Fasciola hepatica* infection: a systematic review. *Rev Gastroenterol Peru.* 2020;40(2):155-161.
76. Sarkari B, Khabisi SA. Immunodiagnosis of human fascioliasis: an update of concepts and performances of the serological assays. *J Clin Diagn Res.* 2017;11(6):OE05-OE10.
77. Sadaow L, Yamasaki H, Morishima Y, et al. Effectiveness of *Fasciola gigantica* excretory-secretory and recombinant cathepsin L antigens for rapid diagnosis of human fascioliasis using immunochromatographic devices. *Parasitol Res.* 2020;119(11):3691-3698.
78. Espinoza JR, Maco V, Marcos L, et al. Evaluation of Fas2-ELISA for the serological detection of *Fasciola hepatica* infection in humans. *Am J Trop Med Hyg.* 2007;76(5):977-982.
79. Shin SH, Hsu A, Chastain HM, et al. Development of two FhSAP2 recombinant-based assays for immunodiagnosis of human chronic fascioliasis. *Am J Trop Med Hyg.* 2016;95(4):852-855.
80. World Health Organization. *Report of the WHO Informal Meeting on use of triclabendazole in fascioliasis control.* Geneva: WHO Headquarters; 2006. Available at: https://apps.who.int/iris/bitstream/handle/10665/333543/WHO-CDS-NTD-PCT-2007.1-eng.pdf. Accessed March 28, 2023.
81. Lopez M, Morales ML, Konana M, et al. Kato-Katz and Lumbreras rapid sedimentation test to evaluate helminth prevalence in the setting of a school-based deworming program. *Pathog Glob Health.* 2016; 110(3):130-134.

82. Zárate-Rendón DA, Vlaminck J, Levecke B, Briones-Montero A, Geldhof P. Comparison of Kato-Katz thick smear, mini-FLOTAC, and Flukefinder for the detection and quantification of *Fasciola hepatica* eggs in artificially spiked human stool. *Am J Trop Med Hyg*. 2019;101(1):59-61.
83. Cabada MM, Malaga JL, Castellanos-Gonzalez A, et al. Recombinase polymerase amplification compared to real-time polymerase chain reaction test for the detection of *Fasciola hepatica* in human stool. *Am J Trop Med Hyg*. 2017;96(2):341-346.
84. Amiri S, Shemshadi B, Shirali S, Kheirandish F, Fallahi S. Accurate and rapid detection of *Fasciola hepatica* copro-DNA in sheep using loop-mediated isothermal amplification (LAMP) technique. *Vet Med Sci*. 2021;7(4):1316-1324.
85. Martínez-Valladares M, Rojo-Vázquez FA. Loop-mediated isothermal amplification (LAMP) assay for the diagnosis of fasciolosis in sheep and its application under field conditions. *Parasit Vectors*. 2016;9:73.
86. Robles-Pérez D, Martínez-Pérez JM, Rojo-Vázquez FA, Martínez-Valladares M. The diagnosis of fasciolosis in feces of sheep by means of a PCR and its application in the detection of anthelmintic resistance in sheep flocks naturally infected. *Vet Parasitol*. 2013;197(1-2):277-282.
87. Salahshour F, Tajmalzai A. Imaging findings of human hepatic fascioliasis: a case report and review of the literature. *J Med Case Rep*. 2021;15(1):324.
88. Leon M, Alave J, Alvarado R, Gotuzzo E, Terashima A, Seas C. A 52-year-old woman with a subcapsular liver hematoma. *Clin Infect Dis*. 2011;52(9):1137, 1195-1196.
89. Chang Wong MR, Pinto Elera JO, Guzman Rojas P, Terashima Iwashita A, Samalvides Cuba F. Demographic and clinical aspects of hepatic fascioliasis between 2013–2010 in National Hospital Cayetano Heredia, Lima, Peru. *Rev Gastroenterol Peru*. 2016;36(1):23-28.
90. Cantisani V, Cantisani C, Mortelé K, et al. Diagnostic imaging in the study of human hepatobiliary fascioliasis. *Radiol Med*. 2010;115(1):83-92.
91. Richter J, Freise S, Mull R, Millán JC. Fascioliasis: sonographic abnormalities of the biliary tract and evolution after treatment with triclabendazole. *Trop Med Int Health*. 1999;4(11):774-781.
92. WHO. *Report of the WHO Expert Consultation on Foodborne Trematode Infections and Taeniasis/Cysticercosis*. 2011. Available at: https://apps.who.int/iris/bitstream/handle/10665/75209/WHO_HTM_NTD_PCT_2011.3_eng.pdf?sequence=1&isAllowed=y.
93. FDA. *Drug Approval Package: Egaten (Triclabendazole)*. New Hampshire: U.S. Food and Drug Administration; 2019 Available at: https://www.accessdata.fda.gov/drugsatfda_docs/nda/2018/208711Orig1s000TOC.cfm.
94. Bennett JE, Dolin R, Blaser MJ. Mandell, Douglas, and Bennett's principles and practice of infectious diseases. 9th ed. Philadelphia: Elsevier; 2020.
95. Gandhi P, Schmitt EK, Chen CW, Samantray S, Venishetty VK, Hughes D. Triclabendazole in the treatment of human fascioliasis: a review. *Trans R Soc Trop Med Hyg*. 2019;113(12):797-804.
96. Villegas F, Angles R, Barrientos R, et al. Administration of triclabendazole is safe and effective in controlling fascioliasis in an endemic community of the Bolivian Altiplano. *PLoS Negl Trop Dis*. 2012; 6(8):e1720.
97. Kabil SM, Ashry ESHE, Ashraf NK. An open-label clinical study of nitazoxanide in the treatment of human fascioliasis. *Curr Ther Res Clin Exp*. 2000;61:339-345.
98. Favennec L, Jave Ortiz J, Gargala G, Lopez Chegne N, Ayoub A, Rossignol JF. Double-blind, randomized, placebo-controlled study of nitazoxanide in the treatment of fascioliasis in adults and children from northern Peru. *Aliment Pharmacol Ther*. 2003;17(2):265-270.
99. Ramadan HK, Hassan WA, Elossily NA, et al. Evaluation of nitazoxanide treatment following triclabendazole failure in an outbreak of human fascioliasis in Upper Egypt. *PLoS Negl Trop Dis*. 2019; 13(9):e0007779.
100. Zumaquero-Ríos JL, Sarracent-Pérez J, Rojas-García R, et al. Fascioliasis and intestinal parasitoses affecting schoolchildren in Atlixco, Puebla State, Mexico: epidemiology and treatment with nitazoxanide. *PLoS Negl Trop Dis*. 2013;7(11):e2553.
101. Fairweather I, Brennan GP, Hanna REB, Robinson MW, Skuce PJ. Drug resistance in liver flukes. *Int J Parasitol Drugs Drug Resist*. 2020;12:39-59.
102. Gil LC, Díaz A, Rueda C, Martínez C, Castillo D, Apt W. Resistant human fasciolasis: report of four patients. *Rev Med Chil*. 2014;142(10):1330-1333.
103. Branco EA, Ruas R, Nuak J, Sarmento A. Treatment failure after multiple courses of triclabendazole in a Portuguese patient with fascioliasis. *BMJ Case Rep*. 2020;13(3):e232299.

104. Winkelhagen AJ, Mank T, de Vries PJ, Soetekouw R. Apparent triclabendazole-resistant human *Fasciola hepatica* infection, the Netherlands. *Emerg Infect Dis*. 2012;18(6):1028-1029.
105. Belgin G, S KY, H T, et al. Partial hepatectomy for the resistant *Fasciola hepatica* infection in a child. *APSP J Case Rep*. 2015;6(3):27.
106. Mollinedo S, Gutierrez P, Azurduy R, et al. Mass drug administration of triclabendazole for *Fasciola hepatica* in Bolivia. *Am J Trop Med Hyg*. 2019;100(6):1494-1497.

CHAPTER 12

Opisthorchis and Clonorchis

Prasert Saichua ■ Banchob Sripa

KEY POINTS

- *Opisthorchis viverrini*, *Opisthorchis felineus*, and *Clonorchis sinensis* are foodborne trematodes endemic in Southeast Asia, Eastern Europe, and eastern Asia, with over 30 million people infected
- Stool examination for the parasite's eggs is the gold-standard diagnosis
- Acute opisthorchiasis felineus, sporadically reported, is not uncommon in endemic areas
- Hepatobiliary diseases associated with chronic infections include cholangitis, cholelithiasis, periductal fibrosis, and cholangiocarcinoma
- Praziquantel is a drug of choice, administered at a dose of 25 mg/kg three times daily for 2 to 3 consecutive days or a single administration at 40 mg/kg
- Integrated control using EcoHealth/One Health approach targeting components of the life cycle and multi-sectoral involvement is recommended by WHO

Introduction

Human liver fluke infections caused by *Opisthorchis viverrini*, *Opisthorchis felineus*, and *Clonorchis sinensis* are major public health problems in many parts of the world, ranging from eastern and southeastern Asia to Europe.[1] The liver flukes are designated by WHO as neglected tropical diseases that affect the poorest in endemic countries. Opisthorchiasis caused by *O. viverrini* is endemic in Thailand, Lao People's Democratic Republic (Lao PDR), Cambodia, Myanmar, and central-southern Vietnam.[1,2] *O. felineus* is endemic in the Russian Federation, particularly in Western Siberia, and in Central-Eastern Europe.[3-6] Clonorchiasis caused by *C. sinensis* is endemic in northern Vietnam, southern and northeastern China, Korea, and eastern Siberia. Throughout the world, 30 million are infected and over 700 million people are at risk of infection with these liver flukes.[3,7] The infections are associated with hepatobiliary diseases including hepatomegaly, cholangitis, fibrosis of the periportal system, cholecystitis, and gallstones.[6,8,9] Moreover, there is strong evidence from epidemiological, laboratory animal, and human studies implicating *O. viverrini* and *C. sinensis* in the development of cholangiocarcinoma (CCA).[10-12] Thus the International Agency for Research on Cancer, World Health Organization (WHO), classified *O. viverrini* and *C. sinensis* as Group 1 biological carcinogens.[13,14] The Khon Kaen Province in Northeast Thailand has reported the highest incidence of liver fluke–associated CCA in the world.[15-17]

Epidemiology

LIFE CYCLE AND TRANSMISSION

The life cycle of the *Opisthorchis* spp. and *C. sinensis* parasites involves multiple stages of development.[1] A mammalian definitive host (such as humans, cats, dogs, and various fish-eating mammals) is infected by eating undercooked or raw freshwater fish containing infective metacercariae (Figure 12.1). Once ingested, the metacercariae will excyst in the duodenum, and the juvenile worms migrate to the bile ducts in the liver. Adult flukes lay eggs in the bile of an infected definitive host, pass through the host's feces, and are eventually released into the environment. Once the eggs enter the freshwater environment (e.g., streams, rivers, and lakes) and are ingested by suitable freshwater snails (the first intermediate host), the eggs release miracidia, which undergo several developmental stages in the snails. The miracidia develop into cercariae, release from the snails, and penetrate freshwater cyprinoid fish (the second intermediate host), encysting as metacercariae in the muscles or under the scales. Humans consume the raw fish, get infected, and complete the cycle.

GEOGRAPHICAL DISTRIBUTION AND RISK OF INFECTION

Distribution of *Opisthorchis* spp. is very distinct; *O. viverrini* lives in tropical areas, whereas *O. felineus* lives in temperate zones. The first human cases of *O. viverrini* infection were

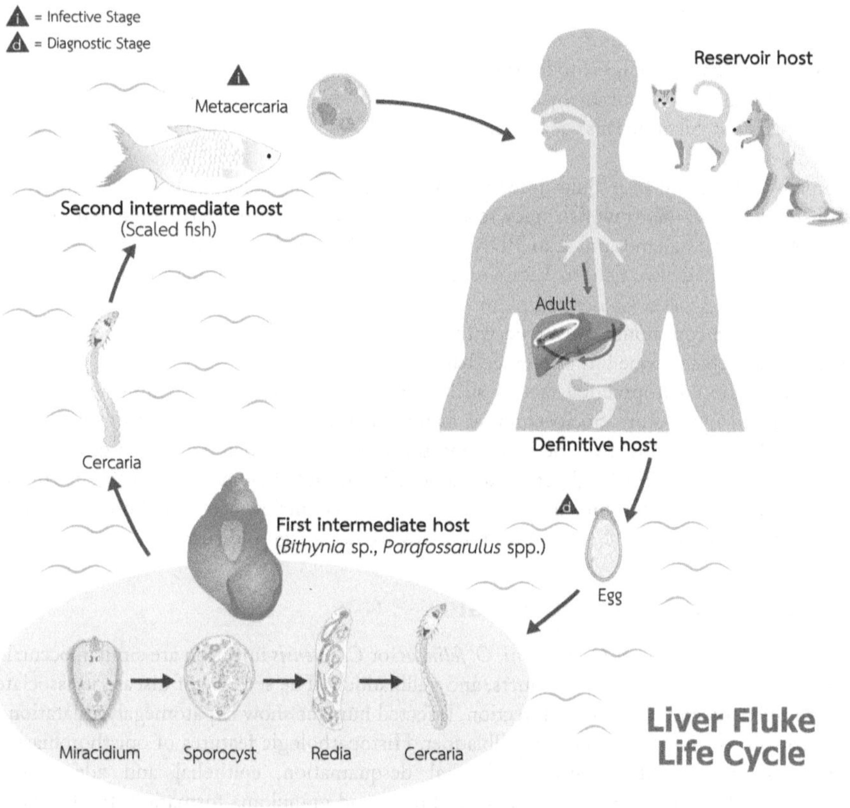

Figure 12.1 Life cycle of *Opisthorchis* spp. and *Clonorchis sinensis*. (Modified from Ref. [18].)

reported in Thailand, more than 100 years ago (1915).[11] To date, *O. viverrini* infection has been reported from Mekong River basin countries including Lao PDR, Cambodia, Vietnam, and, recently, Myanmar, with sporadic case reports from Malaysia, Singapore, and the Philippines.[18,19] A total of 12 million people were recently estimated to be infected with *O. viverrini* (in 2018) in four major endemic countries, namely Thailand (6.71 million), Lao PDR (2.45 million), Vietnam (2.07 million), and Cambodia (1.00 million).[20] *O. felineus* was first discovered in a cat (1884) and in humans from Tomsk, Russia (1891), and was named the "Siberian liver fluke."[5,21] *O. felineus* is endemic in Russian Federation, Eastern Europe, and Central Asia. A recent report revealed more than 60% prevalence of *O. felineus* infection in rural districts along the Ob and Irtysh river junction in Western Siberia.[6] Several outbreaks have been reported in Italy due to recent trends of consuming raw fish dishes. Sporadic outbreaks are reported in German and Greece.[22] Moreover, opisthorchiasis is commonly noted in Lao immigrants in Europe and the United States.

It has been estimated that up to 18 million people are infected with *C. sinensis* in China alone.[23-25] Heavy *C. sinensis* infection has been reported in southern and northeastern China. A national surveillance in 70 counties spread across 15 provinces of China in 2016 revealed an average prevalence of *C. sinensis* infection of 2.04%, with 89.37% of the infected people distributed among Jilin, Heilongjiang, Guangdong, and Guangxi provinces.[26] Clonorchiasis has long been known to be endemic in northern Vietnam, with prevalence at the commune level ranging between 26.5% and 53.3%.[27] South Korea used to have a high prevalence of *C. sinensis* infection, particularly in the four major river basins, with an average prevalence of 21.5% nationwide in 1981.[28] Due to socioeconomic development in Korea, several parasites have been eliminated, but *C. sinensis* remains a major foodborne disease with up to 5.3% prevalence recently reported along the river basin in southern part of the country.[29] Clonorchiasis is also reported in the southern Far East Siberia, Russia, especially near the Amur River basin, with approximately 3000 people infected.[30]

Humans acquire the liver fluke infection by eating raw or inadequately cooked freshwater scaled fish, such as *koi pla* (raw fish spicy salad) and *pla som* (short sour fermented fish), particularly in Northeast Thailand and Lao PDR; *pra hok* in Cambodia; *Gỏi cá* (raw fish salad) and *Gỏi cá nhảy* (eat small alive fish) in Vietnam; raw pickled fishes in Myanmar; and other raw fish dishes such as *Cao yu* and *Ci yan yu* in China and frozen fish slices in Siberia. These traditional raw fish dishes are commonly consumed with alcohol, which not only enhances the excystation of the parasite metacercariae but also exacerbates the liver damage.

Other risks are environmental factors such as wetland ecology and proximity of people to water bodies and aquaculture. Socioeconomic factors such as deficiency in sanitation and a proper latrine also play a role. Poor hygiene habits and practices such as open defecation or disposal of wastes into the water bodies, "night soil," and other circumstantial factors such as absence of food inspections are commonly found in endemic developing countries. Most of those who are infected live in agricultural rural areas consuming raw fish as an age-old custom.

Pathology and Pathogenesis

Pathological consequences of *O.viverrini*, *O.felineus*, or *C. sinensis* infection are similar, occurring mainly in the liver, extrahepatic bile ducts, and gallbladder.[1] The severity of disease is associated with both intensity and duration of infection. Infected humans show hepatomegaly, dilatation of subcapsular bile ducts, and thickened gallbladder. Histopathologic features of opisthorchiasis or clonorchiasis include inflammation, epithelial desquamation, epithelial and adenomatous hyperplasia, goblet cell metaplasia, periductal fibrosis, and granuloma formation. In chronic inflammation, infiltrations of lymphocytes, monocytes, eosinophils, and plasma cells are common. Granulomatous inflammation around the parasite eggs is occasionally observed along the bile ducts of infected livers. Epithelial hyperplasia, adenomatous hyperplasia, and goblet cell metaplasia can be seen in chronic opisthorchiasis and clonorchiasis. Periductal fibrosis is the most prominent histological feature of chronic liver fluke infection. The fibrosis corresponds to periportal echoes detected by ultrasonography. Gallstone is a common complication of the human liver fluke infections, particularly clonorchiasis. Parasite eggs have been observed in the nidus of the stones in the gallbladder and intrahepatic ducts. Poor function of the gallbladder may cause calcium/bilirubin precipitation on fluke eggshell, admixed with mucin and other bile constituents, leading to stone formation.[31]

Pathogenesis of liver fluke–mediated tissue damage may be direct via mechanical or chemical irritation and/or is immune mediated.[8] Mechanical injury caused by parasite's suckers during feeding activities and migration contributes to biliary ulceration. The metabolic products from infection are strongly immunogenic and can induce host innate and adaptive immune responses leading to inflammation. Repeated anthelminthic treatment with praziquantel (PZQ) may induce more oxidative DNA damage of the biliary cells and is thought to enhance cholangiocarcinogenesis.[32] However, this hypothesis is still controversial. Increased endogenous nitrosation from the liver fluke infection and exogenous *N*-nitroso compounds from dietary fermented fish may enhance mutagenic conditions for the chronically inflamed and proliferating bile duct epithelium.[8] Together, these pathological conditions form an ideal environment for cancer development in the infected bile ducts.[8,10] Recent studies suggest that co-infection with cagA-positive *Helicobacter pylori* in opisthorchiasis orchestrates severe pathology and may increase carcinogenic potential of infected bile ducts.[33-36]

Clinical Presentation

Acute *O. felineus* is sporadically reported in outbreaks in non-endemic Europe or new immigrants to endemic Siberian state of the former USSR. The major symptoms include high fever (3–12 days), abdominal pain, headache, asthenia, arthralgia, diarrhea, and nausea.[37] Jaundice has been described in certain cases. The median onset of signs and symptoms is 20 days after infection (range 7–37 days). Majority of those with symptoms show eosinophilia and increased liver enzymes. Most of the infected people are symptomatic from the third and fourth weeks after infection.[37] Acute opisthorchiasis viverrini and acute clonorchiasis are rarely observed.[38]

Most chronic human opisthorchiasis and clonorchiasis cases show few specific signs or symptoms, except an increased frequency of palpable liver, as shown in community-based studies.[1,39] Hematological and biochemical features are generally unremarkable, even in heavy infections.[40] By contrast, ultrasonography reveals a high frequency of gallbladder enlargement, sludge, and gallstones in asymptomatic individuals.[41,42] These gallbladder abnormalities usually resolve to a large extent after treatment with PZQ, usually within a year or two after treatment.[43] Periductal fibrosis seen as periportal echoes along the intrahepatic biliary trees is a predominant ultrasonographic feature in chronic liver fluke infections.[41,44] Upon ultrasonographic grading, positive advanced periductal fibrosis (APF) has been observed in chronic opisthorchiasis in over 30% of cases.[44] Resolved APF is found in about 30% of cases, while persistent APF occurs more than half of the time in positive periductal fibrosis cases post-PZQ treatment over a 5-year follow-up.[45]

Symptomatic cases of opisthorchiasis and clonorchiasis generally report pain in the right upper quadrant, diarrhea, loss of appetite, indigestion, and fullness. For opisthorchiasis, 5% to 10% of infected individuals had weakness or malaise, flatulence or dyspepsia, and abdominal pain, and 5% had hepatomegaly.[46] Complications may include cholangitis, obstructive jaundice, intra-abdominal mass, cholecystitis, and gallbladder or intrahepatic stones. Stones are particularly common in clonorchiasis.[39,47]

The most important clinical complication of liver fluke infection is an enhanced susceptibility to CCA. Heavily *O. viverrini*–infected people may approach a 15-fold risk compared with the uninfected populations in Thailand.[48] Moreover, up to 27-fold increased risk has been reported using antibody to the liver fluke in a case-control study in this region.[49] For clonorchiasis, an increased risk of CCA with an odds ratio of up to 8.62 has been reported.[50] Patients with liver fluke–associated CCA present with variable clinical manifestations. Jaundice is the main clinical manifestation that accounts for 60% of a hospital series of opisthorchiasis-related CCA in Northeast Thailand.[51]

O. viverrini and *C. sinensis* are designated as "Group I biological carcinogens" by the WHO International Agency for Research on Cancer. However, there is not enough evidence to support the carcinogenic of *O. felineus* in humans.

Diagnosis

Gold-standard diagnoses of *O. viverrini, O. felineus,* and *C. sinensis* are conventional fecal examination and adult worm detection. Eggs can be detected either in feces, bile from endoscopic retrograde cholangiopancreatography (ERCP), or percutaneous transhepatic biliary drainage (PTBD) during treatment of bile duct obstruction.[52] Fecal examination is routinely used for diagnosis of liver fluke infections due to its noninvasiveness and ease of sample collection. This method includes modified formalin ether concentration technique (FECT), modified thick Kato smear, and Stoll's dilution egg count technique. Kato-Katz technique, the preferred diagnostic tool, allows quantitative estimation of infection. Single stool examination has low sensitivity, so there is a need for multiple stool examinations to increase sensitivity. Three consecutive Kato-Katz thick smears were reported to be more sensitive than a single examination by FECT.[53] The FECT is presently considered the gold standard for diagnosing opisthorchiasis using a microscope to detect the eggs.

Structurally, *O. viverrini* is basically similar to *O. felineus* and *C. sinensis*. The body of an adult liver fluke is flat (dorsoventrally flattened) like a leaf. The main difference among the three liver flukes is the different branch testis of *C. sinensis* from those of *O. viverrini* and *O. felineus*, which have lobed testes. The adult *O. viverrini* is the smallest among the three species (5–7 mm by 1.5 mm) (Figure 12.2A), whereas the size of *O. felineus* and *C. sinensis* measure 2 to 13 mm by 1 to 3.5 mm and 10 to 25 by 3 to 5 mm, respectively. The liver fluke egg is ovoid with a maximum width at abopercular side and yellowish in color, as well as measuring 27 to 35 μm by 15 to 17 μm (*C. sinensis*), 26 μm by 10 μm (*O. felineus*), and 30 μm by 12 μm (*O. viverrini*) for the three liver flukes (Figure 12.2B). Given that geographical distribution of the liver flukes is different, identification of the adult flukes is not difficult. However, the eggs of the liver flukes are similar in shape and size to several species of small intestinal foodborne trematodes (MIF) belonging to the families Heterophyidae and Lecithodendriidae, which are co-endemic, particularly in Asian countries.[54-56] This makes the diagnosis even more difficult. Differentiation of *O. viverrini* eggs from MIF eggs is possible with the use of stains such as iodine, potassium permanganate, or methylene blue and done by a skilled microscopist.[55] Stool analysis is not capable of differentiating the eggs of *Opisthorchis* spp. and those of *C. sinensis*. These liver flukes, which can be co-endemic in Vietnam, are difficult to differentiate based on egg morphology by microscopy and need an experienced laboratory technician.

DNA-based methods can also be used for diagnosis. A variety of PCR techniques (including conventional PCR, real-time PCR, multiplex PCR, PCR-RFLP) have been employed. Sensitive and specific target genes, such as internal transcribed spacers (ITS-1 or ITS-2) of nuclear ribosomal DNA (rDNA), cox1, Rn1, and nad2, have been documented.[52] These methods are alternatives to microscopic methods where limitations are noted in low-intensity settings and in differentiating the liver flukes from MIF eggs.[57]

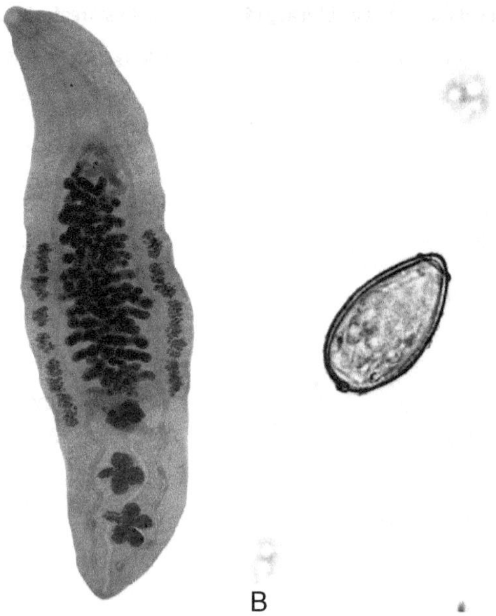

Figure 12.2 Adult *Opisthorchis viverrini* worm with lobed testis (A) and an egg with prominent shoulder and knob (B).

Treatment

PZQ remains the drug of choice for its high degree of efficacy.[58] WHO recommends a dose of 25 mg/kg three times daily for 2 to 3 consecutive days or a single administration at 40 mg/kg. No drug resistance to PZQ has been reported so far for these liver flukes. Table 12.1 shows recommended regimen and efficacy of PZQ for treatment of human liver flukes. While cure rates can be as high as 96 to 100%, PZQ does not provide immunity against reinfection. Single-dose PZQ has been widely used in large-scale control programs in Thailand for >40 years.[59,60] Rim[39] recommended that the most effective regimen, particularly for clonorchiasis, is 25 mg/kg three times over a day (total dose: 75 mg/kg). Side effects, such as dizziness, vomiting, and abdominal pain, occur frequently but are transient and rarely severe.[61,62]

Other drugs such as artemether, artesunate, 1,2,4-trioxolane (OZ78), and mebendazole have also been evaluated for treating *O. viverrini*, *O. felineus*, and *C. sinensis* infection in animals and humans with varying degree of efficacy.[63,64] Tribendimidine originally developed for nematode treatment by the Chinese National Institute of Parasitic Diseases has proven to be highly effective for treating the liver flukes in vitro and in animals. Recent clinical studies demonstrated that tribendimidine is as efficacious for the treatment of *C. sinensis* and *O. viverrini* infection as PZQ, with slightly less adverse events.[61,65-67]

Control of Opisthorchiasis and Clonorchiasis

Given that liver flukes are foodborne zoonotic diseases with a complex life cycle involving several hosts (snails, fish, human, and animal reservoirs), environments, socioeconomic status, human behaviors, culture, and belief,[35,68,69] they are difficult to control by conventional methods. Infected individuals may also not be aware of the infection. In addition, infection typically does not reduce

TABLE 12.1 ■ **Recommended Regimen and Efficacy of Praziquantel for Treatment of Human Liver Flukes**

Parasite	Regimen of Praziquantel	Cure Rate (%)	Egg Reduction Rate (%)
Opisthorchis viverrini	30 mg/kg, single	80.0–98.5	98.4–100.0
	40 mg/kg, single	81.7–98.6	99.0–100.0
	50 mg/kg, single	81.3–98.6	99.3–100.0
	2 × 25 mg/kg × 1 day	88.5	ND
	75 mg/kg (first dose 50 mg/kg, second dose 25 mg/kg, 6 hours apart)	96·9%	99·9–100·0
	75 mg/kg (25 mg/kg, 3 doses × 4 hours)	80.0–98.5	98.8–100.0
Opisthorchis felineus	40 mg/kg, single	97.0	ND
	3 × 25 mg/kg × 1 day	100.0	100.0
Clonorchis sinensis	40 mg/kg, single	87.1	97.6
	3 × 25 mg/kg × 1 day	85.7	99.7
	3 × 25 mg/kg × 2 day	100.0	100.0
	75 mg/kg (4 doses within 2 days)	56.8	98.0

ND = not done.
Modified from Refs. [58, 61, 62, 64, and 66].

work capacity, making individuals unaware of their infection. As a result, >60% of those who are infected report that they intend to keep eating raw fish despite knowing the risk of liver fluke infection.[70] Another major risk factor for liver fluke infection is the "raw attitudes" culture of eating raw food, particularly in the Mekong region, where people have strong livelihood and lifestyle associations within wetland ecosystems. Raw fish consumption is deeply rooted in local cultures, beliefs, and collective rituals of people in the region.[68] Therefore integrative control measures including multisectoral, interdisciplinary, and transdisciplinary approaches must be met. Incorporation of parasite ecology, human behavior, socioeconomics, public health awareness, and active community participation should be employed for effective and sustainable control.[35,71] The control principle is consistent with EcoHealth or One Health approach recommended by WHO/SEARO.[71] Control strategies include case finding by stool examination and selective treatment of infected individuals using PZQ, health education in schools for both children and adults in the community aiming at changing from eating raw to cooked fish, and the practice of proper disposal of waste.[35,72] Extended measures include enhancement in food safety such as issuance of certificates to well-maintained fish farms by national agriculture and aquaculture authorities, development of (information-education-communication) IEC materials regarding food safety practices, latrine construction and utilization to reduce fecal contamination of freshwater bodies, and snail control.

References

1. Sripa B, Kaewkes S, Intapan PM, et al. Food-borne trematodiases in Southeast Asia epidemiology, pathology, clinical manifestation and control. *Adv Parasitol.* 2010;72:305-350.
2. Doanh PN, Nawa Y. Clonorchis sinensis and Opisthorchis spp. in Vietnam: current status and prospects. *Trans R Soc Trop Med Hyg.* 2016;110(1):13-20.
3. Keiser J, Utzinger J. Emerging foodborne trematodiasis. *Emerg Infect Dis.* 2005;11(10):1507-1514.

4. Armignacco O, Caterini L, Marucci G, et al. Human illnesses caused by Opisthorchis felineus flukes, Italy. *Emerg Infect Dis*. 2008;14(12):1902-1905.
5. Fedorova OS, Fedotova MM, Sokolova TS, et al. Opisthorchis felineus infection prevalence in Western Siberia: a review of Russian literature. *Acta Trop*. 2018;178:196-204.
6. Fedorova OS, Fedotova MM, Zvonareva OI, et al. Opisthorchis felineus infection, risks, and morbidity in rural Western Siberia, Russian Federation. *PLoS Negl Trop Dis*. 2020;14(6):e0008421.
7. Keiser J, Utzinger J, Xiao SH, et al. Opisthorchis viverrini: efficacy and tegumental alterations following administration of tribendimidine in vivo and in vitro. *Parasitol Res*. 2008;102(4):771-776.
8. Sripa B, Tangkawattana S, Brindley PJ. Update on pathogenesis of Opisthorchiasis and Cholangiocarcinoma. *Adv Parasitol*. 2018;102:97-113.
9. Qian MB, Li HM, Jiang ZH, et al. Severe hepatobiliary morbidity is associated with Clonorchis sinensis infection: the evidence from a cross-sectional community study. *PLoS Negl Trop Dis*. 2021;15(1):e0009116.
10. Sripa B, Kaewkes S, Sithithaworn P, et al. Liver fluke induces cholangiocarcinoma. *PLoS Med*. 2007;4(7):e201.
11. Sripa B, Brindley PJ, Mulvenna J, et al. The tumorigenic liver fluke Opisthorchis viverrini—multiple pathways to cancer. *Trends Parasitol*. 2012;28(10):395-407.
12. Na BK, Pak JH, Hong SJ. Clonorchis sinensis and clonorchiasis. *Acta Trop*. 2020;203:105309.
13. Bouvard V, Baan R, Straif K, et al. A review of human carcinogens—Part B: biological agents. *Lancet Oncol*. 2009;10(4):321-322.
14. IARC. A review of human carcinogens part B: biological agents. *IARC Monogr Eval Carcinog Risks Hum*. 2011;100(B):457.
15. Vatanasapt V, Uttaravichien T, Mairiang EO, et al. Cholangiocarcinoma in north-east Thailand. *Lancet*. 1990;335(8681):116-117.
16. Shin HR, Oh JK, Masuyer E, et al. Epidemiology of cholangiocarcinoma: an update focusing on risk factors. *Cancer Sci*. 2010;101(3):579-585.
17. Bertuccio P, Malvezzi M, Carioli G, et al. Reply to: "Global trends in mortality from intrahepatic and extrahepatic cholangiocarcinoma." *J Hepatol*. 2019;71(6):1262-1263.
18. Sripa B, Suwannatrai AT, Sayasone S, et al. Current status of human liver fluke infections in the Greater Mekong Subregion. *Acta Trop*. 2021;224:106133.
19. Sithithaworn P, Andrews RH, Nguyen VD, et al. The current status of opisthorchiasis and clonorchiasis in the Mekong Basin. *Parasitol Int*. 2012;61(1):10-16.
20. Zhao TT, Feng YJ, Doanh PN, et al. Model-based spatial-temporal mapping of opisthorchiasis in endemic countries of Southeast Asia. *Elife*. 2021;10:e59755.
21. Sripa B, Tesana S, Yurlova N, et al. A historical review of small liver fluke infections in humans. *Parasitol Int*. 2017;66(4):337-340.
22. Pozio E, Armignacco O, Ferri F, et al. Opisthorchis felineus, an emerging infection in Italy and its implication for the European Union. *Acta Trop*. 2013;126(1):54-62.
23. Furst T, Keiser J, Utzinger J. Global burden of human food-borne trematodiasis: a systematic review and meta-analysis. *Lancet Infect Dis*. 2012;12(3):210-221.
24. Lai YS, Zhou XN, Pan ZH, et al. Risk mapping of clonorchiasis in the People's Republic of China: a systematic review and Bayesian geostatistical analysis. *PLoS Negl Trop Dis*. 2017;11(3):e0005239.
25. Brattig NW, Bergquist R, Qian MB, et al. Helminthiases in the People's Republic of China: status and prospects. *Acta Trop*. 2020;212:105670.
26. Zhu TJ, Chen YD, Qian MB, et al. Surveillance of clonorchiasis in China in 2016. *Acta Trop*. 2020;203:105320.
27. Nguyen TTB, Dermauw V, Dahma H, et al. Prevalence and risk factors associated with Clonorchis sinensis infections in rural communities in northern Vietnam. *PLoS Negl Trop Dis*. 2020;14(8):e0008483.
28. Hong ST, Yong TS. Review of successful control of parasitic infections in Korea. *Infect Chemother*. 2020;52(3):427-440.
29. Lee SE, Shin HE, Lee MR, et al. Risk factors of Clonorchis sinensis human infections in endemic areas, Haman-Gun, Republic of Korea: a case-control study. *Korean J Parasitol*. 2020;58(6):647-652.
30. Tang ZL, Huang Y, Yu XB. Current status and perspectives of Clonorchis sinensis and clonorchiasis: epidemiology, pathogenesis, omics, prevention and control. *Infect Dis Poverty*. 2016;5(1):71.
31. Sripa B, Kanla P, Sinawat P, et al. Opisthorchiasis-associated biliary stones: light and scanning electron microscopic study. *World J Gastroenterol*. 2004;10(22):3318-3321.

32. Pinlaor S, Prakobwong S, Hiraku Y, et al. Oxidative and nitrative stress in Opisthorchis viverrini-infected hamsters: an indirect effect after praziquantel treatment. *Am J Trop Med Hyg.* 2008;78(4):564-573.
33. Dangtakot R, Intuyod K, Chamgramol Y, et al. CagA(+) Helicobacter pylori infection and N-nitrosodimethylamine administration induce cholangiocarcinoma development in hamsters. *Helicobacter.* 2021;26(4):e12817.
34. Deenonpoe R, Mairiang E, Mairiang P, et al. Elevated prevalence of Helicobacter species and virulence factors in opisthorchiasis and associated hepatobiliary disease. *Sci Rep.* 2017;7:42744.
35. Sripa B, Echaubard P. Prospects and challenges towards sustainable liver fluke control. *Trends Parasitol.* 2017;33(10):799-812.
36. Suyapoh W, Tangkawattana S, Suttiprapa S, et al. Synergistic effects of cagA+ Helicobacter pylori co-infected with Opisthorchis viverrini on hepatobiliary pathology in hamsters. *Acta Trop.* 2021;213:105740.
37. Traverso A, Repetto E, Magnani S, et al. A large outbreak of Opisthorchis felineus in Italy suggests that opisthorchiasis develops as a febrile eosinophilic syndrome with cholestasis rather than a hepatitis-like syndrome. *Eur J Clin Microbiol Infect Dis.* 2012;31(6):1089-1093.
38. Liao WC, Wang HP, Chiu HM, et al. Multiple hepatic nodules: rare manifestation of clonorchiasis. *J Gastroenterol Hepatol.* 2006;21(9):1497-1500.
39. Rim HJ. Clonorchiasis: an update. *J Helminthol.* 2005;79(3):269-281.
40. Pungpak S, Chalermrut K, Harinasuta T, et al. Opisthorchis viverrini infection in Thailand: symptoms and signs of infection—A population-based study. *Trans R Soc Trop Med Hyg.* 1994;88(5):561-564.
41. Choi MS, Choi D, Choi MH, et al. Correlation between sonographic findings and infection intensity in clonorchiasis. *Am J Trop Med Hyg.* 2005;73(6):1139-1144.
42. Mairiang E. Ultrasonographic features of hepatobiliary pathology in opisthorchiasis and opisthorchiasis-associated cholangiocarcinoma. *Parasitol Int.* 2017;66(4):378-382.
43. Mairiang E, Haswell-Elkins MR, Mairiang P, et al. Reversal of biliary tract abnormalities associated with Opisthorchis viverrini infection following praziquantel treatment. *Trans R Soc Trop Med Hyg.* 1993; 87(2):194-197.
44. Mairiang E, Laha T, Bethony JM, et al. Ultrasonography assessment of hepatobiliary abnormalities in 3359 subjects with Opisthorchis viverrini infection in endemic areas of Thailand. *Parasitol Int.* 2012; 61(1):208-211.
45. Mairiang E, Laha T, Kaewkes S, et al. Hepatobiliary morbidities detected by ultrasonography in Opisthorchis viverrini-infected patients before and after praziquantel treatment: a five-year follow up study. *Acta Trop.* 2021;217:105853.
46. Upatham ES, Viyanant V, Kurathong S, et al. Relationship between prevalence and intensity of Opisthorchis viverrini infection, and clinical symptoms and signs in a rural community in north-east Thailand. *Bull World Health Organ.* 1984;62(3):451-461.
47. Choi D, Lim JH, Lee KT, et al. Gallstones and Clonorchis sinensis infection: a hospital-based case-control study in Korea. *J Gastroenterol Hepatol.* 2008;23(8 Pt 2):e399-e404.
48. Haswell-Elkins MR, Mairiang E, Mairiang P, et al. Cross-sectional study of Opisthorchis viverrini infection and cholangiocarcinoma in communities within a high-risk area in northeast Thailand. *Int J Cancer.* 1994;59(4):505-509.
49. Honjo S, Srivatanakul P, Sriplung H, et al. Genetic and environmental determinants of risk for cholangiocarcinoma via Opisthorchis viverrini in a densely infested area in Nakhon Phanom, northeast Thailand. *Int J Cancer.* 2005;117(5):854-860.
50. Choi D, Lim JH, Lee KT, et al. Cholangiocarcinoma and Clonorchis sinensis infection: a case-control study in Korea. *J Hepatol.* 2006;44(6):1066-1073.
51. Mairiang E, Mairiang P. Clinical manifestation of opisthorchiasis and treatment. *Acta Trop.* 2003; 88(3):221-227.
52. Johansen MV, Sithithaworn P, Bergquist R, et al. Towards improved diagnosis of zoonotic trematode infections in Southeast Asia. *Adv Parasitol.* 2010;73:171-195.
53. Lovis L, Mak TK, Phongluxa K, et al. PCR diagnosis of Opisthorchis viverrini and Haplorchis taichui infections in a Lao Community in an area of endemicity and comparison of diagnostic methods for parasitological field surveys. *J Clin Microbiol.* 2009;47(5):1517-1523.
54. Chai JY, Darwin Murrell K, Lymbery AJ. Fish–borne parasitic zoonoses: status and issues. *Int J Parasitol.* 2005;35(11-12):1233-1254.
55. Kaewkes S. Taxonomy and biology of liver flukes. *Acta Trop.* 2003;88(3):177-186.

56. De NV, Le TH. Human infections of fish-borne trematodes in Vietnam: prevalence and molecular specific identification at an endemic commune in Nam Dinh province. *Exp Parasitol.* 2011;129(4):355-361.
57. Buathong S, Phaiphilai K, Ruang-Areerate T, et al. Genetic differentiation of Opisthorchis-like eggs in northern Thailand using stool specimens under National Strategic Plan to Control Liver Fluke Infection and Cholangiocarcinoma. *Am J Trop Med Hyg.* 2020;103(3):1118-1124.
58. Chai JY. Praziquantel treatment in trematode and cestode infections: an update. *Infect Chemother.* 2013;45(1):32-43.
59. Jongsuksuntigul P, Imsomboon T. Opisthorchiasis control in Thailand. *Acta Trop.* 2003;88(3):229-232.
60. Thinkhamrop K, Khuntikeo N, Sithithaworn P, et al. Repeated praziquantel treatment and Opisthorchis viverrini infection: a population-based cross-sectional study in northeast Thailand. *Infect Dis Poverty.* 2019;8(1):18.
61. Sayasone S, Keiser J, Meister I, et al. Efficacy and safety of tribendimidine versus praziquantel against Opisthorchis viverrini in Laos: an open-label, randomised, non-inferiority, phase 2 trial. *Lancet Infect Dis.* 2018;18(2):155-161.
62. Sayasone S, Meister I, Andrews JR, et al. Efficacy and safety of praziquantel against light infections of Opisthorchis viverrini: a randomized parallel single-blind dose-ranging trial. *Clin Infect Dis.* 2017; 64(4):451-458.
63. Keiser J, Vargas M. Effect of artemether, artesunate, OZ78, praziquantel, and tribendimidine alone or in combination chemotherapy on the tegument of Clonorchis sinensis. *Parasitol Int.* 2010;59(3):472-476.
64. Soukhathammavong P, Odermatt P, Sayasone S, et al. Efficacy and safety of mefloquine, artesunate, mefloquine-artesunate, tribendimidine, and praziquantel in patients with Opisthorchis viverrini: a randomised, exploratory, open-label, phase 2 trial. *Lancet Infect Dis.* 2011;11(2):110-118.
65. Qian MB, Yap P, Yang YC, et al. Efficacy and safety of tribendimidine against Clonorchis sinensis. *Clin Infect Dis.* 2013;56(7):e76-e82.
66. Xu LL, Jiang B, Duan JH, et al. Efficacy and safety of praziquantel, tribendimidine and mebendazole in patients with co-infection of Clonorchis sinensis and other helminths. *PLoS Negl Trop Dis.* 2014; 8(8):e3046.
67. Sayasone S, Odermatt P, Vonghachack Y, et al. Efficacy and safety of tribendimidine against Opisthorchis viverrini: two randomised, parallel-group, single-blind, dose-ranging, phase 2 trials. *Lancet Infect Dis.* 2016;16(10):1145-1153.
68. Grundy-Warr C, Andrews RH, Sithithaworn P, et al. Raw attitudes, wetland cultures, life-cycles: socio-cultural dynamics relating to Opisthorchis viverrini in the Mekong Basin. *Parasitol Int.* 2012;61(1):65-70.
69. Tangkawattana S, Sripa B. Integrative EcoHealth/One Health approach for sustainable liver fluke control: the Lawa model. *Adv Parasitol.* 2018;102:115-139.
70. Xin H, Yang Y, Jiang Z, et al. An investigation of Human Clonorchiasis prevalence in an Endemic County in Guangxi Zhuang Autonomous Region, China, 2016. *Food Waterborne Parasitol.* 2021;22:e00109.
71. WHO/WPRO. Expert Consultation to Accelerate Control of Foodborne Trematode Infections, Taeniasis and Cysticercosis, Seoul, Republic of Korea, 17–19 May 2017: Meeting report. 2017 [cited July 20, 2021]. Available at: https://apps.who.int/iris/handle/10665/260007.
72. Sripa B, Tangkawattana S, Laha T, et al. Toward integrated opisthorchiasis control in northeast Thailand: the Lawa project. *Acta Trop.* 2015;141(Pt B):361-367.

CHAPTER 13

Hepatic Tuberculosis

Vishal Sharma ■ Vineet Ahuja

KEY POINTS

- Hepatic tuberculosis is an uncommon form of gastrointestinal tuberculosis
- The morphologic forms include localized (mass or abscess forming) or diffuse patterns (granulomatous hepatitis)
- The diagnosis is difficult because it is often not considered, and histology is often nonspecific
- The evaluation should include histology (granulomas, caseating necrosis, which is specific) and microbiology (AFB stain, mycobacterial culture or PCR)
- Standard 6 months ATT is usually sufficient, but it is prudent to follow up with these patients for biochemical and radiological resolution.

Introduction

Tuberculosis (TB) is recognized as a cause of pulmonary disease but can involve virtually any organ of the human body. While it is preventable and treatable, TB affects 10 million individuals every year and is a leading infectious killer globally.[1] The involvement of the liver by TB is less commonly recognized and can have variable clinical presentation.[2] Clinicians in TB endemic regions should be aware of the patterns of hepatic TB, clinical situations in which the diagnosis should be considered and the appropriate diagnostic and management approach in these patients.

Pathogenesis

The involvement of the liver by the mycobacterial infection is usually of hematogenous origin. The liver receives blood supply from two major sources: hepatic arterial supply from the aorta and from the portal vein. A possible spread of TB to the liver could be from pulmonary infection through hematogenous route. This would usually occur through the arterial route. Another possible path is from the gastrointestinal tract through the portal vein. While arterial spread is implicated in the multifocal or miliary pattern of involvement of the liver, the portal venous route is blamed for the localized hepatic TB.[2] An uncommon phenomenon occurring in congenital TB results in liver as the primary focus of TB due to dissemination through placental route (umbilical vein).[3] Broadly the morphologic patterns of hepatic tubercular involvement may also involve two forms: a more diffuse involvement, which is usually in association with disseminated TB; or a more localized involvement, which could be due to reactivation of a previous hepatic focus.

Epidemiology

Most case series on hepatic TB have originated from the continents of Asia and Africa.[2] This possibly is related to the higher frequency of pulmonary TB in these regions. The most frequent mechanism of hepatic involvement is related to systemic disease in which the liver is one of the organs affected.

The risk factors for hepatic TB include HIV infection, alcohol intake, intravenous drug use, past TB, and smoking. These risk factors are largely similar to those of TB infection in general. The reported overall frequency of hepatic TB is extremely variable depending on the definition used (systemic or localized), clinical spectrum (isolated hepatic TB, disseminated TB or pulmonary TB), and whether HIV infection is present or not. Many of these factors also drive the clinical outcomes. The miliary involvement is characterized by small lesions all over the hepatic parenchyma, which are usually smaller than 2 mm.[2] Hepatic involvement may accompany 50% to 80% of patients who die of pulmonary TB, but this is usually silent and undiagnosed.

Clinical Presentation

The clinical presentation may be variable and related to the pattern of involvement. No age or gender is immune to TB, although the majority of reported cases are in young to middle-age individuals. Systemic symptoms like fever and loss of weight and of appetite may dominate the clinical presentation in cases where the liver involvement is secondary to disseminated TB. In these cases hepatic involvement is characterized by hepatomegaly and deranged liver functions tests (mild elevations in transaminases but significant increases in alkaline phosphatase) (Table 13.1).[4-9] In addition, these patients may have pulmonary symptoms in the form of cough and expectoration, associated splenomegaly, ascites, and lymphadenopathy.

Localized hepatic TB (Table 13.2) could be in the form of a single or multiple hepatic masses, often termed tuberculomas, or nodular or pseudo-tumoral form. The clinical presentation may include fever, abdominal pain, and hepatomegaly. These lesions are less frequently associated with active pulmonary disease as compared to the miliary involvement. These masses may later form a liver abscess. Liver abscess typically presents with fever, abdominal pain, and palpable and tender hepatomegaly. Hepatic TB should be considered in the differential diagnosis of non-resolving liver abscess in an endemic region. Non-resolution of liver abscess after antibiotics and amoebicidal drugs along with drainage procedures should prompt evaluation for TB as a possible cause.[10,11]

Granulomatous hepatitis is a diffuse involvement of the hepatic parenchyma by an infiltrative process that usually accompanies systemic TB. Typically, the presentation is with fever and hepatomegaly and the liver functions demonstrate impressive elevations of alkaline phosphatase and slight elevations of aminotransferases. The diagnosis is usually achieved by a liver biopsy, and clinicians must send the tissue also for microbiological tests (culture and polymerase chain reaction [PCR]). The causes of hepatic granulomas are diverse, but TB is an important consideration in endemic areas (Table 13.3).[12]

Imaging

Chest roentgenogram may demonstrate changes of past or active pulmonary TB in a substantial number of patients (up to 65% in some series).[5] Computed tomography (CT) of the chest may be considered along with abdominal CT, as presence of pulmonary lesions may increase the confidence in the diagnosis of underlying TB.[13-16]

Ultrasound is the modality of choice for initial evaluation of lesions in the liver.[13-16] It is an easily available modality that also provides an opportunity to sample the lesions for microbiological and histological evaluation. In granulomatous hepatitis, hepatomegaly without any

TABLE 13.1 ■ **Major Series of Hepatic Tuberculosis: Clinical and Investigative Findings**[4-9]

Reference	Amarapurkar et al.	Alvarez et al.	Essop et al.	Hersch et al.	Maharaj et al.	Gounder
Region	Western India	Philippines	South Africa	South Africa	South Africa	South Africa
Population	38 with hepatobiliary TB	130 patients with hepatobiliary TB	96 patients of tuberculous hepatitis	200 patients (143 adults)	41 Black patients	20 HIV-associated hepatic TB
Age	38.1 ± 12.5		Bimodal peak	Both pediatric and adult Adults (44–46 years)	44.5 ± 15.8 years	34.5 years
Gender, Male	27 (71%)	86 (66%)	NA	NA	24 (58.5%)	6 (30%)
Period	1998–2003	1958–1978	1974–1981	1955–1961		2005–2012
Clinical						
Pain	45	25	66	55	46	35
Fever	80	65	70	97	63	85
Weight loss	60	55	NA	75	61	30
Jaundice	0	35	11	22	14	
Hepatomegaly	75	96	80	87	95	
Splenomegaly	30	25	40	35	31.7	
Radiology						
Abnormal CXRPA		65	75	NA	78	
Calcification		50	NA	NA	NA	
Histology						
Caseating granuloma	NA	67	83	NA	51	65%
Granuloma	40	NA	96	NA	NA	100%
Microbiology						
AFB+	50*	7	9	21†	59%	70
Culture +	100				NA	35%
PCR+					NA	NA
Outcomes		Mortality: 12%	Mortality: 42% Only 1 primary hepatic and 9 local; rest were disseminated			Mortality: 30%

*Includes culture positive also
†From those who underwent liver biopsy/autopsy

identifiable individual lesions may be reported. Miliary lesions are usually small (≤2 mm), multiple, studding the hepatic parenchyma, and are typically iso-hypoechoic on ultrasound. These may have associated splenic lesions.[13-18] Ultrasound may demonstrate single or multiple predominantly hypoechoic lesions. Sonographically, the macronodular lesions are typically hypoechoic, although the lesions may show variable echogenicity. They usually do not have a well-defined margin, especially if the lesions are small.[18] Contrast-enhanced ultrasound has also been used, but the findings are not specific to hepatic TB. On arterial phase, rim enhancement or

TABLE 13.2 ■ **Patterns of Hepatic TB and Evaluation**

Patterns	Presentation	LFTs	Diagnosis	Treatment	Follow-up
Miliary TB/ granulomatous hepatitis	Fever weight loss hepatomegaly splenomegaly	Infiltrative pattern (elevated alk. phos.)	Liver biopsy	ATT	LFTs, imaging
Nodular hepatic tuberculosis	Abdominal pain, fever, weight loss	May be normal or abnormal	Imaging-guided fine needle aspiration/biopsy	ATT	Imaging
Hepatic abscess	Fever abdominal pain tender hepatomegaly	May be normal or abnormal	Guided aspiration	ATT, may require drainage	Imaging

TABLE 13.3 ■ **Causes of Hepatic Granulomas**

Infectious	Tuberculosis, Atypical mycobacteria, *Brucella*, *Listeria*, Melioidosis, Syphilis, *Coxiella burnetii*, Cryptococcosis, Histoplasma, CMV, Infectious mononucleosis, Leishmaniasis
Malignancies	Hodgkin disease, Non-Hodgkin lymphoma
Drugs	Allopurinol, Sulfonamide, Carbamazepine, Quinidine, Hydralazine
Hepatic disease	Primary biliary cholangitis, Primary sclerosing cholangitis
Others	Sarcoidosis, Crohn disease, Chronic granulomatous disease, Vasculitis

enhancement of the entire lesion may be noted. The lesions could also be confused with hepatocellular carcinoma.[17]

Hepatic TB, on the basis of CT, is described in one of two forms: parenchymal or sero-hepatic. On the basis of the size of lesions, miliary (2 mm), micronodular (2 cm), macronodular (≥2 cm) or mixed patterns have been reported. On CT, the lesions may be hypo-attenuating and may appear cystic or nodular. Macronodular lesions may appear hypo-attenuating on CT and have poor rim enhancement. These lesions could be single or multiple and have variable sizes.[13-16] Some areas may show parenchymal calcifications.[13] Over time, some of the lesions may transform into abscess-like lesions. Cluster sign or honeycombing may be seen as a result of multiple small lesions developing liquefaction.

Frosted liver appearance has been described with the sero-hepatic variant wherein the subcapsular area of the liver may demonstrate multifocal thickening and nodularity, showing findings akin to scalloping of the liver.[13,19]

The use of magnetic resonance imaging has been reported in a few studies; tuberculous nodules may appear hypointense on T1-weighted images and hyperintense on T2-weighted images, with the core being more hyperintense. Also, contrast images show peripheral rim enhancement.[14,16]

Differential Diagnosis

The mass-forming hepatic TB could be misdiagnosed as hepatocellular carcinoma, intrahepatic cholangiocarcinoma, gallbladder cancer, and hepatic metastasis.[20-23]

Tubercular liver abscess could be confused with amoebic or pyogenic liver abscess, hepatic hydatid disease, and other cystic diseases of the liver.[11,24]

The differential diagnosis of granulomatous hepatitis is broad (see Table 13.3).

Diagnosis

The diagnostic approach must be guided by radiological investigations.[5] In patients who have demonstrable macroscopic lesions (abscess or mass), ultrasound-guided fine-needle aspiration cytology/biopsy may be helpful in providing tissue. A percutaneous ultrasound-guided liver biopsy may be of help in patients where granulomatous hepatitis is a consideration (Figure 13.1).[5]

The diagnosis of hepatic TB is usually based on either a microbiological diagnosis or characteristic histology. Irrespective of the macroscopic pattern of involvement, presence of granulomas is the histologic hallmark of hepatic TB. Granulomas are localized nodular areas of macrophages that may coalesce to result in formation of Langhans giant cells.[5-9,25] Presence of caseating necrosis where the gross appearance is of cheese-like character provides some degree of specificity to the tubercular origin of the granulomas. In absence of caseating necrosis, the differential diagnosis of hepatic granulomas is wide (see Table 13.3). The tissue must also be evaluated with microbiological tests, with mycobacterial culture being the gold standard. Tissue PCR may be of value in achieving a more rapid diagnosis. Microbiological positivity can be seen in less than 50% of cases, but the yield may be higher in tubercular abscess.[5] However, in one study, 80% positivity was reported with use of PCR on archival samples of liver cytology.[26] The presence of TB elsewhere (sputum for pulmonary lesions, cytology from peripheral lymph nodes) may provide contributory evidence and should be sought. Evaluation for exclusion of possible risk factors is also important, and testing for HIV and exclusion of diabetes should be routinely done.

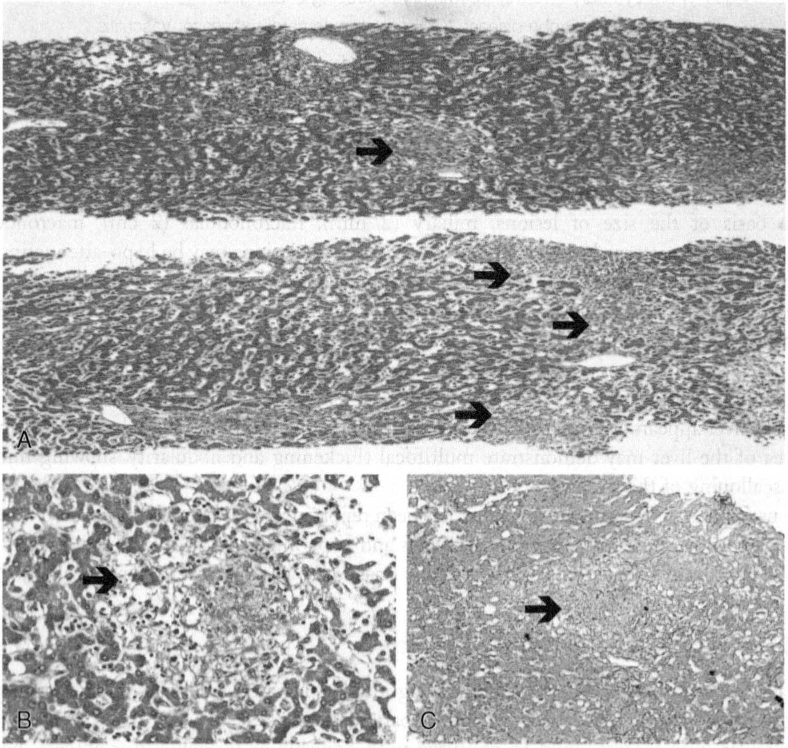

Figure 13.1 A shows liver biopsy with multiple confluent epithelioid cell granulomas in hepatic lobules. B shows a lobular epithelioid cell granuloma with surrounding lymphoid cell layer and Langhan's type of giant cell (arrow). C shows tubercular hepatic granulomas (arrow) which are reticulin-poor and do not show intra or perilesional reticulin condensation.

Management

For nodular TB and granulomatous hepatitis, antitubercular therapy (ATT) is usually sufficient, while drainage could be needed in tubercular abscess. Therapy is usually with four drugs (isoniazid: 5 mg/kg/day; rifampin: 10 mg/kg/day; pyrazinamide: 25 mg/kg/day; ethambutol: 15 mg/kg/day) for the initial 2 months followed by the continuation phase with three drugs (except pyrazinamide) for a minimum of 4 months. The appropriate duration of therapy is uncertain: 6 to 12 months of therapy has been reported in the literature.[5,25,27] Some recent reports describe good results with 6 months of treatment, including radiological resolution of lesions.[25] We suggest that 6 months of therapy may be appropriate if the follow-up demonstrates complete radiological resolution.

Another consideration is the use of less hepatotoxic drugs in patients with deranged liver function tests. In absence of chronic liver disease, the use of modified ATT is usually considered in presence of hyperbilirubinemia (≥3 mg/dL) or significant elevations of aminotransferases (≥5 ULN). Modified ATT typically excludes hepatotoxic agents (isoniazid, rifampin, and pyrazinamide) and replaces these with other drugs (fluoroquinolones, aminoglycosides). In patients with less impressive aminotransferase elevations or sole elevations of alkaline phosphatase, our policy is to use standard therapy with close monitoring of liver function tests. We recommend follow-up of patients with imaging (typically ultrasound) for resolution of the lesions. Occasional reports have suggested use of other modalities (CT, PET-CT, etc.) for follow-up.[28] The follow-up in granulomatous hepatitis is usually with liver function tests (improvements in alkaline phosphatase levels).[29]

Complications

Reported complications of tubercular liver disease include rupture of tubercular liver abscess into the abdominal or pleural cavity or fistulization into adjacent structures like the stomach or biliary system.[30,31] Systemic complications that have been reported include secondary hemophagocytic lymphohistiocytosis and occasional reports have described acute liver failure due to TB.[32]

Congenital Tuberculosis

This is an infrequently reported entity characterized by transplacental or aspirational spread of TB from mother to fetus. In situations wherein the transfer is hematogenous from the placenta, the primary focus could form in the lungs or the liver. Hepatic involvement may occur in one-fifth of cases of congenital TB and presents as fever, jaundice, and hepatomegaly. Although liver biopsy is very sensitive, it is rarely used due to invasive nature. The disease has a high mortality, and early diagnosis could improve outcomes.[3,33]

References

1. World Health Organization. *Global Tuberculosis Report 2020.* Geneva: World Health Organization; 2020. Licence: CC BY-NC-SA 3.0 IGO Available at: https://www.who.int/publications/i/item/9789240013131
2. Hickey AJ, Gounder L, Moosa MY, Drain PK. A systematic review of hepatic tuberculosis with considerations in human immunodeficiency virus co-infection. *BMC Infect Dis.* 2015;15:209.
3. Li C, Liu L, Tao Y. Diagnosis and treatment of congenital tuberculosis: a systematic review of 92 cases. *Orphanet J Rare Dis.* 2019;14(1):131.
4. Amarapurkar DN, Patel ND, Amarapurkar AD. Hepatobiliary tuberculosis in western India. *Indian J Pathol Microbiol.* 2008;51(2):175-181.
5. Alvarez SZ, Carpio R. Hepatobiliary tuberculosis. *Dig Dis Sci.* 1983;28(3):193-200.
6. Essop AR, Posen JA, Hodkinson JH, Segal I. Tuberculosis hepatitis: a clinical review of 96 cases. *Q J Med.* 1984;53(212):465-477.

7. Hersch C. Tuberculosis of the liver: a study of 200 cases. *S Afr Med J.* 1964;38:857-863.
8. Maharaj B, Leary WP, Pudifin DJ. A prospective study of hepatic tuberculosis in 41 black patients. *Q J Med.* 1987;63(242):517-522.
9. Gounder L, Moodley P, Drain PK, Hickey AJ, Moosa MS. Hepatic tuberculosis in human immunodeficiency virus co-infected adults: a case series of South African adults. *BMC Infect Dis.* 2017;17(1):115.
10. Agarwala R, Dhooria S, Khaire NS, et al. Xpert MTB/RIF for diagnosis of tubercular liver abscess. A case series. *Infez Med.* 2020;28(3):420-424.
11. Choudhury A, Shukla J, Mahajan G, Jha DK, Gupta P, Sharma V. Hepatic tuberculosis: Myriad of hues. *Germs.* 2021;11(2):310-13.
12. Choi EK, Lamps LW. Granulomas in the liver, with a focus on infectious causes. *Surg Pathol Clin.* 2018;11(2):231-250.
13. Schininà V, Albarello F, Cristofaro M, et al. Diagnostic imaging of hepatic tuberculosis: case series. *Int J Tuberc Lung Dis.* 2018;22(7):779-787.
14. Ch'ng LS, Amzar H, Ghazali KC, Siam F. Imaging appearances of hepatic tuberculosis: experience with 12 patients. *Clin Radiol.* 2018;73(3):321.e11-321.e16.
15. Karaosmanoglu AD, Onur MR, Sahani DV, Tabari A, Karcaaltincaba M. Hepatobiliary tuberculosis: imaging findings. *AJR Am J Roentgenol.* 2016;207(4):694-704.
16. Kakkar C, Polnaya AM, Koteshwara P, Smiti S, Rajagopal KV, Arora A. Hepatic tuberculosis: a multimodality imaging review. *Insights Imaging.* 2015;6(6):647-658.
17. Forgione A, Tovoli F, Ravaioli M, et al. Contrast-enhanced ultrasound LI-RADS LR-5 in hepatic tuberculosis: case report and literature review of imaging features. *Gastroenterol Insights* 2021;12:1-9. doi:10.3390/gastroent1201000.
18. Cao BS, Li XL, Li N, Wang ZY. The nodular form of hepatic tuberculosis: contrast-enhanced ultrasonographic findings with pathologic correlation. *J Ultrasound Med.* 2010;29(6):881-888. doi:10.7863/jum.2010.29.6.881.
19. Israrahmed A, Agarwal S, Singh S, Lal H. "Frosted liver" appearance in serohepatic variant of hepatic tuberculosis. *BMJ Case Rep.* 2021;14(3):e241643.
20. Yang C, Liu X, Ling W, Song B, Liu F. Primary isolated hepatic tuberculosis mimicking small hepatocellular carcinoma: a case report. *Medicine (Baltimore).* 2020;99(41):e22580.
21. Maguire C, Sivabalan P, Jhamb S, Palamuthusingam P. Hepatic tuberculosis masquerading as cholangiocarcinoma: an unusual differential for a liver mass. *J Surg Case Rep.* 2020;2020(8):rjaa247.
22. Haque MMU, Whadva RK, Luck NH, Mubarak M. Primary hepaticobiliary tuberculosis mimicking gall bladder carcinoma with liver invasion: a case report. *Pan Afr Med J.* 2019;32:68.
23. Keri VC, Jorwal P, Kodan P, Biswas A. Tuberculosis masquerading as metastasis in liver: a rare and an unusual presentation. *BMJ Case Rep.* 2020;13(2):e233303.
24. Azzaza M, Farhat W, Ammar H, et al. Isolated hepatic tuberculosis presenting as hydatid cyst. *Clin J Gastroenterol.* 2020;13(3):408-412.
25. Kale A, Patil PS, Chhanchure U, et al. Hepatic tuberculosis masquerading as malignancy. *Hepatol Int.* 2022;16(2):463-472. doi:10.1007/s12072-021-10257-9.
26. Sharma K, Gupta N, Goyal K, Duseja AK, Sharma A, Rajwanshi A. Evaluation of polymerase chain reaction in space-occupying lesions of liver reported as granulomatous inflammation/tuberculosis on fine-needle aspiration cytology. *Cytojournal.* 2017;14:1.
27. Wu Z, Wang WL, Zhu Y, et al. Diagnosis and treatment of hepatic tuberculosis: report of five cases and review of literature. *Int J Clin Exp Med.* 2013;6(9):845-850.
28. Jin X, Huo L, Wang T, Liu Y, Li F. Hepatosplenic tuberculosis on pretherapy and posttherapy FDG PET/CT. *Clin Nucl Med.* 2020;45(2):174-176.
29. Dhali A, Dhali GK, Ghosh R, Sarkar A. Primary tubercular granulomatous hepatitis presenting as fluctuating jaundice. *Int J Mycobacteriol.* 2021;10:320-323.
30. Bansal M, Dalal P, Kadian Y, Malik N. Tubercular liver abscess rupturing into the pleural cavity: a rare complication. *Trop Doct.* 2019;49(4):320-322.
31. Sharma V, Ahmed SU, Prasad KK, Mandavdhare HS, Singh H, Rana SS. Tubercular gastric fistula: apropos of two cases. *Trop Doct.* 2018;48(1):46-48.
32. Hussain W, Mutimer D, Harrison R, Hubscher S, Neuberger J. Fulminant hepatic failure caused by tuberculosis. *Gut.* 1995;36(5):792-794.
33. Yeh JJ, Lin SC, Lin WC. Congenital tuberculosis in a neonate: a case report and literature review. *Front Pediatr.* 2019;7:255.

CHAPTER 14

Malaria and the Liver

Perry J.J. van Genderen ■ Isaie J. Reuling

KEY POINTS

- Malaria is a deadly parasitic disease, but it is preventable and treatable if diagnosed promptly. It particularly affects children under the age of 5 years living in the poorest countries in sub-Saharan Africa.
- The liver is the initial target organ for parasite reproduction of malaria.
- Symptomatic disease is only observed when the parasite reproduces itself in red blood cells, leading to their lysis and dumping toxic parasite constituents into the circulation.
- The liver may be involved in symptomatology of malaria disease by two different processes: (1) sequestration of RBCs causing microcirculatory obstruction of vital organs (i.e. kidney, lungs, liver) and (2) toxins from RBC lysis being dumped in the liver (more notable in malaria-naive persons).
- The liver inflammation and hepatic dysfunction of severe malaria are usually reversible, with timely treatment and lacks well-defined long-term sequelae.

Epidemiology of Malaria

The WHO global malaria strategy has shown a successful period in malaria control for the past 20 years, with 1.5 billion cases and 7.6 million deaths averted.[1] However, the fight against malaria is currently undermined by the spread of parasite resistance against artemisinins, mosquito resistance against insecticides, and fragile health systems hampering overall progress and threatening global strategies for malaria elimination.[1]

Unfortunately, each year, still more than 600,000 people die of malaria, a preventable and treatable disease. More than 90% of malaria cases occur in the WHO African Region, where transmission is dominated by the parasite *Plasmodium falciparum*. This specific parasite is responsible for most malaria-related deaths, particularly in children under the age of 5 years living in the poorest countries in sub-Saharan Africa.[1]

Life Cycle of Malaria

Malaria is caused by *Plasmodium* parasites that are transmitted to the human host by a bite of an infected female *Anopheles* mosquito. Six different principal *Plasmodium* species (spp.) possess the ability to infect humans: *P. falciparum*, *P. vivax*, *P. malariae*, *P. ovale*, *P. knowlesi*, and the recently identified simian parasite *P. cynomolgi*.[2] After blood ingestion, sporozoites colonizing the mosquito salivary glands are egested in the human skin together with saliva when the mosquito is probing skin during a blood meal (Figure 14.1). The majority of injected parasites migrate through the skin, enter the blood circulation, and travel to the liver. Subsequently, these sporozoites invade

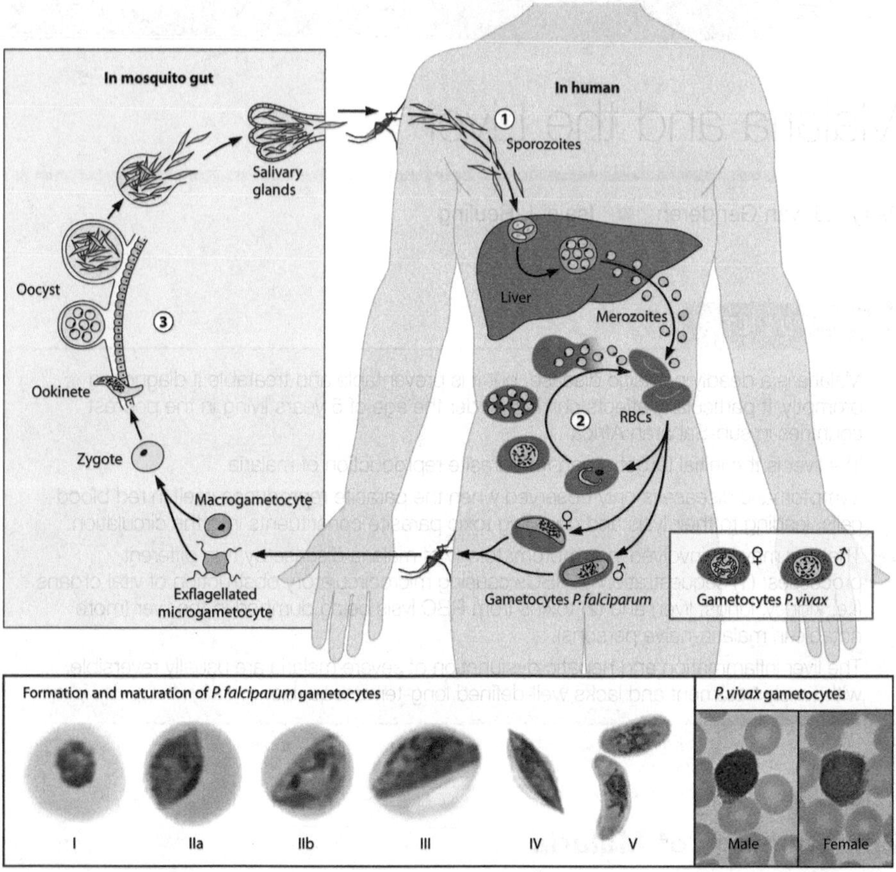

Figure 14.1 Life cycle of malaria. After blood ingestion, sporozoites colonizing the mosquito salivary glands are egested in the human skin together with saliva when the mosquito is probing the skin during a blood meal. The majority of injected parasites migrate through the skin, enter the blood circulation, and travel to the liver. Subsequently, these sporozoites invade hepatocytes and start to replicate, resulting in thousands of merozoites within liver schizonts (liver stage). After approximately 6–20 days of development inside hepatocytes, the schizonts burst, releasing the merozoites into the blood stream. These merozoites then rapidly invade the red blood cells (RBCs). Inside the RBCs the merozoites multiply until the erythrocytic membrane ruptures, releasing them into the blood circulation. Merozoites are capable of infecting and invading new RBCs.

A small percentage of the asexual parasites develop into a sexual form, gametocytes. If these sexual stages are taken up by uninfected *Anopheles* mosquitoes, male and female gametes can fuse to form zygotes and develop in oocysts. As the oocysts grow and rupture inside the mosquito's mid-gut, sporozoites are released and migrate to the salivary glands of the mosquito. The mosquitoes then become infective with the ability to transmit malaria to new human individuals during a subsequent blood meal. (Figure reproduced from *Clin Microbiol Rev*. 2011 Apr;24(2):377-410. doi:10.1128/CMR.00051-10 with permission of the publisher.)

hepatocytes and start to replicate, resulting in thousands of merozoites within liver schizonts. The parasite developmental phase from sporozoite in the skin until schizogony in the liver is referred to as the pre-erythrocytic phase (liver stage). After approximately 6 to 20 days of development inside hepatocytes, the schizonts burst, releasing the merozoites into the blood stream. These merozoites then rapidly invade red blood cells (RBCs) through different ligand-receptor interactions, where they mark the beginning of the erythrocytic phase (blood stage). Inside the RBCs, the merozoites multiply until the erythrocytic membrane ruptures releasing merozoites into the blood circulation. These merozoites are capable of infecting and invading new RBCs and entering a new erythrocytic cycle of parasite reproduction. Depending on the Plasmodium species, this cycle may take approximately 1 to 3 days. *P. vivax*, *P. ovale*, and *P. malariae* target specific RBC subsets for invasion, causing a natural restriction to its eventual parasite load. This preference for certain RBC subsets is lacking for *P. falciparum* and *P. knowlesi* parasites, with higher parasite burdens as a consequence.[2]

A small percentage of the asexual parasites develop into a sexual form, gametocytes. If these sexual stages are taken up by uninfected *Anopheles* mosquitoes, male and female gametes can fuse to form zygotes and develop in oocysts. As the oocysts grow and rupture inside the mosquito's mid-gut, sporozoites are released and migrate to the salivary glands of the mosquito. The mosquitoes then become infective with the ability to transmit malaria to new human individuals during a subsequent blood meal.

Pathogenesis of Malaria

CYTO-ADHERENCE AND SEQUESTRATION OF (INFECTED) RED BLOOD CELLS

As a consequence of the infection of RBCs with *P. falciparum* knobs emerge on the surface extruding high-molecular-weight, strain-specific, adhesive proteins.[2] Infected RBCs may not only adhere to the vessel walls but sometimes also to each other (platelet-mediated agglutination) and even to uninfected RBCs (rosetting). The ultimate consequence of cytoadherence of (parasitized) RBCs is sequestration of RBCs into vital organs. By clumping together, the parasitized RBCs clog the microcirculatory flow of small blood vessels of vital organs, thereby hampering oxygen delivery and metabolism as well as the functioning of vascular endothelium.[2] It is certainly interesting to note that the *Plasmodium* species other than *P. falciparum* do not exhibit significant cyto-adhesion and sequestration and therefore rarely cause life-threatening disease.[2]

INFLAMMATORY HOST RESPONSE TO MALARIA PARASITES AND RED BLOOD CELL CONSTITUENTS

When the parasite develops during the erythrocytic phase, all kinds of waste substances such as hemozoin (malaria pigment) and other toxic products will accumulate in infected RBCs. These substances are subsequently dumped into the circulation when the infected cells lyse at the end of their erythrocytic cycle with the aim to liberate invasive merozoites. Hemozoin gives rise to a pro-inflammatory environment in the host by locally stimulating macrophages and other immune cells to secrete cytokines and other inflammatory mediators, eventually leading to fever.[3,4]

During lysis of the RBCs, other substituents like hemoglobin and hemin are released in the circulation. They are bound by haptoglobin and hemopexin, respectively, and subsequently removed from the circulation by the liver. Excess of these products may, however, give rise to oxidative damage to cells present in the liver leading to apoptosis or lysis. These released constituents of infected RBCs together with parasite antigens may not only amplify immune responses but may also result in accumulation of hemolytic products in the liver that may impact the function of hepatocytes.[5] The elevated levels of nuclear factor kappa-light-chain-enhancer of activated B cells (NF-$\kappa\beta$) and tumor necrosis factor-alpha (TNF-α) in Kupffer cells may generate inflammatory response against cells in the liver during malaria.[6] Hepcidin-mediated iron delocalization in hepatocytes may also contribute to potential liver damage. Some animal studies additionally suggest a role of free radicals generated as a consequence of oxidative stress in inducing dysfunction of hepatocytes.[4]

Clinical Features of Malaria

It is certainly noteworthy that the pre-erythrocytic phase (liver stage) of malaria is not associated with clinical signs or symptoms in infected individuals.[2] All the clinical signs and symptoms associated with malaria are caused by blood stage parasites (asexual parasitemia). Infection with malaria parasites may result in a wide variety of symptoms, ranging from absent or very mild symptoms to severe and complicated disease, and even death if left untreated. Malaria disease can be categorized as uncomplicated or severe (complicated).[2] Severe malaria is diagnosed when *Plasmodium* infections are complicated by evidence of vital organ dysfunction occurring in the absence of an identified alternative cause. The manifestations of severe malaria depend in part on age and immune status. Severe anemia and hypoglycemia are more common in children, whereas pulmonary edema, acute kidney injury, and jaundice are more common in adults. Coma (cerebral malaria) and acidosis may occur in both children and adults.[5] Severe disease has also been described for *P. vivax* and *P. knowlesi* infections, indicating that severe malaria is not exclusively related to *P. falciparum* infections.[2,5]

The Liver in Severe Malaria

The most frequently occurring manifestation of severe malaria in relation to liver involvement is jaundice.[3,7] Hepatic involvement has been demonstrated for both *P. falciparum* and *P. vivax* malaria. Severe jaundice may result from a combination of hemolysis (unconjugated bilirubin fraction), hepatocyte dysfunction, and cholestasis (conjugated bilirubin fraction).[3,8] Jaundice is more common in adults than in children and is frequently accompanied by impairment of renal function. Between 2.5% and 62% of malaria patients suffer from some kind of liver dysfunction and may develop jaundice, depending on the region where they live and endemicity of *P. falciparum* malaria.[3] Some authors have described *malarial hepatopathy* or *malarial hepatitis* as a separate disease manifestation being characterized by increased levels ($\geq$ three fold increase of the upper limit of normal) of serum bilirubin and serum aminotransferases.[9] Malarial hepatopathy is not uncommon during severe malaria and is estimated to contribute to mortality in up to 2% to 5% of the cases. Actual inflammation of the liver parenchyma is, however, not frequently seen.[10] Hepatocellular dysfunction in severe malaria has been linked in particular to hypoglycemia (decreased hepatic blood flow and suppressed gluconeogenesis) and lactic acidosis (impaired hepatic clearance).[11,12] Interestingly, pure hepatic encephalopathy is considered to be rare in severe malaria.[4] The frequently occurring altered mental status in severe malaria is more readily explained by the occurrence of cerebral malaria, hypoglycemia, and/or uremia in case of coexisting acute kidney failure.[2,4]

In some patients with severe malaria inflammatory infiltrates, hepatocyte swelling, hemozoin deposition, loss of microvilli at the sinusoidal pole, and centrizonal necrosis have been observed in liver tissues.[13] However, in most *P. falciparum*–infected patients histological evidence of liver injury is limited.[3] Sequestration of parasitized RBCs is also a common finding in liver tissue depending on the malaria parasite burden. In a well-designed study involving postmortem liver tissues from patient with severe *falciparum* malaria with and without clear jaundice and controls, the histopathological changes in the liver of those with severe *falciparum* malaria were characterized by hyperplastic Kupffer cells, portal tract inflammation, sinusoidal congestion, hemozoin pigment deposition in Kupffer cells, and central veins containing numerous parasitized RBCs.[6] These histopathological changes were more pronounced in severe malaria patients with jaundice as compared to severe malaria patients without jaundice or to normal controls. These findings are in line with the general observation that the hepatic dysfunction in severe malaria is often reversible and lack well-defined long-term sequelae in those patients who respond favorably to antimalarial treatment.[7]

The Liver in Uncomplicated Malaria

Liver injury can also occur in uncomplicated malaria but is often limited and seems fully reversible after parasitological cure.[14] Nevertheless, severe elevations in serum transaminases (up to ≥3 × ULN) can be found in uncomplicated disease, specifically in nonimmune (malaria-naive) individuals. The reported incidence of liver injury varies to a large extent but seems rather underreported in general.[15] The organ damage seems hepatocellular based, as relative higher elevations in serum transaminases are found compared to alkaline phosphatase and gamma-lutamyltransferase. There are no clear signs of clinically significant functional liver impairment in uncomplicated disease. Increased bilirubin levels can be found but are likely reflecting hemolysis and not functional liver impairment as conjugation of bilirubin is frequently normal. The dynamics of liver enzyme elevations seem to gradually rise over the course of infection, tending to peak after initiation of antimalarial treatment.[16] This particular timing of peak damage could suggest hepatotoxicity of antimalarials. However, it is more likely caused by a maximized and enduring pro-inflammatory response post-treatment.[15] Incorrect attribution of liver injury to an antimalarial drug can lead to unnecessary discontinuation or shifts in drug regimens.

The pathophysiology of liver injury in uncomplicated malaria seems at least partly different to severe malaria. In severe *falciparum* malaria tissue damage is often thought to be largely related to decreased oxygen supply and disturbed metabolisms due to parasite sequestration in the microvascular capillary system.[17] However, data from Controlled Human Malaria Infection (CHMI) models in malaria-naive individuals show severe elevations in serum transaminases despite low parasite burdens (uncomplicated malaria). These studies demonstrate strong associations between pro-inflammatory and oxidative stress markers and liver enzyme elevations.[15,16] This suggests a more inflammation-based mechanism of liver injury.

The Effect of Preexisting Immunity on Liver Damage

Large observed differences in incidence of liver injury in uncomplicated malaria exist between study populations and are thought to depend on malaria endemicity and preexisting immunity. Liver injury is a very common feature in malaria-naive individuals, such as returning travelers with uncomplicated malaria (~69%).[15] In contrast, the degree of liver injury in malaria-endemic population can be significantly lower.[18] A study in South-East Asia showed a roughly three times lower incidence of liver enzyme elevations (≥3 × ULN) compared to malaria-naive CHMI participants. Furthermore, CHMI conducted with individuals with preexisting immunity against malaria showed much less liver enzyme elevations compared to malaria-naive individuals from Europe. Interestingly, when malaria-naive CHMI participants were repeatedly infected over a course of 12 months, no liver injury was observed after the third infection.[19] This disease tolerance seems related to host control of T-cell activation. Preexisting immune responses may therefore mitigate inflammatory responses to malaria and subsequently reduce liver injury.

MANAGEMENT OF HEPATIC INVOLVEMENT IN MALARIA

No specific therapy to prevent liver injury has been proven effective. Treatment should remain focused on rapid parasite clearance through antimalarial drugs.[2] An expectative approach might be warranted to prevent unnecessary discontinuation or shifts in antimalarials due to supposed drug-induced liver injury. Supportive drugs with hepatotoxic potential should be limited or given with close care only. Furthermore, other specific management of malaria treatment should be directed toward hypoglycemia, shock, pulmonary edema, secondary infections, maintenance of renal function, and an associated hemorrhagic diathesis.[2]

References

1. WHO. *World Malaria Report 2022.* Geneva: World Health Organization; 2022. Licence: CC BY-NC-SA 3.0 IGO.
2. WHO. *WHO Guidelines for Malaria.* Geneva: World Health Organization; 2021. (WHO/UCN/GMP/2021.01). Licence: CC BY-NC-SA 3.0 IGO.
3. Anand A, Puri P. Jaundice in malaria. *J Gastroenterol Hepatol.* 2005;20:1322-1332.
4. Balaji SN, Deshmukh R, Trivedi V. Severe malaria: biology, clinical manifestations, pathogenesis and consequences. *J Vector Borne Dis.* 2020;57:1-13.
5. Viriyavejakul P, Khachonsaksumet V, Punsawad C. Liver changes in severe *Plasmodium falciparum* malaria: histopathology, apoptosis and nuclear factor kappa B expression. *Malar J.* 2014;13:106.
6. Wassmer SC, Taylor TE, Rathod PK, et al. Investigating the pathogenesis of severe malaria: a multidisciplinary and cross-geographical approach. *Am J Trop Med Hyg.* 2015;93:42-56.
7. Cook GC. Malaria in the liver. *Postgrade Med J.* 1994;70:780-784.
8. Vasa VK, Rao TMV, Paturi N, et al. Liver dysfunction in malaria: an observational study. *Int Arch Integr Med.* 2019;6:150-155.
9. Bhalla A, Suri V, Singh V. Malarial hepatopathy. *J Postgrad Med.* 2006;52:315-320.
10. Anand AC, Garg HK. Approach to clinical syndrome of jaundice and encephalopathy in tropics. *J Clin Exp Hepatol.* 2015;5:S116-S130.
11. Fazil A, Vernekar PV, Geriani D, et al. Clinical profile and complication of malaria hepatopathy. *J Infect Public Health.* 2013;6:383-388.
12. Possemiers H, Vandermosten L, van den Steen P. Etiology of lactic acidosis in malaria. *PLoS Pathog.* 2021;17:e1009122.
13. Kochar DK, Singh P, Agarwal P, et al. Malarial hepatitis. *J Assoc Phys India.* 2003;51:1069-1072.
14. Silva-Pinto A, Ruas R, Almeida F, et al. Artemether-lumefantrine and liver enzyme abnormalities in non-severe *Plasmodium falciparum* malaria in returned travellers: a retrospective comparative study with quinine-doxycycline in a Portuguese centre. *Malar J.* 2017;16(1):43.
15. Reuling IJ, de Jong GM, Yap XZ, et al. Liver injury in uncomplicated malaria is an overlooked phenomenon: an observational study. *EBioMedicine.* 2018;36:131-139.
16. Woodford J, Shanks GD, Griffin P, Chalon S, McCarthy JS. The dynamics of liver function test abnormalities after malaria infection: a retrospective observational study. *The Am J Trop Med Hyg.* 2018; 98(4):1113-1119.
17. Molyneux ME, Looareesuwan S, Menzies IS, et al. Reduced hepatic blood flow and intestinal malabsorption in severe falciparum malaria. *Am J Trop Med Hyg.* 1989;40(5):470-476.
18. van der Pluijm RW, Tripura R, Hoglund RM, et al. Triple artemisinin-based combination therapies versus artemisinin-based combination therapies for uncomplicated plasmodium falciparum malaria: a multicentre, open-label, randomised clinical trial. *Lancet.* 2020;395:1345-1360.
19. Salkeld J, Themistocleous Y, Barrett JR, et al. Repeat controlled human malaria infection of healthy UK adults with blood-stage Plasmodium falciparum: safety and parasite growth dynamics. *Front Immunol.* 2022;13:984323.

CHAPTER 15

HIV and Liver Disease

Francesca Cainelli ■ Sandro Vento

KEY POINTS

- Liver disease is a leading cause of non-AIDS-related death in people living with HIV.
- HIV *per se* favors liver fibrosis, the detection of which at early stages is difficult, being based on transient elastography, which is often unavailable in resource-limited settings.
- Alcohol related and nonalcoholic steatohepatitis are frequent and deserve more attention.
- Prevalence of HBV infection is high in tropical and resource-limited countries. Diagnosis is based on HBsAg, HBeAg, and anti-HBe detection, and, if available, HBV-DNA levels.
- Tenofovir disoproxil fumarate or tenofovir alafenamide are first-line HBV treatments in PLWH.
- HDV infection is underdiagnosed and linked to high rates of liver disease progression to decompensated cirrhosis and HCC in PLWH.
- HCV infection is diagnosed on the basis of HCV-RNA positivity. Direct-acting antivirals against HCV are very effective in PLWH.
- Although all classes of antiretrovirals can cause liver toxicity, nevirapine and efavirenz have been more often implicated.

Introduction

Liver diseases account for 10% of all-cause mortality in people living with HIV (PLWH) and are among the leading causes of non-AIDS-related deaths.[1] Liver damage can be due to hepatitis B, C, or D viruses; alcohol consumption; and nonalcoholic fatty liver disease; however, toxicity of antiretroviral drugs and of traditional herbal medicine should not be disregarded, especially in tropical and resource-limited settings (Table 15.1).

Role of HIV in Liver Damage

HIV can replicatively infect cells in the liver; in fact, Kupffer cells and, to a lesser extent, hepatocytes can be positive by *in situ* hybridization for HIV-1 RNA.[2,3] Interestingly, HIV stimulates hepatic stellate cells via the gp120 receptor and activates pathways that result in free reactive oxygen species, leading to increased production of profibrotic cytokines.[4] Lower CD4 lymphocyte count and higher HIV load are significantly associated with progression to advanced hepatic fibrosis (as measured by the Fibrosis-4 index) in a count-dependent manner (Figure 15.1).[5]

TABLE 15.1 ■ **Frequent Causes of Elevated Liver Enzymes in PLWH**

Hepatitis B
Hepatitis C
NAFLD or ALD
Medication side effects
Herbals
AIDS cholangiopathy
MAC infection
Lymphoma
Kaposi's sarcoma

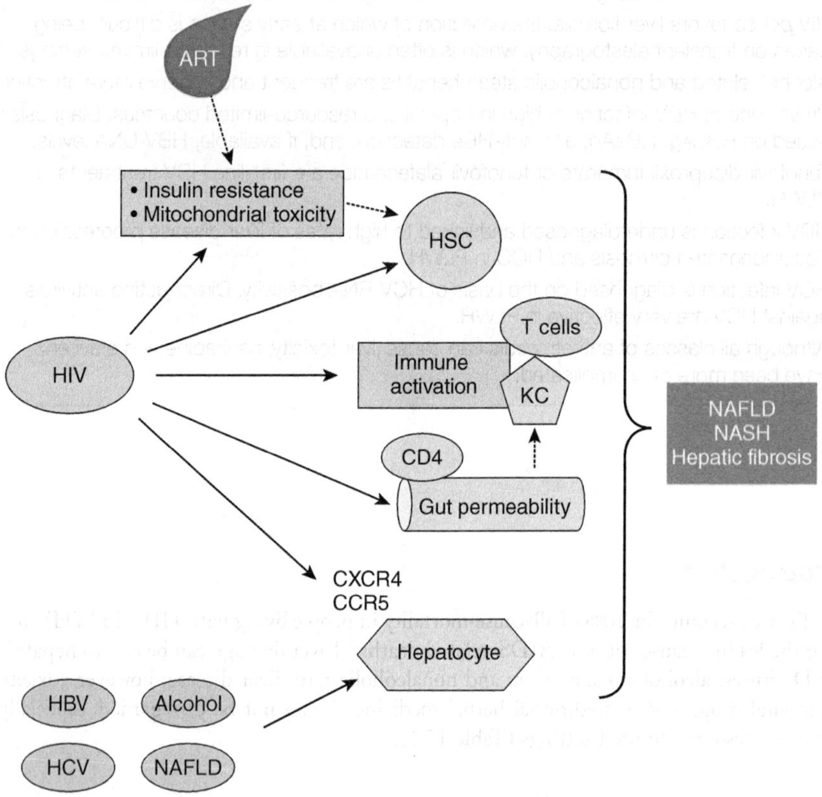

Figure 15.1 Factors affecting liver fibrosis and steatosis during HIV infection. HIV can induce a direct effect on hepatic stellate cells (HSC) and affect T cells and Kupffer cells (KC), hepatocytes, and mitochondrial DNA. HIV can also increase gut permeability through depletion of intestinal CD4 cells. Antiretroviral therapy (ART) can induce insulin resistance and mitochondrial toxicity in the liver. Other factors like HBV, HCV, diet heritage–related NAFLD, and alcohol consumption can affect hepatocytes and worsen liver fibrosis.

Hepatitis B Virus Coinfection

Hepatitis B virus (HBV)-HIV coinfection is frequent, due to the common transmission routes. In a recent meta-analysis estimating the global HBV burden in PLWH, the overall prevalence of

HBV infection was 8.4%, and 26.8% of coinfected people were hepatitis B e antigen positive.[6] About 73.8% of cases were from sub-Saharan Africa and 17.1% from Asia and the Pacific[6]; prevalence of HBV coinfection was higher in sex workers, injection drug users, and men who have sex with men.[6]

INFLUENCE OF HBV COINFECTION ON HIV PROGRESSION AND MORTALITY

In vitro, HBV enhances HIV transcription[7] and coinfection with HBV stimulates HIV replication within mononuclear cells,[8] favoring the idea of a negative role of HBV in the course of HIV infection. However, *in vivo* findings are contradictory; a few studies have shown reduced survival of HBV-HIV coinfected patients,[9-13] while other studies found no effect.[14-17] For unknown reasons, HBV coinfection is associated with slower immunoreconstitution and reduced CD4 cell counts on long-term antiretroviral therapy (ART).[18-21]

INFLUENCE OF HIV INFECTION ON THE NATURAL HISTORY OF HEPATITIS B

HIV coinfection increases the risk of chronicity of HBV infection[22-24] and diminishes the chances of seroconversion from HBeAg to anti-HBe.[25,26] HIV also accelerates liver disease progression and increases mortality in patients with chronic hepatitis B compared with HIV-uninfected patients.[27]

The use of HBV-active ART can lead to high rates of HBeAg seroconversion to anti-HBe and possible HBsAg to anti-HBs seroconversion over 5 years of therapy.[28,29] However, clearance of HBsAg is not common[30] and favored by low HBsAg and HBV-DNA levels, lack of pre-core mutations, and older age.[30] Importantly, ART may reverse liver fibrosis progression in HBV coinfected patients.[31]

HEPATITIS B VACCINATION

Considering the high rate of chronicity, it is important to prevent HBV acquisition in people living with HIV; unfortunately, the responsiveness of PLWH to the hepatitis B vaccine is impaired, and up to one-third of them fail to develop anti-HBs antibodies following three injections.[32-34] Patients who receive more than three doses, with higher CD4 lymphocyte counts, and on ART have higher response rates.[35,36] In an interesting study, a low response rate to the HBV vaccine was detected especially in adolescents with high $CD8^{+}CD38^{+}DR^{+}$ T-lymphocyte levels,[37] suggesting that excessive immune activation decreases the capacity of the immune system of people living with HIV to respond to the HBV vaccine. Regrettably, anti-HBV immunity following vaccination wanes more rapidly in PLWH.[38,39]

ISOLATED ANTI-HBc ANTIBODY POSITIVITY

The isolated presence of IgG antibodies to HBcAg may represent resolved HBV infection (with lack of production or loss of anti-HBs antibodies), occult chronic HBV infection (with HBsAg levels below the limits of detection), or false-positive EIA test result. Isolated anti-HBc-positivity is more frequent in hepatitis C virus (HCV) co-infected patients, while it is much rarer in subjects with HIV alone[40,41]; the association between isolated anti-HBc positivity and HCV infection in PLWH likely reflects a common route of acquisition (intravenous drug use) and the well-known trend of these patients to be exclusively anti-HBc positive without anti-HBs. Should these individuals be vaccinated against HBV? The answer is "yes," as most of them have a primary anti-HBs antibody response to HBV vaccination.[42-46]

TREATMENT OF HBV-RELATED CHRONIC LIVER DISEASE

Tenofovir disoproxil fumarate or tenofovir alafenamide are first-line HBV treatments for co-infected individuals due to their high efficacy and high genetic barrier for resistance. However, either liver fibrosis regression or progression can occur in tenofovir-treated patients, as shown by a study in 167 patients treated with tenofovir-containing ART in France with a median follow-up of 60 months[47] and by a numerically smaller previous study done in Spain.[48]

Hepatitis D and HIV Infection

The prevalence of HDV coinfection in HIV/HBV-coinfected patients in Europe is around 15%,[49,50] and liver fibrosis rates are higher than in HBV-HIV coinfected individuals both in Europe[49,51] and in sub-Saharan Africa.[52] However, HDV infection is underdiagnosed in PLWH,[53] and this contributes to the high rates of liver disease progression to decompensated cirrhosis and HCC in these patients.[53] In fact, a sixfold increased risk of HCC was noted among HIV/HBV/HDV triple-infected patients, compared to HIV/HBV coinfected patients in a recent systematic review and meta-analysis of longitudinal studies.[54]

Treatment results are disappointing; in an open, uncontrolled Italian trial that continues to represent the longest conducted in HDV-HIV coinfected patients, treatment for 2 years with progressively decreasing doses of interferon alpha-2b led to a very poor long-term response rate in 16 PLWH,[55] and as for nucleos(t)ide analogues, only a study done in Spain on 19 patients found significantly reduced serum HDV-RNA and significant improvements in liver fibrosis in HDV-coinfected PLWH on long-term tenofovir treatment.[56] In other studies, nucleos(t)ide analogues had no effect on HDV viremia in PLWH.[57,58]

Hepatitis C Virus Coinfection

The estimated global prevalence of HCV coinfection in PLWH is 6.2%, with the largest burden in Eastern Europe and Central Asia and injecting drug use as the main underlying factor.[59]

INFLUENCE OF HCV INFECTION ON HIV1 DISEASE PROGRESSION

HCV coinfection seems to negatively influence HIV disease; in an Asian cohort of PLWH, HCV coinfection was associated with lower CD4 lymphocyte recovery on ART and increased mortality,[60] and increased mortality was confirmed by a recent study in China.[61]

INFLUENCE OF HIV1 INFECTION ON THE NATURAL HISTORY OF CHRONIC HEPATITIS C

Liver fibrosis progresses more rapidly in HCV-HIV coinfected individuals[62,63] and incidence of hepatic decompensation is higher even in patients treated with ART.[64] The progression rate of liver fibrosis is higher in people with low CD4 cell count[62,63] and high alcohol consumption.[62]

In a study of liver biopsy pairs from 282 largely African American, male, HCV genotype 1, non-cirrhotic patients, almost all with no or minimal fibrosis, after a median of 2.5 years between biopsies, fibrosis progression was observed in 34% of patients.[65] Hepatic steatosis and diabetes were associated with fibrosis progression,[65] indicating an important role of concomitant non-alcoholic fatty liver disease.

HEPATITIS B AND/OR C COINFECTION AND ALL-CAUSE MORTALITY

HBV and HCV coinfection can independently increase all-cause mortality in people living with HIV treated with antiretrovirals,[66] and coinfection with both HCV and HBV has an additive effect on the risk of death.[66,67]

THERAPY OF HCV-RELATED CHRONIC LIVER DISEASE

Direct-acting antivirals against HCV are very effective in PLWH, with sustained responses similar to HIV-uninfected individuals also in cirrhotics, and minimal interactions with antiretrovirals.[68]

Alcohol Use Disorder

Hazardous alcohol use is common in people living with HIV and associated with important liver fibrosis,[69] with an even higher impact in HBV-coinfected individuals.[69] In a recent systematic review and meta-analysis, daily alcohol consumption >50 g was an important risk factor for liver fibrosis among PLWH.[70] This is a still overlooked and important issue with more attention needed by physicians caring for PLWH.

Non-Alcoholic Steatohepatitis

Metabolic syndrome and non-alcoholic steatohepatitis have long been noted in both ART-naive and ART-treated PLWH.[71,72] In a US study performed a few years ago, liver biopsy identified non-alcoholic steatohepatitis and fibrosis in most PLWH with chronic elevation of aminotransferase levels on ART, in the absence of alcohol abuse or viral hepatitis.[73] A more recent multicenter European study examining a large cohort of PLWH over 40 years of age at risk of nonalcoholic fatty liver disease (because of metabolic syndrome, and/or persistently raised liver enzymes, and/or lipodystrophy) found that steatosis was present in 64% of individuals, and 11% had advanced fibrosis.[74] Studies in low- and middle-income countries are needed as it is likely that a "Westernized" lifestyle in these areas becomes more prevalent, and so will the interaction of NAFLD-NASH and HIV.

Hepatocellular Carcinoma

In sub-Saharan Africa hepatocellular carcinoma (HCC) develops at a younger age in PLWH than in HIV-uninfected individuals, particularly in women,[75] and is associated with HBV coinfection.[76] Unfortunately, in these countries many HBV and HCV infections are only diagnosed after the patients present with advanced HCC, with multiple and/or large, untreatable liver lesions.

Herbal Medicines

In a study in Rakai, Uganda, HIV was associated with a 50% increase in liver fibrosis, as measured by transient elastography.[77] Traditional herbal medicine, the use of which is associated with a substantial increase in liver fibrosis in both PLWH and HIV-uninfected people in sub-Saharan Africa,[78] is likely to play a role, as it can also lead to jaundice and liver dysfunction, with a high associated risk of death.[79]

Autoimmune Hepatitis

A few cases of autoimmune hepatitis have occurred after initiation of ARVs in PLWH, and females of African descent seem more likely to be affected.[80-82]

Antiretroviral Drug–Induced Liver Injury

Most antiretroviral drugs are safe and rarely cause severe liver damage or liver fibrosis.[83]

However. ART-induced liver injury ranges from 8% to 23% and up to one-third of the patients can require change of regimen or treatment discontinuation.[84-86] Although all classes of ARTs can cause liver toxicity, first-generation non-nucleoside reverse transcriptase inhibitors are implicated in most cases. Nevirapine (NVP) has been especially involved, as liver injury occurs in up to 17% of treated patients,[87] with severe liver toxicity reported in 1.3% to 12%.[88-90] Efavirenz can also induce liver injury and occasionally lead to submassive necrosis, presenting with jaundice and coagulopathy,[91,92] with ensuing death in up to 14% of cases[93,94]; female sex, young age, and high CD4 cell counts are risk factors.[91,92]

Other Liver Diseases

AIDS cholangiopathy can occur in severely immunocompromised (CD4 cell count below 100/μL) patients and is characterized by strictures in the biliary tract due to opportunistic infections, with consequent biliary obstruction and cholestatic liver damage.[95] *Cryptosporidium parvum* is the most commonly associated pathogen, followed by cytomegalovirus and microsporidia (especially *Enterocytozoon bieneusi*). The most common presentation is severe right upper quadrant pain associated with nausea, vomiting, and diarrhea; treatment is problematic and includes endoscopic approach when appropriate, use of ursodeoxycholic acid (in patients with elevated liver tests and intrahepatic disease), and therapy of underlying infection.

Mycobacterium avium complex can cause disseminated infections in patients with AIDS and CD4 lymphocyte counts below 100/μL, often with hepatic granulomatosis.[96] Treatment is complex (at least two medications) and often requires 12-month therapy.

Kaposi's sarcoma, although rarely reported, can affect the liver in AIDS patients; cutaneous involvement is present in most cases and may help with the diagnosis.[97,98]

Lymphomas involve the liver quite frequently in PLWH.[99] Interestingly, primary hepatic lymphomas (i.e., lymphomas limited to the liver or with major liver involvement at presentation without evidence of extrahepatic involvement within 6 months)[100] can also be observed and are generally,[101] but not always,[102] non-Hodgkin's lymphomas.

Conclusions

A few practical conclusions can be reached from the published work related to HIV and liver diseases. Hepatitis B is a potentially controllable disease that occurs very frequently in people living with HIV in the very area of the world (sub-Saharan Africa)[103,104] most affected by HIV infection. These patients are at risk of developing HBV-related chronic hepatitis—associated outcomes, such as cirrhosis, hepatocellular carcinoma, and death. Treatment with antiretroviral drugs concurrently acting on HIV and HBV reduces morbidity and mortality associated with both HBV and HIV infections. In addition, people living with HIV and the population at large must be made aware of the need to abstain from alcohol, as its fundamental role in the development of liver cirrhosis is still overlooked and must be clearly stressed, especially in developing regions, where alcohol consumption is increasing and often far higher than commonly assumed.

In HIV-HCV coinfection the two main cofactors associated with progression to cirrhosis and mortality in PLWH are low (<200/μL) CD4 lymphocyte counts and alcohol consumption above 50 g daily. As CD4 lymphocyte decline depends on continuing HIV replication, effective antiretroviral therapies can slow HCV disease progression. However, in countries where direct-acting antivirals are available, they will of course allow HCV elimination and considerably lessen the risk of cirrhosis and HCC.

Finally, severe hepatotoxicity due to antiretroviral drugs can occur throughout the course of treatment and is more common among patients coinfected with HBV or HCV and treated with nevirapine or efavirenz. Hence frequent monitoring of transaminases should be done, particularly for these patient subgroups.

Unfortunately, liver diseases and liver-related mortality are still overlooked in people living with HIV, especially in developing countries with limited resources. In an important cohort study of 301 HIV-infected patients observed at the Division of Hepatology, Groote Schuur Hospital, Cape Town, and biopsied between 2000 and 2013, drug-induced liver injury was the most common finding, followed by granulomatous inflammation (largely due to tuberculosis immune reconstitution syndrome), hepatitis B, and nonalcoholic steatohepatitis; 16% of patients had more than one pathology.[92] Monitoring of hepatitis B, C, and D co-infections and of aminotransferase levels should become part of routine assessment, as should abdominal ultrasound. Transient elastography should be made available in referral centers to diagnose and monitor liver fibrosis. Liver biopsies should also be done more widely in referral centers to make a diagnosis in cases where noninvasive investigations have failed.

References

1. Smith CJ, Ryom L, Weber R, et al. Trends in underlying causes of death in people with HIV from 1999 to 2011 (D:A:D): a multicohort collaboration. *Lancet*. 2014;384:241-248.
2. Cao YZ, Dieterich D, Thomas PA, Huang YX, Mirabile M, Ho DD. Identification and quantitation of HIV-1 in the liver of patients with AIDS. *AIDS*. 1992;6:65-70.
3. Housset C, Lamas E, Courgnaud V, et al. Presence of HIV-1 in human parenchymal and *non-parenchymal* liver cells in vivo. *J Hepatol*. 1993;19:252-258.
4. Mastroianni CM, Lichtner M, Mascia C, et al. Molecular mechanisms of liver fibrosis in HIV/HCV coinfection. *Int J Mol Sci*. 2014;15:9184-9208.
5. Kim HN, Nance R, Van Rompaey S, et al. Poorly controlled HIV infection: an independent risk factor for liver fibrosis. *J Acquir Immune Defic Syndr*. 2016;72:437-443.
6. Leumi S, Bigna JJ, Amougou MA, Ngouo A, Nyaga UF, Noubiap JJ. Global burden of hepatitis B infection in people living with human immunodeficiency virus: a systematic review and meta-analysis. *Clin Infect Dis*. 2020;71:2799-2806.
7. Twu J, Chu K, Robinson W. Hepatitis B virus X gene activates kappa B-like enhancer sequences in the long terminal repeat of human immunodeficiency virus 1. *Proc Natl Acad Sci U S A*. 1989;86:5168-5172.
8. Gomez-Gonzalo M, Carretero M, Rullas J, et al. The hepatitis B virus X protein induces HIV-1 replication and transcription in synergy with T-cell activation signals. *J Biol Chem*. 2001;276:35435-35443.
9. McGovern BH. The epidemiology, natural history and prevention of hepatitis B: implications of HIV coinfection. *Antivir Ther*. 2007;12(suppl 3):H3-H13.
10. Nikolopoulos GK, Paraskevis D, Hatzitheodorou E, et al. Impact of hepatitis B virus infection on the progression of AIDS and mortality in HIV-infected individuals: a cohort study and meta-analysis. *Clin Infect Dis*. 2009;48:1763-1771.
11. Thornton AC, Jose S, Bhagani S, et al. Hepatitis B, hepatitis C, and mortality among HIV-positive individuals. *AIDS*. 2017;31:2525-2532.
12. Kouamé GM, Gabillard D, Moh R, et al. Higher risk of mortality in HIV-HBV co-infected patients from sub-Saharan Africa is observed at lower CD4+ cell counts. *Antivir Ther*. 2021;26:25-33.
13. Jia J, Zhu Q, Deng L, et al. Treatment outcomes of HIV patients with hepatitis B and C virus co-infections in Southwest China: an observational cohort study. *Infect Dis Poverty*. 2022;11:7.
14. Zhang F, Zhu H, Wu Y, et al. HIV, hepatitis B virus, and hepatitis C virus co-infection in patients in the China National Free Antiretroviral Treatment Program, 2010–12: a retrospective observational cohort study. *Lancet Infect Dis*. 2014;14:1065-1072.
15. Ladep NG. Hepatitis B co-infection is associated with poorer survival of HIV-infected patients on highly active antiretroviral therapy in West Africa. *JAIDS Clin Res*. 2013;(suppl 3):006. doi:10.4172/2155-6113.S3-006.

16. Chen M, Wong WW, Law MG, et al. Hepatitis B and C co-infection in HIV patients from the TREAT Asia HIV observational database: analysis of risk factors and survival. *PLoS One.* 2016;11:1-17.
17. Umutesi J, Nsanzimana S, Yingkai Liu C, Vanella P, Ott JJ, Krause G. Long-term effect of chronic hepatitis B on mortality in HIV-infected persons in a differential HBV transmission setting. *BMC Infect Dis.* 2022;22:500.
18. Idoko J, Meloni S, Muazu M, et al. Impact of hepatitis B virus infection on human immunodeficiency virus response to antiretroviral therapy in Nigeria. *Clin Infect Dis.* 2009;49:1268-1273.
19. Wandeler G, Gsponer T, Bihl F, et al. Hepatitis B virus infection is associated with impaired immunological recovery during antiretroviral therapy in the Swiss HIV cohort study. *J Infect Dis.* 2013;208:1454-1458.
20. Hawkins C, Christian B, Ye J, et al. Prevalence of hepatitis B co-infection and response to antiretroviral therapy among HIV-infected patients in Tanzania. *AIDS.* 2013;27:919-927.
21. Anderson M, Gaseitsiwe S, Moyo S, et al. Slow CD4+ T-cell recovery in human immunodeficiency virus/hepatitis B virus-coinfected patients initiating Truvada-based combination antiretroviral therapy in Botswana. *Open Forum Infect Dis.* 2016;3:ofw140.
22. Hadler SC. Hepatitis B prevention and human immunodeficiency virus (HIV) infection. *Ann Intern Med.* 1988;109:92-94.
23. Bodsworth NJ, Cooper DA, Donovan B. The influence of human immunodeficiency virus type 1 infection on the development of the hepatitis B virus carrier state. *J Infect Dis.* 1991;163:1138-1140.
24. Sinicco A, Raiteri R, Sciandra M, et al. Co-infection and superinfection of hepatitis B virus in patients infected with human immunodeficiency virus: no evidence of faster progression to AIDS. *Scand J Infect Dis.* 1997;29:111-115.
25. Krogsgaard K, Lindhardt BO, Nielson JO, et al. The influence of HTLV-III infection on the natural history of hepatitis B virus infection in male homosexual HBsAg carriers. *Hepatology.* 1987;7:37-41.
26. Gilson RJ, Hawkins AE, Beecham MR, et al. Interactions between HIV and hepatitis B virus in homosexual men: effects on the natural history of infection. *AIDS.* 1997;11:597-606.
27. Thio CL, Seaberg EC, Skolasky Jr R, et al. Multicenter AIDS Cohort Study. HIV-1, hepatitis B virus, and risk of liver-related mortality in the Multicenter Cohort Study (MACS). *Lancet.* 2002;360:1921-1926.
28. de Vries-Sluijs TE, Reijnders JG, Hansen BE, et al. Long-term therapy with tenofovir is effective for patients co-infected with human immunodeficiency virus and hepatitis B virus. *Gastroenterology.* 2010;139:1934-1941.
29. Psevdos Jr G, Kim JH, Suh JS, Sharp VL. Predictors of loss of hepatitis B surface antigen in HIV infected patients. *World J Gastroenterol.* 2010;16:1093-1096.
30. Boyd A, Dezanet LNC, Lacombe K. Functional cure of hepatitis B virus infection in individuals with HIV-coinfection: a literature review. *Viruses.* 2021;13:1341.
31. Yang R, Gui X, Ke H, Xiong Y, Gao S. Combination antiretroviral therapy is associated with reduction in liver fibrosis scores in patients with HIV and HBV co-infection. *AIDS Res Ther.* 2021;18:98.
32. Carne CA, Weller IVD, Waite J, et al. Impaired responsiveness of homosexual men with HIV antibodies to plasma derived hepatitis B vaccine. *Br Med J.* 1987;294:866-868.
33. Collier AC, Corey L, Murphy VL, Handsfield HH. Antibody to human immunodeficiency virus (HIV) and suboptimal response to hepatitis B vaccination. *Ann Intern Med.* 1988;109:101-105.
34. Odaka N, Eldred L, Cohn S, et al. Comparative immunogenicity of plasma derived and recombinant hepatitis B virus vaccines in homosexual men. *JAMA.* 1988;260:3635-3637.
35. Rey D, Krantz V, Partisani M, et al. Increasing the number of hepatitis B vaccine injections augments anti-HBs response rate in HIV-infected patients: effects on HIV-1 viral load. *Vaccine.* 2000;18:1161-1165.
36. Landrum ML, Huppler Hullsiek K, Ganesan A, et al. Hepatitis B vaccine responses in a large U.S. military cohort of HIV-infected individuals: another benefit of HAART in those with preserved CD4 count. *Vaccine.* 2009;27:4731-4738.
37. Wilson CM, Ellenberg JH, Sawyer MK, et al. Serologic response to hepatitis B vaccine in HIV infected and high-risk HIV uninfected adolescents in the REACH cohort. Reaching for Excellence in Adolescent Care and Health. *J Adolesc Health.* 2001;29:123-129.
38. O'Bryan TA, Rini EA, Okulicz JF, et al. HIV viraemia during hepatitis B vaccination shortens the duration of protective antibody levels. *HIV Med.* 2015;16:161-167.

39. Nicolini LA, Magne F, Signori A, et al. Hepatitis B Virus vaccination in HIV: immunogenicity and persistence of seroprotection up to 7 years following a primary immunization course. *AIDS Res Hum Retroviruses*. 2018;34:922-928.
40. Gandhi RT, Wurcel A, Lee H, et al. Isolated antibody to hepatitis B core antigen in human immunodeficiency virus type 1-infected individuals. *Clin Infect Dis*. 2003;36:1602-1605.
41. Bhattacharya D, Tseng CH, Tate JP, et al. Isolated hepatitis B core antibody is associated with advanced hepatic fibrosis in HIV/HCV infection but not in HIV infection alone. *J Acquir Immune Defic Syndr*. 2016;72:e14-e17.
42. Gandhi RT, Wurcel A, Lee H, et al. Response to hepatitis B vaccine in HIV-1-positive subjects who test positive for isolated antibody to hepatitis B core antigen: implications for hepatitis B vaccine strategies. *J Infect Dis*. 2005;191:1435-1441.
43. Jongjirawisan Y, Ungulkraiwit P, Sungkanuparph S. Isolated antibody to hepatitis B core antigen in HIV-1 infected patients and a pilot study of vaccination to determine the anamnestic response. *J Med Assoc Thai*. 2006;89:2028-2034.
44. Chakvetadze C, Bani-Sadr F, Le Pendeven C, et al. Serologic response to hepatitis B vaccination in HIV-infected patients with isolated positivity for antibodies to hepatitis B core antigen. *Clin Infect Dis*. 2010;50:1184-1186.
45. Kaech C, Pache I, Bürgisser P, Elzi L, Darling KE, Cavassini M. Immune response to hepatitis B vaccination in HIV-positive adults with isolated antibodies to HBV core antigen. *J Infect*. 2012;65:157-164.
46. Piroth L, Launay O, Michel ML, et al. Vaccination against hepatitis B virus (HBV) in HIV-1-infected patients with isolated anti-HBV core antibody: the ANRS HB EP03 CISOVAC Prospective Study. *J Infect Dis*. 2016;213:1735-1742.
47. Boyd A, Bottero J, Miailhes P, et al. Liver fibrosis regression and progression during controlled hepatitis B virus infection among HIV-HBV patients treated with tenofovir disoproxil fumarate in France: a prospective cohort study. *J Int AIDS Soc*. 2017;20:21426.
48. Martín-Carbonero L, Teixeira T, Poveda E, et al. Clinical and virological outcomes in HIV-infected patients with chronic hepatitis B on long-term nucleos(t)ide analogues. *AIDS*. 2011;25:73-79.
49. Soriano V, Grint D, d'Arminio Monforte A, et al. Hepatitis delta in HIV-infected individuals in Europe. *AIDS*. 2011;25:1987-1992.
50. Béguelin C, Moradpour D, Sahli R, et al. Hepatitis delta-associated mortality in HIV/HBV-coinfected patients. *J Hepatol*. 2017;66:297-303.
51. Fernández-Montero JV, Vispo E, Barreiro P, et al. Hepatitis delta is a major determinant of liver decompensation events and death in HIV-infected patients. *Clin Infect Dis*. 2014;58:1549-1553.
52. Jaquet A, Wandeler G, Nouaman M, et al. Alcohol use, viral hepatitis and liver fibrosis among HIV-positive persons in West Africa: a cross-sectional study. *J Int AIDS Soc*. 2017;19:21424.
53. Brancaccio G, Shanyinde M, Puoti M, et al. Hepatitis delta coinfection in persons with HIV: misdiagnosis and disease burden in Italy. *Pathog Glob Health*. 2022:1-9.
54. Kamal H, Fornes R, Simin J, et al. Risk of hepatocellular carcinoma in hepatitis B and D virus co-infected patients: a systematic review and meta-analysis of longitudinal studies. *J Viral Hepat*. 2021;28:1431-1442.
55. Puoti M, Rossi S, Forleo MA, et al. Treatment of chronic hepatitis D with interferon alpha-2b in patients with human immunodeficiency virus infection. *J Hepatol*. 1998;29:45-52.
56. Soriano V, Vispo E, Sierra-Enguita R, et al. Efficacy of prolonged tenofovir therapy on hepatitis delta in HIV-infected patients. *AIDS*. 2014;28:2389-2394.
57. Boyd A, Miailhes P, Brichler S, et al. Effect of tenofovir with and without interferon on hepatitis D virus replication in HIV-hepatitis B virus-hepatitis D virus-infected patients. *AIDS Res Hum Retroviruses*. 2013;29:1535-1540.
58. Béguelin C, Friolet N, Moradpour D, et al. Impact of tenofovir on hepatitis delta virus replication in the Swiss human immunodeficiency Virus Cohort Study. *Clin Infect Dis*. 2017;64:1275-1278.
59. Platt L, Easterbrook P, Gower E, et al. Prevalence and burden of HCV co-infection in people living with HIV: a global systematic review and meta-analysis. *Lancet Infect Dis*. 2016;16:797-808.
60. Chen M, Wong WW, Law MG, et al. Hepatitis B and C co-infection in HIV patients from the TREAT Asia HIV Observational Database: analysis of risk factors and survival. *PLoS One*. 2016;11:e0150512.
61. Jia J, Zhu Q, Deng L, et al. Treatment outcomes of HIV patients with hepatitis B and C virus co-infections in Southwest China: an observational cohort study. *Infect Dis Poverty*. 2022;11:7.

62. Benhamou Y, Bochet M, Di Martino V, et al. Liver fibrosis progression in human immunodeficiency virus and hepatitis C virus coinfected patients. The Multivirc Group. *Hepatology*. 1999;30:1054-1058.
63. Mohsen AH, Easterbrook PJ, Taylor C, et al. Impact of human immunodeficiency virus (HIV) infection on the progression of liver fibrosis in hepatitis C virus infected patients. *Gut*. 2003;52:1035-1040.
64. Lo Re V III, Kallan MJ, Tate JP, et al. Hepatic decompensation in antiretroviral-treated patients co-infected with HIV and hepatitis C virus compared with hepatitis C virus-monoinfected patients: a cohort study. *Ann Intern Med*. 2014;160:369-379.
65. Konerman MA, Mehta SH, Sutcliffe CG, et al. Fibrosis progression in human immunodeficiency virus/hepatitis C virus coinfected adults: prospective analysis of 435 liver biopsy pairs. *Hepatology*. 2014;59:767-775.
66. Jia J, Zhu Q, Deng L, et al. Treatment outcomes of HIV patients with hepatitis B and C virus co-infections in Southwest China: an observational cohort study. *Infect Dis Poverty*. 2022;11:7.
67. Chen M, Wong WW, Law MG, et al. Hepatitis B and C co-infection in HIV patients from the TREAT Asia HIV observational database: analysis of risk factors and survival. *PLoS One*. 2016;11(3):e0150512.
68. Wyles DL, Ruane PJ, Sulkowski MS, et al. Daclatasvir plus sofosbuvir for HCV in patients coinfected with HIV-1. *N Engl J Med*. 2015;373:714-725.
69. Jaquet A, Wandeler G, Nouaman M, et al. Alcohol use, viral hepatitis and liver fibrosis among HIV-positive persons in West Africa: a cross-sectional study. *J Int AIDS Soc*. 2017;19:21424.
70. Lyu H, Tang H, Liang Y, et al. Alcohol consumption and risk of liver fibrosis in people living with HIV: a systematic review and meta-analysis. *Front Immunol*. 2022;13:841314.
71. Ingiliz P, Valantin MA, Duvivier C, et al. Liver damage underlying unexplained transaminase elevation in human immunodeficiency virus-1 monoinfected patients on antiretroviral therapy. *Hepatology*. 2009; 49:436-442.
72. Price JC, Seaberg EC, Latanich R, et al. Risk factors for fatty liver in the Multicenter AIDS Cohort Study. *Am J Gastroenterol*. 2014;109:695-704.
73. Morse CG, McLaughlin M, Matthews L, et al. Non-alcoholic steatohepatitis and hepatic fibrosis in HIV-1-monoinfected adults with elevated aminotransferase levels on antiretroviral therapy. *Clin Infect Dis*. 2015;60:1569-1578.
74. Lemoine M, Assoumou L, Girard PM, et al. ANRS-ECHAM group. Screening HIV patients at risk for NAFLD using MRI-PDFF and transient elastography: a European multicenter prospective study. *Clin Gastroenterol Hepatol*. 2023;21:713-722.e3.
75. Tanon A, Jaquet A, Ekouevi DK, et al. The spectrum of cancers in West Africa: associations with human immunodeficiency virus. *PLoS One*. 2012;7:e48108.
76. Maponga TG, Glashoff RH, Vermeulen H, et al. Hepatitis B virus-associated hepatocellular carcinoma in South Africa in the era of HIV. *BMC Gastroenterol*. 2020;20:226.
77. Stabinski L, Reynolds SJ, Ocama P, et al. High prevalence of liver fibrosis associated with HIV infection: a cross-sectional study in rural Rakai, Uganda. *Antivir Ther*. 2011;16:405-411.
78. Auerbach BJ, Reynolds SJ, Lamorde M, et al. Traditional herbal medicine use associated with liver fibrosis in rural Rakai, Uganda. *PLoS One*. 2012;7:e41737.
79. Luyckx VA, Steenkamp V, Rubel JR, Stewart MJ. Adverse effects associated with the use of South African traditional folk remedies. *Cent Afr J Med*. 2004;50:46-51.
80. Puius YA, Dove LM, Brust DG, et al. Three cases of autoimmune hepatitis in HIV-infected patients. *J Clin Gastroenterol*. 2008;42:425-429.
81. Murunga E, Andersson M, van Rensburg C. Autoimmune hepatitis: a manifestation of immune reconstitution inflammatory syndrome in HIV infected patients? *Scand J Gastroenterol*. 2016;51:814-818.
82. Chaiteerakij R, Sanpawat A, Avihingsanon A, Treeprasertsuk S. Autoimmune hepatitis in human immunodeficiency virus-infected patients: a case series and review of the literature. *World J Gastroenterol*. 2019;25:5388-5402.
83. Bakasis AD, Androutsakos T. Liver fibrosis during antiretroviral treatment in HIV-infected individuals: truth or tale.? *Cells*. 2021;10:1212.
84. Núñez M. Clinical syndromes and consequences of antiretroviral-related hepatotoxicity. *Hepatology*. 2010;52:1143-1155.
85. Jones M, Núñez M. Liver toxicity of antiretroviral drugs. *Semin Liver Dis*. 2012;32:167-176.
86. Yimer G, Gry M, Amogne W, et al. Evaluation of patterns of liver toxicity in patients on antiretroviral and anti-tuberculosis drugs: a prospective four arm observational study in Ethiopian patients. *PLoS One*. 2014;9:e94271.

87. Sanne I, Mommeja-Marin H, Hinkle J, et al. Severe hepatotoxicity associated with nevirapine use in HIV-infected subjects. *J Infect Dis.* 2005;191:825-829.
88. Martín-Carbonero L, Núñez M, González-Lahoz J, Soriano V. Incidence of liver injury after beginning antiretroviral therapy with efavirenz or nevirapine. *HIV Clin Trials.* 2003;4:115-120.
89. Shubber Z, Calmy A, Andrieux-Meyer I, et al. Adverse events associated with nevirapine and efavirenz-based first-line antiretroviral therapy: a systematic review and meta-analysis. *AIDS.* 2013;27:1403-1412.
90. Giacomelli A, Riva A, Falvella FS, et al. Clinical and genetic factors associated with increased risk of severe liver toxicity in a monocentric cohort of HIV positive patients receiving nevirapine-based antiretroviral therapy. *BMC Infect Dis.* 2018;18:556.
91. Sonderup MW, Wainwright H, Maughan D, Setshedi M, Spearman CWN. Characteristics of efavirenz drug induced liver injury: a cohort analysis. 65th Annual Meeting of the American Association for the Study of Liver Diseases; Boston, MA, USA; Nov 7–11, 2014. Abstract 1056.
92. Sonderup MW, Wainwright H, Hall P, Hairwadzi H, Spearman CWN. A clinicopathological cohort study of liver pathology in 301 patients with human immunodeficiency virus/acquired immune deficiency syndrome. *Hepatology.* 2015;61:1721-1729.
93. Segamwenge IL, Bernard MK. Acute liver failure among patients on efavirenz-based antiretroviral therapy. *Case Reports Hepatol.* 2018;2018:1270716.
94. Maughan D, Sonderup M, Gogela N, et al. A natural history of efavirenz drug-induced liver injury. *S Afr Med J.* 2021;111:1190-1196.
95. Naseer M, Dailey FE, Juboori AA, Samiullah S, Tahan V. Epidemiology, determinants, and management of AIDS cholangiopathy: a review. *World J Gastroenterol.* 2018;24:767-774.
96. Lizardi-Cervera J, Soto Ramírez LE, Poo JL, Uribe M. Hepatobiliary diseases in patients with human immunodeficiency virus (HIV) treated with non highly active anti-retroviral therapy: frequency and clinical manifestations. *Ann Hepatol.* 2005;4:188-191.
97. Tappero JW, Conant MA, Wolfe SF, Berger TG. Kaposi's sarcoma. Epidemiology, pathogenesis, histology, clinical spectrum, staging criteria and therapy. *J Am Acad Dermatol.* 1993;28:371-395.
98. Restrepo CS, Martinez S, Lemos JA, et al. Imaging manifestations of Kaposi sarcoma. *Radiographics.* 2006;26:1169-1185.
99. Grogg KL, Miller RF, Dogan A. HIV infection and lymphoma. *J Clin Pathol.* 2007;60:1365-1372.
100. El-Fattah MA. Non-Hodgkin lymphoma of the liver: a US population-based analysis. *J Clin Transl Hepatol.* 2017;5:83-91.
101. Scerpella EG, Villareal AA, Casanova PF, Moreno J. Primary lymphoma of the liver in AIDS: report of one new case and review of the literature. *J Clin Gastroenterol.* 1996;22:51-53.
102. Muthukrishnan S, Amudhan A, Rajendran S. Primary Hodgkin's lymphoma of liver in HIV—A case report and review of literature. *AME Case Rep.* 2018;2:21.
103. Lodenyo H, Schoub B, Ally R, Kairu S, Segal I. Hepatitis B and C virus infections and liver function in AIDS patients at Chris Hani Baragwanath Hospital, Johannesburg. *East Afr Med J.* 2000;77:13-15.
104. Nakwagala FN, Kagimu MM. Hepatitis B virus and HIV infections among patients in Mulago hospital. *East Afr Med J.* 2002;79:68-72.

CHAPTER 16

Amebic Liver Abscess

Amir S. Seid

KEY POINTS

- Amebic liver abscess is a common extraintestinal manifestation of *Entamoeba histolytica*.
- In nonendemic areas it is commonly seen in travelers where clinical manifestations might occur a few weeks after return.
- Imaging modalities are the most common modes of diagnosis, with the (single) abscess typically having a distinct appearance.
- Treatment typically is with metronidazole followed by a luminal agent; a high success rate can be achieved with oral therapy.
- Complications like rupture into adjacent structures can happen, in which the mortality rate significantly increases.

Introduction

Amebiasis is caused by a protozoan infection, typically *Entamoeba histolytica*.[1] Infections with *Entamoeba* are rampant in the tropics; however, the main clinical manifestations are intestinal. The organism is usually transmitted feco-orally and is commonly seen in communities with low socioeconomic conditions.[2] After gaining entry into the body, the infective cyst forms of the protozoa develop in the colon to become mature trophozoites. The trophozoites are the invasive forms of the parasite and are responsible for the colonic symptoms of the infection as well as extraintestinal disease.[3] Specifically, invasion into the portal vein is considered to be the pathogenesis of the development of an amebic liver abscess. The process is thought to involve invasion of the intestinal mucosa and transportation of the ameba to the liver, where small hepatic vessel thrombosis occurs. Subsequently, amebae proliferate in the liver in a small foci fashion and later coalesce to form a larger abscess.[4]

EPIDEMIOLOGY

Amebiasis is characteristically endemic in the tropics and subtropics, particularly in areas of low socioeconomic status and suboptimal sanitary practices. High rates of infection are reported in Mexico, Bangladesh, parts of India, and sub-Saharan Africa.[5] In contrast, in more resource-rich parts of the world the condition is rare and usually reported in travelers only.[6,7] In endemic parts of the world amebic liver abscess is usually seen among adults, typically male patients. The factors that predispose to abscess development are not well elucidated, although impairment of cell-mediated immunity might play a role.[8] Of all patients with intestinal amebiasis, the risk of developing a liver abscess is estimated to be 2% to 5%.

Clinical Presentation

In endemic environments the typical clinical presentation usually occurs approximately 2 weeks after the acquisition of infection. Around 50% of patients might have concomitant bowel symptoms with the onset of the liver symptoms. Common symptoms include right upper quadrant pain, fever, loss of appetite, and nausea.[9] In some patients the pain might localized to the right shoulder due to diaphragmatic irritation. Pleuritic as well as epigastric pain might also be present. Fever is very common in amebic liver abscess, occurring in most patients. However, due to the occasional intermittent nature of the fever in some patients, serial monitoring of temperature is warranted. Jaundice, albeit rare, can also be present. On physical examination, findings include hepatomegaly and tenderness in the right upper quadrant which occurs in 50% of patients.

If there is an extension into adjoining structures or rupture of the abscess into the peritoneal or pericardial cavities, clinical manifestations could be significantly different.[10] With rupture, patients could present with rapidly progressing symptoms depending on the location of the site. There might be leukocytosis on a complete blood count; however, it should be noted that usually significant eosinophilia is not typical of amebic liver abscess, unlike other parasitic infections. Transaminases and alkaline phosphatase could be elevated, ranging from 5 to 10 times from baseline. Significant hyperbilirubinemia is uncommon, occurring in less than 10% of patients.[11]

Diagnosis

Typically, an amebic liver abscess in the tropics is diagnosed using ultrasound. Ultrasound is commonly available in many parts of the world and can make an accurate diagnosis in a significant proportion of patients. Characteristic findings include a single hypoechoic, well-defined, round lesion, usually located in the periphery of the right hepatic lobe.[12] A highly suggestive finding is a focal liver lesion with a disruption of the diaphragmatic edge (Figure 16.1).

CT is also used to diagnose the condition; however, the availability of a CT scan machines might be limited in many resource-limited settings. On CT, the abscess appears as a hypodense lesion with peripheral contrast enhancement, typically in the right lobe. Unusually, a target pattern might be seen with a dense echogenic center and a peripheral hypoechoic rim. Lesions located in the left lobe are prone to extension into the pericardium and adjacent structures.[13]

In nonendemic areas 92% to 97% of patients develop detectable levels of antibody with the onset of symptoms. However, in most places in the tropics up to one-third of patients with no

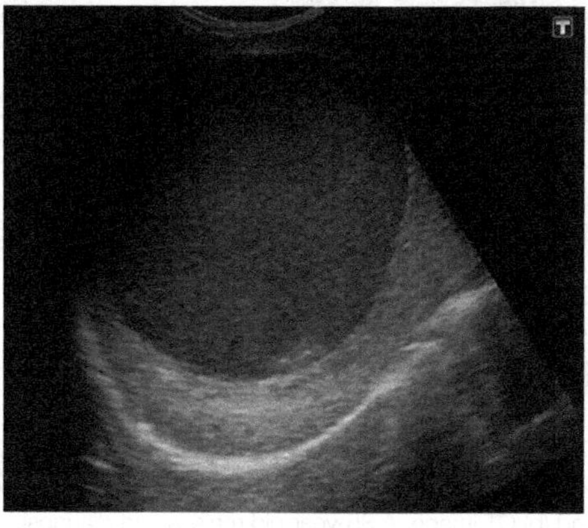

Figure 16.1 Ultrasound image of amebic liver abscess in a 28-year-old female patient from Addis Ababa. A distinct, well-rounded hypoechoic lesion is seen. (Image courtesy of Dr Tesfaye Kebede, Addis Ababa University.)

active infection could have a positive test, making the utility of the tests less helpful. Regardless, a negative test could be used in ruling out the condition if it is available.[14]

In the past, aspiration was used as a diagnostic tool, with the characteristic chocolate-colored "anchovy paste" appearance of the abscess content. This has been supplanted by the currently available imaging modalities, even though it is sometimes used in indeterminate situations.

Potential differential diagnoses for the condition include pyogenic liver abscess, echinococcal infection, and malignancy. Particularly, a pyogenic liver abscess is often confused with amebic liver abscess, and the difference between the two conditions is described in Table 16.1. Imaging findings of the two conditions might appear similar occasionally, but pyogenic liver abscesses typically present with multiple lesions (Figure 16.2a and b). In endemic settings an echinococcal infection could present with an imaging finding similar to an abscess, but the lack of clinical features of infection could be used to differentiate the two conditions. In addition, an echinococcal infection usually causes multiloculated cyst, with visible daughter cysts and sandy appearance. These features can help differentiate the two conditions.

TABLE 16.1 ■ **Comparison of Amebic Liver Abscess and Pyogenic Liver Abscess**

	Amebic Liver Abscess	Pyogenic Liver abscess
Etiology	*Entamoeba histolytica*	Gram-negatives, usually *Escherichia coli*
Risk factors	Endemic area residence, recent travel	Diabetes, stone disease
Location	Typically right lobe, subcapsular	Could be on both lobes of the liver
Number	Single	Usually multiple
Clinical course	Acute	Subacute
Liver enzymes	Could be normal	Usually elevated
Diagnosis	Ultrasound or CT; serology in non-endemic settings	Ultrasound or CT
Treatment	Metronidazole/tinidazole	Antibiotics with drainage in most cases

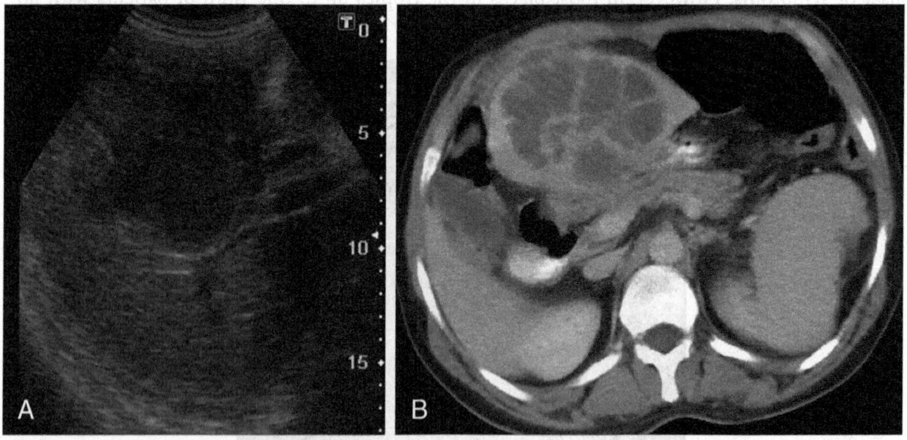

Figure 16.2 (a) Ultrasound and (b) CT image. A 35-year-old male with a diagnosis of pyogenic liver abscess. Note the non-distinct appearing borders of the mass with multiloculated appearance. (Images courtesy of Dr Tesfaye Kebede, Addis Ababa University.)

Treatment

The standard treatment of an amebic liver abscess is metronidazole, usually given 500 to 750 mg three times a day for a total of 7 to 10 days. Oral treatment is preferred, as there is adequate absorption with excellent bioavailability. Patients should be advised about potential side effects of metallic taste and disulfiram-like effect when taken concomitantly with alcohol. An alternative drug used is tinidazole, given 2 g once daily for 5 days. With these tissue agents, cure rates approach 90%.[1] Typically, patients show a marked clinical improvement with the decrement of pain and fever. In the first 2 weeks of therapy worsening of ultrasound features could occur despite a very good clinical response. Hence usage of ultrasound and other imaging findings as surrogates of improvement is limited. Median time for a radiologic resolution is around 7 months according to one study, and some patients might have persistent cystic or calcified lesions as residual findings.[15]

After completion of therapy with tissue agents, patients should be given luminal agents, as there is a need to eradicate the protozoa from the body. Agents used for this purpose include paromomycin, diloxanide furoate, and iodoquinol. Sometimes these drugs might not be available in the tropics, and consideration of recurrence risk should be well understood with the absence of luminal agents.[1]

Therapeutic drainage of the abscess is not warranted in most patients, as medical therapy is usually adequate. However, there is a role for drainage in patients with an abscess size of more than 10 cm or in the case of an imminent rupture and lack of response despite medical therapy.[16] With the effective institution of therapy, the mortality rate is 1% in uncomplicated cases. However, a mortality rate of up to 17% has been reported in those with complications and rupture.[17]

References

1. Haque R, Huston CD, Hughes M, Houpt E, Petri WAJ. Amebiasis. *N Engl J Med.* 2009;348(16): 1565-1573. doi:10.1056/NEJMRA022710.
2. Stanley SL. Amoebiasis. *Lancet.* 2003;361(9362):1025-1034. doi:10.1016/S0140-6736(03)12830-9.
3. Salles JM, Salles MJ, Moraes LA, Silva MC. Invasive amebiasis: an update on diagnosis and management. *Expert Rev Anti Infect Ther.* 2007;5(5):893-901. doi:10.1586/14787210.5.5.893.
4. Aikat BK, Bhusnurmath SR, Pal AK, Chhuttani PN, Datta DV. The pathology and pathogenesis of fatal hepatic amoebiasis: a study based on 79 autopsy cases. *Trans R Soc Trop Med Hyg.* 1979;73(2): 188-192. doi:10.1016/0035-9203(79)90209-8.
5. Shirley DAT, Farr L, Watanabe K, Moonah S. A review of the global burden, new diagnostics, and current therapeutics for amebiasis. *Open Forum Infect Dis.* 2018;5(7):ofy161. doi:10.1093/OFID/OFY161.
6. Cordel H, Prendki V, Madec Y, et al. Imported amoebic liver abscess in France. *PLoS Negl Trop Dis.* 2013;7(8):e2333. doi:10.1371/JOURNAL.PNTD.0002333.
7. Lachish T, Wieder-Finesod A, Schwartz E. Amebic liver abscess in Israeli travelers: a retrospective study. *Am J Trop Med Hyg.* 2016;94(5):1015-1019. doi:10.4269/AJTMH.15-0576.
8. Hung CC, Ji D Der, Sun HY, et al. Increased risk for *Entamoeba histolytica* infection and invasive amebiasis in HIV seropositive men who have sex with men in Taiwan. *PLoS Negl Trop Dis.* 2008;2(2):e175. doi:10.1371/JOURNAL.PNTD.0000175.
9. Anesi JA, Gluckman S. Amebic liver abscess. *Clin Liver Dis.* 2015;6(2):41-43. doi:10.1002/CLD.488.
10. Adams EB, MacLeod IN. Invasive amebiasis. I. Amebic dysentery and its complications. *Medicine (Baltimore).* 1977;56(4):315-323. doi:10.1097/00005792-197707000-00003.
11. Maltz G, Knauer CM. Amebic liver abscess: a 15-year experience. *Am J Gastroenterol.* 1991;86(6): 704-710.
12. Park MS, Kim KW, Ha HK, Lee DH. Intestinal parasitic infection. *Abdom Imaging.* 2008;33(2): 166-171. doi:10.1007/S00261-007-9324-Z.
13. Benedetti NJ, Desser TS, Brooke Jeffrey R. Imaging of hepatic infections. *Ultrasound Q.* 2008;24(4): 267-278. doi:10.1097/RUQ.0B013E31818E5981.

14. Stanley SL, Jackson TFHG, Foster L, Singh S. Longitudinal study of the antibody response to recombinant *Entamoeba histolytica* antigens in patients with amebic liver abscess. *Am J Trop Med Hyg*. 1998; 58(4):414-416. doi:10.4269/AJTMH.1998.58.414.
15. Ralls PW, Quinn MF, Boswell WD, Colletti PM, Radin DR, Halls J. Patterns of resolution in successfully treated hepatic amebic abscess: sonographic evaluation. *Radiology*. 1983;149(2):541-543. doi:10.1148/RADIOLOGY.149.2.6622702.
16. Ghosh JK, Goyal SK, Behera MK, et al. Efficacy of aspiration in amebic liver abscess. *Trop Gastroenterol.* 2015;36(4):251-255. doi:10.7869/TG.299.
17. Sharma MP, Dasarathy S, Verma N, Saksena S, Shukla DK. Prognostic markers in amebic liver abscess: a prospective study. *Am J Gastroenterol.* 1996;91(12):2584-2588.

CHAPTER 17

Cystic Echinococcosis—Hydatid Liver Disease

Tommaso Manciulli ■ Enrico Brunetti

KEY POINTS

- Cystic echinococcosis (CE) is a zoonotic infection caused by the cestode *Echinococcus granulosus*. Dogs and other canids are definitive hosts, while sheep and other ungulates are intermediate hosts. Man is an accidental intermediate host. CE is most prevalent in sheep-raising areas around the world and affects mainly poor communities.
- The larval form is responsible for the formation of cysts in the body of the intermediate host, mostly in the liver and lungs, but any organ can be affected.
- Ultrasound allows the diagnosis and staging of CE.
- Serology has an ancillary role in the diagnosis and follow-up.
- Choice of treatment should be made based on the location, size, and stage of the cyst.
- CE patients should be managed with a multidisciplinary approach.

Introduction

The genus *Echinococcus* comprises four species known to be pathogenic to man: *Echinococcus granulosus, Echinococcus multilocularis, Echinococcus vogeli,* and *Echinococcus shiquicus. E. granulosus* is the causal agent of cystic echinococcosis (CE). This disease has a cosmopolitan distribution and it is present in all continents except Antarctica.[1] *E. multilocularis* is the causal agent of alveolar echinococcosis (AE). AE is found mainly in the northern hemisphere and in the northern part of China.[1] *E. vogeli* is the causal agent of polycystic echinococcosis (PC). This very rare form of echinococcosis is present in South America, with currently less than 150 cases described in humans.[1] *E. shiquicus* is the latest discovered species in the genus and the causal agent of a disease similar to AE, currently confined to the Tibetan plateaus of China and Mongolia.[2,3] *E. granulosus* is the most widespread species in the genus, and although its pathogenicity is lower than that of *E. multilocularis*, the diffusion of the parasite makes it a notable public health problem.[1,4-6] Echinococcoses are zoonoses and affect predominantly poor communities in resource-limited settings.[1,7,8]

From a phylogenetic standpoint, 10 genotypes are distinguished. Genotypes G1 to G3 constitute the *E. ganulosus sensu strictu* complex and genotypes G3 to G10 constitute the *E. granulosus sensu latu* complex.[2,9,10] Genotype G9 has recently been eliminated and considered to be part of the G8 genotype.[2,11,12,13] While these genotypes have shown a preference for different intermediate hosts, there are no differences in clinical presentation in patients infected with different genotypes.[2,9]

E. granulosus can infect several organs but liver is the one most frequently affected.[9] The loss of disability-adjusted life years (DALYs) in humans is estimated at 1,000,000 each year.[5] Animal losses and human expenses account for damages up to USD 356,000,000 each year.[5]

Life Cycle and Natural History

In *E. granulosus* life cycle, dogs and other canids act as definitive hosts.[14] The adult worm living in the intestine of the dog releases eggs in the environment: an adult worm can shed eggs for around 2 weeks and eggs dispersed in the environment can resist for months in appropriate conditions. Eggs are better preserved in humid environments, suffer from contact with direct sunlight, and can resist temperatures between −10°C and 40°C.[15] When an intermediate host ingests food or water contaminated by eggs, these hatch into the intestine, forming an exacant larva, which subsequently hatches and penetrates the intestinal wall.[15] Here, the exacant larvae enter the portal circulation and are carried to organs. Liver and lungs are reached first. Then, larvae can develop into the echinococcal cyst.[14] After encystment, the metacestode develops over a period of years.[14,16] Once formed, the cyst develops brood capsules containing protoscoleces. These can be ingested by suitable definitive hosts when they eat offals or carcasses of parasitized intermediate hosts (Figure 17.1). The protoscoleces reach the intestine and the cycle starts over. Given this life cycle, humans are often "dead-end" hosts and there is no risk of interhuman transmission. A number of ungulates can act as hosts for *E. granulosus*: sheep

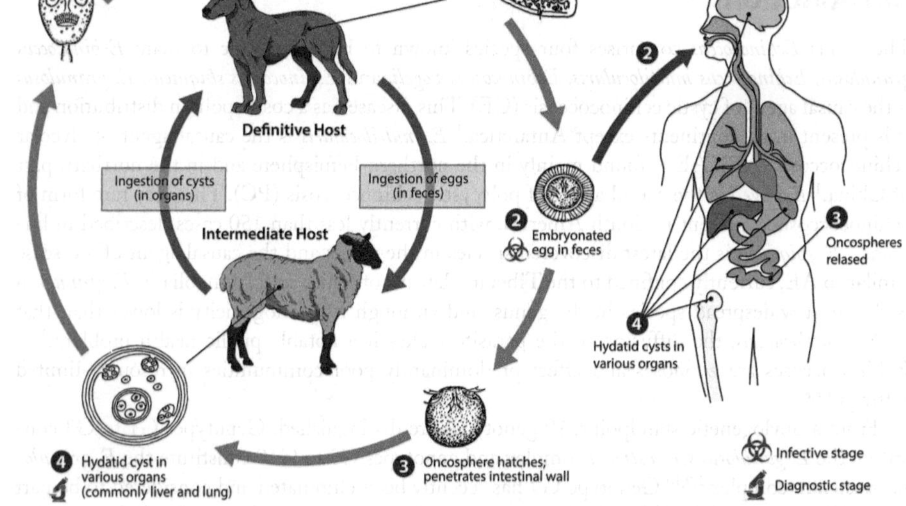

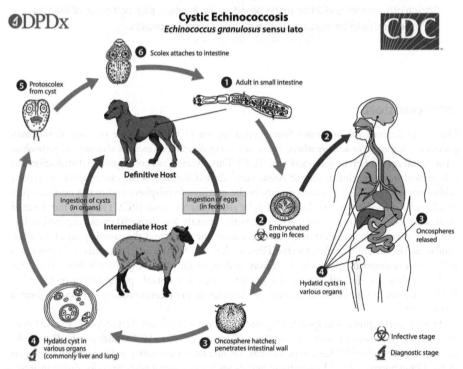

Figure 17.1 *E. granulosus s.l.* life cycle. (From CDC - Centers for Disease Control and Prevention. Echinococcosis - Biology n.d. https://www.cdc.gov/parasites/echinococcosis/biology.html (accessed September 9, 2019)).

are the most competent host with cysts showing fertility rates of up to 80%, while cows, donkeys, horses, and goats show a reduced fertility rate and carry a lower transmission risk to canids.[1,9,14]

The cyst is composed of the endocyst (the larval component) and the pericyst (the host tissue surrounding the endocyst), and it contains a clear fluid (hydatid fluid, HF). The endocyst has an inner germinal layer (GL), from which brood capsules arise, and an outer layer, called laminated layer (LL), mainly composed of glycoproteins.[10] The latter shields the parasite from the host's immune response and has immunomodulatory properties. The external pericyst is host derived.[17,18] Figure 17.2 is a schematic representation of an echinococcal cyst. Over time, the endocyst can detach from the pericyst,[16,18-20] and the cyst fluid becomes increasingly dense, conferring a "solid" appearance to the cyst on ultrasound at the final stages of the process.[20] However, in some instances protoscoleces can produce daughter cysts within the main cyst.[9,16,19]

Most primary CE cysts (60%–70%) are in the liver, the first organ encountered by oncospheres as they are carried by the portal flow.[10,18] The second most frequent location (10%–20%) is the lung, followed by the spleen (5%–15%) and other organs (1%–5%), such as bones and muscles (0.5%–2%) as well as brain (around 1% of cases).[21] Multiple organ involvement is also possible, with the liver and lungs being affected at the same time most frequently. Cysts located outside the abdomen tend to be more symptomatic due to their development in an enclosed space.[21,22] In the lung, cysts tend to grow more rapidly thanks to the reduced resistance by pulmonary parenchyma.[23] Around 70% of the cysts spontaneously inactivate and remain asymptomatic throughout the patient's life.[24]

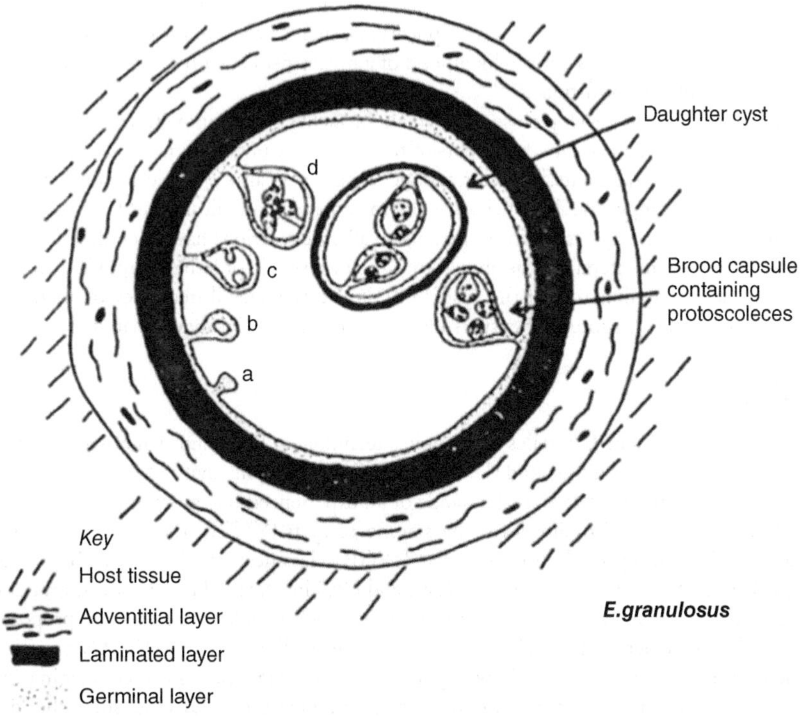

Figure 17.2 Diagrammatic representation of structure of the echinococcal cyst.

Epidemiology

CE has a global distribution, with cases reported from all continents except Antarctica. A specific area is considered endemic if the incidence rate is above 5 out of 100,000.[1] Despite estimates by the World Health Organization (WHO) considering several parts of the world to be hyperendemic, the distribution of CE is patchy, with data missing from most geographic areas.[14,25,26] The disease is underreported due to a lack of knowledge and poor disease surveillance.[26-29] Traditionally, China and most of Central Asia are considered hyperendemic regions, as well as large parts of the Middle East and the Mediterranean basin.[9,30-33] In Europe the disease is a notifiable condition, but cases reported by the European Centre for Disease Prevention and Control (ECDC) are outnumbered by the patients currently enrolled in the European Register of Cystic Echinococcosis (ERCE).[25] In the United States the disease is sporadically diagnosed and most cases are imported by migrants from endemic regions, while *E. granulosus* is endemic in Canada. South America is hyperendemic as well, although many countries in the region are likely to underreport the disease.[1,29,11,33,34] CE is a serious public health problem for poor, pastoral communities in resource-limited settings where scarce access to clean water and practices related to the management of dogs and offal disposal enhance the probability of transmission, but CE is also present in resource-rich countries where it is often an orphan disease, scarcely known by the medical community.[1,35-38]

Clinical Manifestations

CE clinical manifestations depend on cyst number, location, and stage. Around 70% of patients are asymptomatic at diagnosis, and the detection of cysts is accidental.[7,16,18,39] The most frequent symptom is abdominal discomfort or right upper quadrant pain (in around 70% of symptomatic patients),[19,40] due to the cyst mass or to complications, such as rupture into the biliary tree.[19] In fact, the larger the cyst, the higher the likelihood of a biliary fistula, with cysts larger than 7.5 cm carrying a >70% chance of fistulae.[19,41]

In the lungs cysts that develop close to the main bronchi can present with cough.[23,40] If a cyst ruptures into the bronchial system, fragments of the endocyst can be coughed out, usually round-shaped, pearl-colored fragments.[42] Bacterial superinfection is also possible in lung cysts, with ensuing abscesses or empyema. Anaphylaxis is the most feared complication of CE cysts, as cases of spontaneous or traumatic cyst ruptures leading to allergic reactions have been described.[43,44] A systematic review of the literature has shown that the occurrence of lethal anaphylaxis following accidental or deliberate puncture of the cyst is 0.03% and the overall frequency of allergic reactions due to spontaneous rupture of cysts is likely lower than previously estimated.[43]

CE Diagnosis

Imaging. The diagnosis of CE relies on imaging techniques. The main diagnostic tool for the liver and upper abdomen is ultrasound (US),[18] which has a high sensitivity (>90% for cysts larger than 2 cm) and specificity (>95% in the hands of an experienced operator) in the diagnosis and staging of CE.[39,45,46] US also allows for the staging of cysts.[18,47,48] In the standardized WHO Informal Working Group on Echinococcosis (IWGE) classification, CE1 and CE2 cysts are active, CE3a transitional, CE3b active, and CE4 and CE5 inactive.[18] This classification is a rearrangement of a previous one proposed by Gharbi, is much simpler than the one proposed by Caremani,[49,50] and is increasingly being used in the scientific literature on CE.[51] Cysts with fluid components are generally active, as shown by a study using magnetic resonance imaging (MRI) spectroscopy.[52] Some of the cyst stages have pathognomonic signs: CE1 cysts show the "double wall" sign (endocyst and pericyst). CE2 cysts have multiple daughter vesicles with a honeycomb pattern, which needs to be distinguished from that seen in benign lesions and liver tumors.[21] Daughter cysts are round and well defined and, when in contact with each other, they have a double wall appearance.[20] CE3a cyst present with the water lily sign, as the endocyst floats in the HF,[20] after detachment from the endocysts[18,52]: 50% are biologically active. CE3b cysts feature daughter cysts in a solid matrix. However, mimics of daughter vesicles can be seen in both benign and malignant lesions, and the ultrasound appearance of CE3b cyst is not pathognomonic.[18] CE4 and CE5 cysts may present with a "ball of wool" pattern due to the folded endocyst on ultrasound.[20] CE5 cysts have a more marked cyst wall calcification. These (calcifications), however, can be present in any stage.[53,54] In extra-hepatic localizations or in the case of abdominal cysts not seen on US because of anatomical reasons (i.e., gas in the bowel), MRI is the method of choice.[54] Computed tomography (CT) has low specificity but high sensitivity. It is still widely used for pre-surgical examinations but should not be used for diagnosing or staging CE.[54]

Serology. Serological tests have been used in the diagnosis of CE since the late seventies.[45] The first antigens in use came from purified hydatid fluid (HF),[55] a substrate still used in some commercial kits and in-house assays.[55] HF has the highest sensitivity for CE, while specificity has been increased using purified native and recombinant antigens.[55-58] However, the diagnostic yield is hindered by false negative results in early CE1[59-61] and in CE4 and CE5 cysts. The sequestration of antigens due to the adherence of endocyst to the pericyst (early CE1) prevents the immune system from producing antibodies against the antigen itself.[17] In the case of CE4 and CE5 cysts, the lack of immune response can be due to parasite inactivity.[59-61] The results of serology are influenced by several other variables, including cyst size and previous treatment.[62] Also, given the lack of standardization, intra- and inter-laboratory variability make uniform interpretation of results difficult.[55,59,63] Cross-reactions, mostly with *E. multilocularis* but also with other cestodes, have been reported.[55,59,63,64] For all these reasons, the best approach would be to: (1) never employ a serological test in the absence of a suggestive lesion on imaging; (2) avoid serology as a screening tool; (3) use a specific test (e.g., western blot) as a single test. If this is not feasible, two paired first-line tests should be used, and the result should be considered reliable if they are concordant. If this is not the case, a third confirmatory test with good specificity (>90%) would be needed. A recent systematic review and meta-analysis on serological assays has been published, to which readers are referred.[55,59,63,64]

Serological assays are not indicated in the follow-up of patients, as no clear-cut correlation between seroconversion and inactivation has been established, and tests can remain positive for years.[65] Moreover, previously seronegative patients who undergo surgical treatment can become positive after the immunological exposure caused by cyst opening or handling during surgery.[65]

Other diagnostic techniques. Molecular biology plays a minor role, if any, in the diagnosis of CE, as circulating DNA has been detected in patients after cyst rupture but is normally absent otherwise.[66,67] The detection of micro-RNAs (miRNAs) has been proposed by some authors, but it is used only for research purposes.[68,69] Assays based on the detection of cytokine profile induced by the presence of active CE cysts have also been developed, but their use is confined to research studies at the moment.[70-72] In the case of lesions of undetermined nature located in explorable organs, the diagnosis can be made by verifying treatment response with US or MRI. This can be achieved by administering albendazole for 1 to 3 months and monitoring changes in the cyst structure. This approach works best with liquid cysts (CL in the WHO-IWGE classification) that, when treated with albendazole, respond with a detachment in the endocyst, as discussed above.[18] In such cases, if the patient was seronegative, detachment of the endocyst is also followed by seroconversion, best detected with western blot.[59] CE2 or CE3b should respond with a reduction in the number and size of daughter cysts.

Microscopical examination of the fluid aspirated during Puncture, Aspiration, Injection, Re-aspiration (PAIR) technique allows to check for viable protoscolices before proceeding to the intracystic injection of a scolicidal agent. Biopsy is rarely, if ever, performed on CE cysts in the abdomen. Biopsy is not indicated in lung cysts, but it is sometimes used in extra-hepatic abdominal localizations, such as bone CE.[73-75]

Clinical Management

Uncomplicated cysts. Clinical management for liver cysts should be based on a stage-specific approach and each case should be managed with a multidisciplinary team. Figure 17.3 summarizes therapeutic options by stage. Other indications are discussed in the following paragraphs.

Management includes medical treatment with albendazole at a dose of 400 mg BID: albendazole is a benzimidazole, it is absorbed orally without food, and it is administered continuously for 3 to 6 months.[76,77] This is indicated in CE1 or CE3a cysts smaller than 5 cm located in abdominal organs and lungs.[18] Longer treatment courses are used for bone and muscle CE, with low response rates and frequent reactivations.[73] Shortages of the drug have been reported.[78]

Several countries still recommend 15-day breaks every 28 days of drug administration, based on a presumed hepatotoxicity of the drug.[76] Per expert advice, however, elevation of liver transaminases, while not infrequent, is often the expression of parenchymal inflammation due to the cyst degeneration and immune activation.[76,79] Monitoring of liver function tests is indicated, with treatment suspension warranted if transaminases rise above five times the upper limit of normality. Albendazole can sometimes be myelotoxic, although this side effect is idiopathic and rarely seen.[18] Complete blood count is warranted during treatment. Alopecia is a reversible side effect. The use of albendazole is contraindicated in pregnant patients, although data from the mass deworming campaigns where albendazole is used in a single administration have not shown fetal toxicity.[80] Should albendazole be unavailable, mebendazole can be used as a substitute, 50 mg/kg daily, in three takes. Given its lower oral bioavailability linked to poor fasting absorption, it should be taken with a fatty meal. Mebendazole requires the same patient monitoring as albendazole.[76]

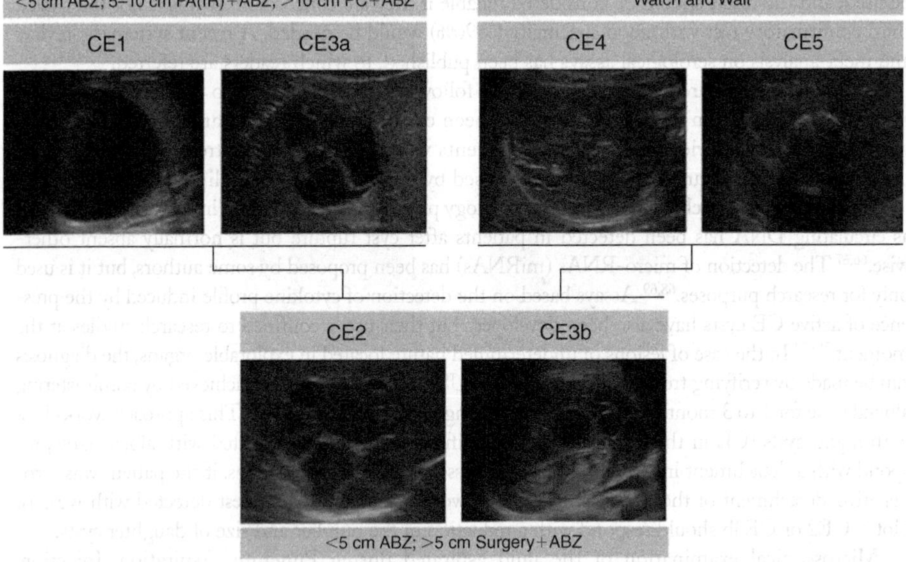

Figure 17.3 Management algorithm for uncomplicated liver cysts in the abdomen. ABZ, albendazole; PA(IR), Puncture, Aspiration (Injection, Re-aspiration); PC, Percutaneous Catheterization. (From Firpo G, Vola A, Lissandrin R, Tamarozzi F, Brunetti E. Preliminary Evaluation of Percutaneous Treatment of Echinococcal Cysts without Injection of Scolicidal Agent. Am J Trop Med Hyg 2017;97:1818–26. https://doi.org/10.4269/ajtmh.17-0468).

Percutaneous procedures include the classical PAIR approach and its several variations.[81-83] This needle-based approach consists of cyst puncture, aspiration of around half the cyst content, and injection of a scolicidal agent (20% hypertonic saline or 90% alcohol have been used with good response rates in CE1 and CE3a stages). The WHO-IWGE considers the technique safe and effective for hepatic CE1 and CE3a cysts 5 to 10 cm in diameter. The procedure is performed in an inpatient setting in the presence of a resuscitation team. The injection of a scolicidal agent should be preceded by the exclusion of biliary communications to avoid chemical cholangitis.[81-83] To avoid this step, a simplified procedure using just the puncture and aspiration steps followed by an extended 3-month cycle of albendazole has been proposed but has not been tested in clinical trials.[84]

Percutaneous procedures using catheters left *in situ* until the daily drainage is less than 50 mL have been used for cysts larger than 10 cm.[18,85]

A modified catheterization approach performed under fluoroscopic guidance has been tried at a single center on CE1, CE3a, CE2, and CE3b cysts, with satisfactory results in a retrospective cases series. However, much like in the case of PAIR, its applicability is limited by local expertise.[86] Although a study from a single center has questioned the use of albendazole as adjuvant treatment after percutaneous procedures on CE cysts, expert recommendations maintain that the drug should be administered at the usual dose of 400 mg BID for 1 month following the procedure. The drug can be started a few days before the procedure or even on the same morning.[18,87]

Surgery is the approach of choice in the treatment of abdominal CE2 and CE3b cysts.[9,18] Removal of all biologically active portions of the cyst (endocyst, daughter vesicles) is the critical step to avoid relapse. A standardized nomenclature for surgical procedures has recently been introduced by the World Association of Hydatidology, to which the readers are referred for further details.[88] Various approaches have been proposed for the surgical treatment of CE cysts. The pericyst can be used as a surgical reference plane, and the cyst can be cautiously separated from the surrounding tissues, without the need to open the cyst itself. This should be avoided unless proper precautions are taken, given the risk of spillage of cyst content, and peritoneal seeding leading to dissemination.[18,89,90] Another approach relies on cyst opening and irrigation with hypertonic saline, allowing endocyst sterilization.[18,89,90] Surgeries for CE in the liver have been carried out with open, laparoscopic and robotic techniques. Conservative approaches versus more invasive ones are associated with decreased morbidity.[18,89,90] While it was previously believed that more invasive surgeries (e.g., hepatectomies) were associated with a decreased rate of relapses due to the avoidance of contact with the cyst, a recent systematic review has disputed this claim.[18,89,90] The level of available local expertise plays a major role in the choice of surgical approach.

Complicated Cysts in the Abdomen

Complications of CE cysts include cyst rupture, including into the biliary tree, superinfection, and anaphylaxis. As per WHO-IWGE, complicated cysts in the abdomen should be evaluated for surgery,[18] with the possible exception of cysts that become superinfected in the liver. These can essentially be treated as abscesses and can be drained percutaneously, if technically feasible.[18]

References

1. Deplazes P, Rinaldi L, Alvarez Rojas CA, et al. Global distribution of alveolar and cystic echinococcosis. *Adv Parasitol.* 2017;95:315-493. Available at: https://doi.org/10.1016/bs.apar.2016.11.001.
2. Romig T, Deplazes P, Jenkins D, et al. Ecology and life cycle patterns of Echinococcus species. *Adv Parasitol.* 2017;95. Available at: https://doi.org/10.1016/bs.apar.2016.11.002.
3. Jenkins DJ, Romig T, Thompson RCA. Emergence/re-emergence of *Echinococcus* spp.—A global update. *Int J Parasitol.* 2005;35:1205-1219. Available at: https://doi.org/10.1016/j.ijpara.2005.07.014.

4. Craig PS, Budke CM, Schantz PM, et al. Human echinococcosis: a neglected disease. *Trop Med Health.* 2007;35:283-292.
5. Budke CM, Deplazes P, Torgerson PR. Global socioeconomic impact of cystic echinococcosis. *Emerg Infect Dis.* 2006;12:296-303. Available at: https://doi.org/10.3201/eid1202.050499.
6. Torgerson PR, Devleesschauwer B, Praet N, et al. World Health Organization Estimates of the Global and Regional Disease Burden of 11 Foodborne Parasitic Diseases, 2010: a data synthesis. *PLoS Med.* 2015;12:e1001920. Available at: https://doi.org/10.1371/journal.pmed.1001920.
7. Brunetti E, Garcia HH, Junghanss T. Cystic echinococcosis: chronic, complex, and still neglected. *PLoS Negl Trop Dis.* 2011;5:3-7. Available at: https://doi.org/10.1371/journal.pntd.0001146.
8. Junghanss T, da Silva AM, Horton J, Chiodini PL, Brunetti E. Clinical management of cystic echinococcosis: state of the art, problems, and perspectives. *Am J Trop Med Hyg.* 2008;79:301-311.
9. Wen H, Vuitton L, Tuxun T, et al. Echinococcosis: advances in the 21st century. *Clin Microbiol Rev.* 2019;32:1-39. Available at: https://doi.org/10.1128/CMR.00075-18.
10. Thompson RCA. Biology and systematics of Echinococcus. *Adv Parasitol.* 2017;95. Available at: https://doi.org/10.1016/bs.apar.2016.07.001.
11. Cucher MA, Macchiaroli N, Baldi G, et al. Cystic echinococcosis in South America: systematic review of species and genotypes of *Echinococcus* granulosus sensu lato in humans and natural domestic hosts. *Trop Med Int Heal.* 2016;21:166-175. Available at: https://doi.org/10.1111/tmi.12647.
12. Kinkar L, Laurimäe T, Simsek S, et al. High-resolution phylogeography of zoonotic tapeworm *Echinococcus* granulosus sensu stricto genotype G1 with an emphasis on its distribution in Turkey, Italy and Spain. *Parasitology.* 2016;143:1790-1801. Available at: https://doi.org/10.1017/S0031182016001530.
13. Kinkar L, Laurimäe T, Sharbatkhori M, et al. New mitogenome and nuclear evidence on the phylogeny and taxonomy of the highly zoonotic tapeworm *Echinococcus* granulosus sensu stricto. *Infect Genet Evol.* 2017;52:52-58. Available at: https://doi.org/10.1016/j.meegid.2017.04.023.
14. Romig T, Deplazes P, Jenkins D, Giraudoux P, Massolo A. Ecology and life cycle patterns of *Echinococcus* species. *Adv Parasitol.* 2017;95:213-314. Available at: https://doi.org/10.1016/bs.apar.2016.11.002.
15. Eckert J, Deplazes P. Biological, epidemiological, and clinical aspects of echinococcosis, a zoonosis of increasing concern. *Clin Microbiol Rev.* 2004;17:107-135. Available at: https://doi.org/10.1128/CMR.17.1.107.
16. Solomon N, Kachani M, Zeyhle E, Macpherson CNL. The natural history of cystic echinococcosis in untreated and albendazole-treated patients. *Acta Trop.* 2017;171:52-57. Available at: https://doi.org/10.1016/j.actatropica.2017.03.018.
17. Tamarozzi F, Mariconti M, Neumayr A, Brunetti E. The intermediate host immune response in cystic echinococcosis. *Parasite Immunol.* 2016;38:170-181. Available at: https://doi.org/10.1111/pim.12301.
18. Brunetti E, Kern P, Vuitton DA. Expert consensus for the diagnosis and treatment of cystic and alveolar echinococcosis in humans. *Acta Trop.* 2010;114:1-16. Available at: https://doi.org/10.1016/j.actatropica.2009.11.001.
19. Rinaldi F, Brunetti E, Neumayr A, Maestri M, Goblirsch S, Tamarozzi F. Cystic echinococcosis of the liver: a primer for hepatologists. *World J Hepatol.* 2014;6:293-305. Available at: https://doi.org/10.4254/wjh.v6.i5.293.
20. Macpherson CNL, Vuitton DA, Gharbi HA, et al. International classification of ultrasound images in cystic echinococcosis for application in clinical and field epidemiological settings. *Acta Trop.* 2003;85:253-261. Available at: https://doi.org/10.1016/S0001-706X(02)00223-1.
21. Polat P, Kantarci M, Alper F, Suma S, Koruyucu MB, Okur A. Hydatid disease from head to toe. *Radiographics.* 2003;23:475-494; quiz 536-537. Available at: https://doi.org/10.1148/rg.232025704.
22. Lianos GD, Lazaros A, Vlachos K, et al. Unusual locations of hydatid disease: a 33 year's experience analysis on 233 patients. *Updates Surg.* 2015;67:279-282. Available at: https://doi.org/10.1007/s13304-015-0291-6.
23. Santivanez S, Garcia HH. Pulmonary cystic echinococcosis. *Curr Opin Pulm Med.* 2010;16:257-261. Available at: https://doi.org/10.1097/MCP.0b013e3283386282.
24. Larrieu EJ, Frider B. Human cystic echinococcosis: contributions to the natural history of the disease. *Ann Trop Med Parasitol.* 2001;95:679-687. Available at: https://doi.org/10.1080/00034980120094730.
25. Rossi P, Tamarozzi F, Galati F, et al. The European Register of Cystic Echinococcosis, ERCE: state-of-the-art five years after its launch. *Parasit Vectors.* 2020;13:236. Available at: https://doi.org/10.1186/s13071-020-04101-6.

26. Tamarozzi F, Akhan O, Cretu CM, et al. Prevalence of abdominal cystic echinococcosis in rural Bulgaria, Romania, and Turkey: a cross-sectional, ultrasound-based, population study from the HERACLES project. *Lancet Infect Dis.* 2018;18:769-778. Available at: https://doi.org/10.1016/S1473-3099(18)30221-4.
27. Frider B, Moguilensky J, Salvitti JC, Odriozola M, Cantoni G, Larrieu E. Epidemiological surveillance of human hydatidosis by means of ultrasonography: its contribution to the evaluation of control programs. *Acta Trop.* 2001;79:219-223. Available at: https://doi.org/10.1016/S0001-706X(01)00096-1.
28. Larrieu E, Del Carpio M, Mercapide CH, et al. Programme for ultrasound diagnoses and treatment with albendazole of cystic echinococcosis in asymptomatic carriers: 10 years of follow-up of cases. *Acta Trop.* 2011;117:1-5. Available at: https://doi.org/10.1016/j.actatropica.2010.08.006.
29. Deplazes P, Rinaldi L, Alvarez Rojas CA, et al. Global distribution of alveolar and cystic echinococcosis. *Adv Parasitol.* 2017:315-493. Available at: https://doi.org/10.1016/bs.apar.2016.11.001.
30. Manciulli T, Mariconti M, Vola A, Lissandrin R, Brunetti E. Cystic echinococcosis in the Mediterranean. *Curr Trop Med Rep.* 2017;4:235-244. Available at: https://doi.org/10.1007/s40475-017-0129-z.
31. Torgerson PR. The emergence of echinococcosis in central Asia. *Parasitology.* 2013;140:1667-1673. Available at: https://doi.org/10.1017/S0031182013000516.
32. Torgerson PR, Oguljahan B, Muminov AE, et al. Present situation of cystic echinococcosis in Central Asia. *Parasitol Int.* 2006;55(suppl):S207-S212. Available at: https://doi.org/10.1016/j.parint.2005.11.032.
33. Moro P, Schantz PM. Cystic echinococcosis in the Americas. *Parasitol Int.* 2006;55(suppl):S181-S186. Available at: https://doi.org/10.1016/j.parint.2005.11.048.
34. Cerda JR, Buttke DE, Ballweber LR. Echinococcus spp. tapeworms in North America. *Emerg Infect Dis.* 2018;24:230-235. Available at: https://doi.org/10.3201/eid2402.161126.
35. Manciulli T, Serraino R, D'Alessandro GL, et al. Evidence of low prevalence of cystic echinococcosis in the Catanzaro Province, Calabria Region, Italy. *Am J Trop Med Hyg.* 2020;103:1951-1954. Available at: https://doi.org/10.4269/ajtmh.20-0119.
36. John K, Kazwala R, Mfinanga GS. Knowledge of causes, clinical features and diagnosis of common zoonoses among medical practitioners in Tanzania. *BMC Infect Dis.* 2008;8:162. Available at: https://doi.org/10.1186/1471-2334-8-162.
37. Possenti A, Manzano-Román R, Sánchez-Ovejero C, et al. Potential risk factors associated with human cystic echinococcosis: systematic review and meta-analysis. *PLoS Negl Trop Dis.* 2016;10:e0005114. Available at: https://doi.org/10.1371/journal.pntd.0005114.
38. Othieno E, Ocaido M, Mupere E, Omadang L, Oba P, Okwi AL. Knowledge, attitude, and beliefs of communities and health staff about *Echinococcus* granulosus infection in selected pastoral and agropastoral regions of Uganda. *J Parasitol Res.* 2018;2018. Available at: https://doi.org/10.1155/2018/5819545.
39. Macpherson CNL, Mengiste A, Zeyhle E, et al. Cystic Echinococcosis in Turkana, Kenya: the role of cross-sectional screening surveys in assessing the prevalence of human infection. *Am J Trop Med Hyg.* 2017;97:587-595. Available at: https://doi.org/10.4269/ajtmh.16-0643.
40. Budke CM, Carabin H, Ndimubanzi PC, et al. A systematic review of the literature on cystic echinococcosis frequency worldwide and its associated clinical manifestations. *Am J Trop Med Hyg.* 2013;88:1011-1027. Available at: https://doi.org/10.4269/ajtmh.12-0692.
41. Kilic M, Yoldas O, Koc M, et al. Can biliary-cyst communication be predicted before surgery for hepatic hydatid disease: does size matter? *Am J Surg.* 2008;196:732-735. Available at: https://doi.org/10.1016/j.amjsurg.2007.07.034.
42. Dietrich CF, Douira-Khomsi W, Gharbi H, et al. Cystic echinococcosis, review and illustration of non-hepatic manifestations. *Med Ultrason.* 2020;22:319. Available at: https://doi.org/10.11152/mu-2537.
43. Neumayr A, Troia G, de Bernardis C, et al. Justified concern or exaggerated fear: the risk of anaphylaxis in percutaneous treatment of cystic echinococcosis—A systematic literature review. *PLoS Negl Trop Dis.* 2011;5:e1154. Available at: https://doi.org/10.1371/journal.pntd.0001154.
44. Collado-Aliaga J, Romero-Alegría Á, Alonso-Sardón M, et al. Complications associated with initial clinical presentation of cystic echinococcosis: a 20-year cohort analysis. *Am J Trop Med Hyg.* 2019;101:628-635. Available at: https://doi.org/10.4269/ajtmh.19-0019.
45. Shambesh MA, Craig PS, Macpherson CNL, Rogan MT, Gusbi AM, Echtuish EF. An extensive ultrasound and serologic study to investigate the prevalence of human cystic echinococcosis in Northern Libya. *Am J Trop Med Hyg.* 1999;60:462-468.
46. MacPherson CN, Romig T, Zeyhle E, Rees PH, Were JB. Portable ultrasound scanner versus serology in screening for hydatid cysts in a nomadic population. *Lancet.* 1987;2:259-261.

47. Eckert J, Gemmel MA, Meslin FX, Pawlowski Z. *WHO/OIE Manual on Echinococcosis in Humans and Animals: A Public Health Problem of Global Concern.* Geneva: World Organ Animal Health (Office Int Des Epizoot World Heal Organ); 2001.
48. Brunetti E, Tamarozzi F, Macpherson C, et al. Ultrasound and cystic echinococcosis. *Ultrasound Int Open.* 2018;4:E70-E78. Available at: https://doi.org/10.1055/a-0650-3807.
49. Gharbi HA, Hassine W, Brauner MW, Dupuch K. Ultrasound examination of the hydatic liver. *Radiology.* 1981;139:459-463. Available at: https://doi.org/10.1148/radiology.139.2.7220891.
50. Caremani M, Maestrini R, Occhini U, et al. Echographic epidemiology of cystic hydatid disease in Italy. *Eur J Epidemiol.* 1993;9:401-404. Available at: https://doi.org/10.1007/bf00157397.
51. Mirabile E, Solomon N, Fields PJ, Macpherson CNL. Progress towards international adoption of the World Health Organization ultrasound classification of cystic echinococcosis. *Acta Trop.* 2019;189:6-9. Available at: https://doi.org/10.1016/j.actatropica.2018.09.024.
52. Hosch W, Junghanss T, Stojkovic M, et al. Metabolic viability assessment of cystic echinococcosis using high-field 1H MRS of cyst contents. *NMR Biomed.* 2008;21:734-754. Available at: https://doi.org/10.1002/nbm.1252.
53. Hosch W, Stojkovic M, Jänisch T, Kauffmann GW, Junghanss T. The role of calcification for staging cystic echinococcosis (CE). *Eur Radiol.* 2007;17:2538-2545. Available at: https://doi.org/10.1007/s00330-007-0638-6.
54. Stojkovic M, Rosenberger K, Kauczor HU, Junghanss T, Hosch W. Diagnosing and staging of cystic echinococcosis: how do CT and MRI perform in comparison to ultrasound? *PLoS Negl Trop Dis.* 2012;6:1-8. Available at: https://doi.org/10.1371/journal.pntd.0001880.
55. Siles-Lucas M, Casulli A, Conraths FJ, Müller N. Laboratory diagnosis of *Echinococcus* spp. in human patients and infected animals. *Adv Parasitol.* 2017;96:159-257. Available at: https://doi.org/10.1016/bs.apar.2016.09.003.
56. Hernández-González A, Sánchez-Ovejero C, Manzano-Román R, et al. Evaluation of the recombinant antigens B2t and 2B2t, compared with hydatid fluid, in IgG-ELISA and immunostrips for the diagnosis and follow up of CE patients. *PLoS Negl Trop Dis.* 2018;12:e0006741. Available at: https://doi.org/10.1371/journal.pntd.0006741.
57. Hernández-González A, Muro A, Barrera I, Ramos G, Orduña A, Siles-Lucas M. Usefulness of four different *Echinococcus* granulosus recombinant antigens for serodiagnosis of unilocular hydatid disease (UHD) and postsurgical follow-up of patients treated for UHD. *Clin Vaccine Immunol.* 2008;15:147-153. Available at: https://doi.org/10.1128/CVI.00363-07.
58. Manzano-Román R, Sánchez-Ovejero C, Hernández-González A, Casulli A, Siles-Lucas M. Serological diagnosis and follow-up of human cystic echinococcosis: a new hope for the future? *Biomed Res Int.* 2015;2015:428205. Available at: https://doi.org/10.1155/2015/428205.
59. Vola A, Manciulli T, De Silvestri A, et al. Diagnostic performances of commercial ELISA, indirect hemagglutination, and western blot in differentiation of hepatic echinococcal and non-echinococcal lesions: a retrospective analysis of data from a single referral centre. *Am J Trop Med Hyg.* 2019;101:1345-1349. Available at: https://doi.org/10.4269/ajtmh.19-0556.
60. Tamarozzi F, Longoni SS, Vola A, et al. Evaluation of nine commercial serological tests for the diagnosis of human hepatic cyst echinococcosis and the differential diagnosis with other focal liver lesions: a diagnostic accuracy study. *Diagnostics.* 2021;11. Available at: https://doi.org/10.3390/diagnostics11020167.
61. Vola A, Tamarozzi F, Noordin R, et al. Preliminary assessment of the diagnostic performances of a new rapid diagnostic test for the serodiagnosis of human cystic echinococcosis. *Diagn Microbiol Infect Dis.* 2018;92:31-33. Available at: https://doi.org/10.1016/j.diagmicrobio.2018.04.007.
62. Lissandrin R, Tamarozzi F, Piccoli L, et al. Factors influencing the serological response in hepatic *Echinococcus* granulosus infection. *Am J Trop Med Hyg.* 2016;94:166-171. Available at: https://doi.org/10.4269/ajtmh.15-0219.
63. Tamarozzi F, Silva R, Fittipaldo VA, Buonfrate D, Gottstein B, Siles-Lucas M. Serology for the diagnosis of human hepatic cystic echinococcosis and its relation with cyst staging: a systematic review of the literature with meta-analysis. *PLoS Negl Trop Dis.* 2021;15:e0009370. Available at: https://doi.org/10.1371/journal.pntd.0009370.
64. Tamarozzi F, Longoni SS, Vola A, et al. Evaluation of nine commercial serological tests for the diagnosis of human hepatic cyst echinococcosis and the differential diagnosis with other focal liver lesions: a diagnostic accuracy study. *Diagnostics.* 2021;11. Available at: https://doi.org/10.3390/diagnostics11020167.

65. Stojkovic M, Adt HM, Rosenberger K, et al. Follow-up of surgically treated patients with cystic echinococcosis: can novel recombinant antigens compete with imaging? Analysis of a patient cohort. *Trop Med Int Health*. 2017;22:614-621. Available at: https://doi.org/10.1111/tmi.12859.
66. Mendes C, Salgueiro P, Gonzalez V, et al. Genetic diversity and signatures of selection of drug resistance in Plasmodium populations from both human and mosquito hosts in continental Equatorial Guinea. *Malar J*. 2013;12:114. Available at: https://doi.org/10.1186/1475-2875-12-114.
67. Chaya D, Parija SC. Performance of polymerase chain reaction for the diagnosis of cystic echinococcosis using serum, urine, and cyst fluid samples. *Trop Parasitol*. 2014;4:43-46. Available at: https://doi.org/10.4103/2229-5070.129164.
68. Mariconti M, Vola A, Manciulli T, et al. Role of microRNAs in host defense against Echinococcus granulosus infection: a preliminary assessment. *Immunol Res*. 2019;67:93-97. Available at: https://doi.org/10.1007/s12026-018-9041-4.
69. Örsten S, Baysal İ, Yabanoglu-Ciftci S, et al. Can parasite-derived microRNAs differentiate active and inactive cystic echinococcosis patients? *Parasitol Res*. 2021. Available at: https://doi.org/10.1007/s00436-021-07382-7.
70. Ciftci TT, Yabanoglu-Ciftci S, Unal E, et al. Metabolomic profiling of active and inactive liver cystic echinococcosis. *Acta Trop*. 2021;221:105985. Available at: https://doi.org/10.1016/j.actatropica.2021.105985.
71. Petrone L, Tamarozzi F, Vola A, et al. Accuracy of an experimental whole-blood test for detecting reactivation of echinococcal cysts. *PLoS Negl Trop Dis*. 2021;15:e0009648. Available at: https://doi.org/10.1371/journal.pntd.0009648.
72. Petrone L, Albrich WC, Tamarozzi F, et al. Species specificity preliminary evaluation of an IL-4-based test for the differential diagnosis of human echinococcosis. *Parasite Immunol*. 2020;42:e12695. Available at: https://doi.org/10.1111/pim.12695.
73. Cattaneo L, Manciulli T, Cretu CM, et al. Cystic echinococcosis of the bone: a European multicenter study. *Am J Trop Med Hyg*. 2019;100:617-621. Available at: https://doi.org/10.4269/ajtmh.18-0758.
74. Monge-Maillo B, Chamorro Tojeiro S, López-Vélez R. Management of osseous cystic echinococcosis. *Expert Rev Anti Infect Ther*. 2017;15:1075-1082. Available at: https://doi.org/10.1080/14787210.2017.1401466.
75. Monge-Maillo B, Olmedo Samperio M, Pérez-Molina JA, et al. Osseous cystic echinococcosis: a case series study at a referral unit in Spain. *PLoS Negl Trop Dis*. 2019;13:e0007006. Available at: https://doi.org/10.1371/journal.pntd.0007006.
76. Tamarozzi F, Horton J, Muhtarov M, et al. A case for adoption of continuous albendazole treatment regimen for human echinococcal infections. *PLoS Negl Trop Dis*. 2020;14:1-7. Available at: https://doi.org/10.1371/journal.pntd.0008566.
77. Horton J. Albendazole for the treatment of echinococcosis. *Fundam Clin Pharmacol*. 2003;17:205-212. Available at: https://doi.org/10.1046/j.1472-8206.2003.00171.x.
78. Manciulli T, Vola A, Mariconti M, et al. Shortage of albendazole and its consequences for patients with cystic echinococcosis treated at a referral center in Italy. *Am J Trop Med Hyg*. 2018;99:1006-1010. Available at: https://doi.org/10.4269/ajtmh.18-0245.
79. Franchi C, Di Vico B, Teggi A. Long-term evaluation of patients with hydatidosis treated with benzimidazole carbamates. *Clin Infect Dis*. 1999;29:304-309. Available at: https://doi.org/10.1086/520205.
80. Horton J. Albendazole: a review of anthelmintic efficacy and safety in humans. *Parasitology*. 2000;121:S113-S132. Available at: https://doi.org/10.1017/S0031182000007290.
81. Özdil B, Keçe C, Ünalp ÖV. An alternative method for percutaneous treatment of hydatid cysts: PAI technique. *Turkiye Parazitolojii Derg*. 2016;40:77-81. Available at: https://doi.org/10.5152/tpd.2016.4264.
82. Filice C, Brunetti E. Use of PAIR in human cystic echinococcosis. *Acta Trop*. 1997;64:95-107.
83. WHO Informal Working Group on Echinococcosis (IWGE). PAIR: Puncture, Aspiration, Injection, Re-Aspiration. WHO/CDS/CSR/APH/2001. 2001;30:1-10. Available at: https://doi.org/10.5860/CHOICE.41-4081.
84. Firpo G, Vola A, Lissandrin R, Tamarozzi F, Brunetti E. Preliminary evaluation of percutaneous treatment of echinococcal cysts without injection of scolicidal agent. *Am J Trop Med Hyg*. 2017;97:1818-1826. Available at: https://doi.org/10.4269/ajtmh.17-0468.
85. Akhan O, Islim F, Balci S, et al. Percutaneous treatment of simple hepatic cysts: the long-term results of PAIR and catheterization techniques as single-session procedures. *Cardiovasc Intervent Radiol*. 2016;39:902-908. Available at: https://doi.org/10.1007/s00270-015-1283-0.

86. Akhan O, Salik AE, Ciftci T, Akinci D, Islim F, Akpinar B. Comparison of long-term results of percutaneous treatment techniques for hepatic cystic echinococcosis types 2 and 3b. *AJR Am J Roentgenol.* 2017;208:878-884. Available at: https://doi.org/10.2214/AJR.16.16131.
87. Akhan O, Yildiz AE, Akinci D, Yildiz BD, Ciftci T. Is the adjuvant albendazole treatment really needed with PAIR in the management of liver hydatid cysts? A prospective, randomized trial with short-term follow-up results. *Cardiovasc Intervent Radiol.* 2014;37:1568-1574. Available at: https://doi.org/10.1007/s00270-014-0840-2.
88. Karima A, Manel A, Sara B, et al. International consensus on terminology to be used in the field of echinococcoses. *Parasite.* 2020;27. Available at: https://doi.org/10.1051/parasite/2020024.
89. Al-Saeedi M, Khajeh E, Hoffmann K, et al. Standardized endocystectomy technique for surgical treatment of uncomplicated hepatic cystic echinococcosis. *PLoS Negl Trop Dis.* 2019;13(6):1-14.
90. Al-Saeedi M, Ramouz A, Khajeh E, et al. Endocystectomy as a conservative surgical treatment for hepatic cystic echinococcosis: a systematic review with single-arm metaanalysis. *PLoS Negl Trop Dis.* 2021;15:1-21. Available at: https://doi.org/10.1371/journal.pntd.0009365.

SECTION IV

Tropical Non-Infectious Liver Disease

CHAPTER 18

Non-Cirrhotic Portal Hypertension

Ashish Goel ■ Chundamannil E. Eapen

KEY POINTS

- Non-cirrhotic portal hypertension, including both extrahepatic portal venous obstruction (EHPVO) and idiopathic non-cirrhotic intrahepatic portal hypertension (NCIPH), are important causes of pre-sinusoidal portal hypertension in tropical countries
- Both these disorders present with well-tolerated portal hypertension and remarkable splenomegaly.
- While EHPVO presents early (first and second decades), NCIPH presents a bit later (second and third decades) in life. Thrombosed portal vein (often replaced by cavernoma) is essential to diagnose EHPVO. NCIPH, on the other hand, is a diagnosis based on extensive evaluation showing patent hepatic inflow and outflow and absence of cirrhosis.
- Management of EHPVO consists of tackling portal hypertension–related complications and also portal cavernoma cholangiopathy.
- Evaluation and management of associated conditions is important in NCIPH patients.

Introduction

Portal hypertension is usually classified per the site of obstruction to portal flow. Consequently, it can be pre-sinusoidal, sinusoidal (e.g., cirrhosis), and post-sinusoidal (e.g., Budd-Chiari syndrome/hepatic venous outflow tract obstruction).

The current chapter aims to deal with two of the causes of pre-sinusoidal portal hypertension—extrahepatic portal venous obstruction (EHPVO, pre-hepatic thrombosis of the portal vein) and idiopathic non-cirrhotic intrahepatic portal hypertension (NCIPH, intrahepatic occlusion of 3rd/4th order small portal vein radicles) seen in the tropics.

Extrahepatic Portal Venous Obstruction

EHPVO is a common cause of pediatric portal hypertension. The affected child or young adult presents with esophageal variceal bleed or becomes aware of an enlarged spleen. As the hepatic artery inflow to the liver is preserved, the patient is usually well otherwise with normal liver function tests.

DEFINITION

Idiopathic chronic portal vein thrombosis presenting in children or young adults is termed EHPVO.

INCIDENCE

In contrast to resource-rich countries, EHPVO is a common cause of upper GI bleeding in children in resource-poor countries.[1-8] Population-based data on the incidence of EHPVO is not available.

ETIOLOGY

Intriguingly, acute thrombosis of portal vein, which subsequently leads to EHPVO, is only rarely recognized clinically. So the exact causes of the EHPVO remain unclear. Uncommonly, umbilical vein catheterization performed in the newborn[9] or umbilical sepsis may trigger portal venous thrombosis. In studies on EHPVO patients from India, increased plasma factor VIII levels were noted in one study,[10] while factors II and V mutations were not associated with EHPVO.[11-13]

Clinical Features

The child or young adult with EHPVO comes to medical attention typically through one of two presentations: upper GI bleed—large-volume hematemesis-melena from bleeding esophageal varices—or by feeling a lump in the abdomen as the spleen enlarges. Growth impairment is an uncommon presentation of EHPVO.[14,15] Physical examination may reveal pallor and a moderately enlarged spleen.

Investigations

Most patients have pancytopenia due to hypersplenism. In patients who had bleeding from varices, iron deficiency anemia is also seen. Liver function tests are normal or near normal.

Upper GI endoscopy reveals esophageal and/or gastric varices. Ultrasound shows the portal vein to be replaced by a leash of collateral vessels (termed "portal cavernoma"). The presence of thrombosed portal vein differentiates EHPVO from other causes of non-cirrhotic intrahepatic portal hypertension (e.g., NCIPH, schistosomiasis). On cross-sectional imaging, the liver may be normal or less often mildly coarse with irregular surface; the latter may be secondary to chronic portal venous insufficiency (Figure 18.1).

Natural History

Once the bleeding varices are controlled by endotherapy, patients do fairly well.[16] In a study of 193 EHPVO patients who had bleeding esophageal varices treated by endoscopic sclerotherapy, 17% had rebleeding from varices on mean follow-up period of 19.8 years. Rebleeding was uncommon after 10 years of the initial variceal eradication.[17]

Anemia, enlarged spleen (which can become massively large in some patients), and ascites[18] can also occur on follow-up. Portal cavernoma cholangiopathy (also known as portal hypertensive biliopathy) can develop in some patients.

Treatment

At present, most patients bleeding from gastroesophageal varices are managed by endotherapy.[19,20] Endoscopic variceal band ligation is done to treat esophageal variceal bleed and glue injection to treat gastric variceal bleed. Rarely, balloon tamponade with Sengstaken-Blakemore tube (or equivalent) is required for rapid and temporary control of bleeding from esophageal varices. Propranolol, usually at a dose of 10 to 20 mg twice daily (gradually increased to achieve

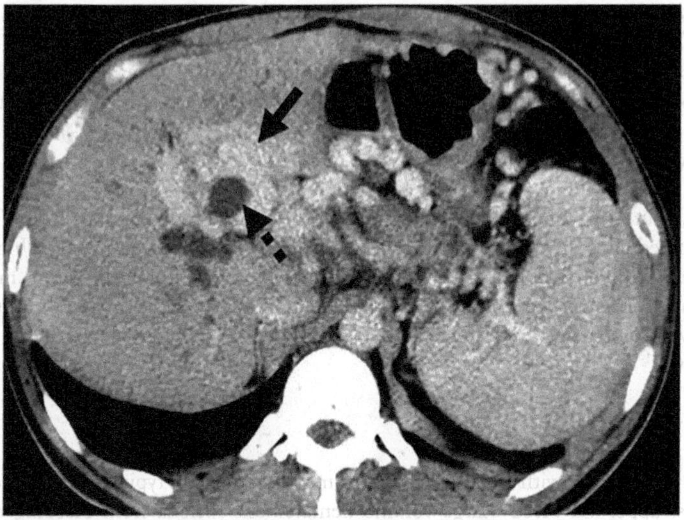

Figure 18.1 Extrahepatic portal vein obstruction. Contrast-enhanced CT image of liver shows a cavernoma at the porta (black arrow) replacing main portal vein and surrounding the proximal common bile duct (dashed black arrow) with mild intrahepatic biliary dilatation in right lobe (portal cavernoma cholangiopathy). (Courtesy of Dr. Anu Eapen, Department of Radiodiagnosis, Christian Medical College, Vellore.)

a target heart rate of ~60 bpm), is given as primary and secondary prophylaxis against variceal bleed. Oral iron supplements are given to correct anemia.

Shunt surgery linking mesenteric vein and left branch of portal vein (termed "Rex" shunt) appears to be a promising option to address the blocked portal venous inflow to the liver[21,22]; however, the atretic portal vein branches and leash of collaterals at the porta represent technical challenges.

Portal cavernoma cholangiopathy (also termed portal hypertensive biliopathy): Some patients with EHPVO, especially in the second or third decade of life, develop features of extrahepatic biliary obstruction.[23] This may be caused by portal venous collaterals compressing the extrahepatic biliary tree or due to ischemia of the biliary tree consequent to portal venous obstruction.

Most patients are asymptomatic and the biliary obstruction is recognized only by raised serum alkaline phosphatase and dilated biliary radicles noted on ultrasound scan. Patients may have symptoms of obstructive jaundice and, uncommonly, have cholangitis and secondary biliary cirrhosis. MRI scan can provide details of the portal venous block and biliary obstruction.

Portal cavernoma cholangiopathy is diagnosed by demonstrating portal cavernoma (a leash of vessels replacing portal vein at the hilum) and typical cholangiopathy on imaging like CT abdomen (Figure 18.1) or magnetic resonance cholangiography[24] and ruling out other causes for the biliary changes like primary sclerosing cholangitis or cholangiocarcinoma. Endoscopic ultrasound may help delineate the collateral channels accurately in this condition.[25] Its natural history suggests that portal cavernoma cholangiopathy is a progressive condition, with symptoms developing only in patients with severe cholangiopathy.[24]

Though various treatment options have been tried, portal cavernoma cholangiopathy remains difficult to treat. In patients with cholangitis, ERCP and sphincterotomy/biliary stent may be attempted; however, because of multiple portal venous collaterals which cannot be visualized during ERCP, this treatment carries the risk of uncontrolled bleeding. Shunt surgery to decompress the portal venous system[26] followed by biliary enteric bypass is not always efficacious. The lack of an adequate portal venous segment makes liver transplant as well as insertion of transjugular intrahepatic portosystemic stent technically challenging or unsuccessful. In view of these challenges with treatment, asymptomatic patients do not warrant treatment and conservative or minimally invasive treatment appears to be the best approach to treat symptomatic disease.

Non-Cirrhotic Intrahepatic Portal Hypertension

HISTORY AND TERMINOLOGY

NCIPH was initially described at great length in India (non-cirrhotic portal fibrosis) and Japan (idiopathic portal hypertension). It remains an important cause of portal hypertension in India and presumably other resource-limited regions of the world, but recent reports have also noted rare occurrence in resource-rich parts of the world (INCPH, idiopathic non-cirrhotic portal hypertension).[27,28]

Multiple histologic equivalents have also been used to describe the disease such as nodular regenerative hyperplasia, hepato-portal sclerosis, obliterative portal venopathy, and incomplete septal cirrhosis.[29,30]

NCIPH terminology denotes presence of portal hypertension and level of blockade (intrahepatic) and also refers to essential criteria of absence of advanced fibrosis/cirrhosis on liver biopsy.[31] In contrast, the recently coined terminology of porto-sinusoidal vascular disease (PSVD) seeks to broaden the disease spectrum. PSVD includes patients with characteristic histology findings, suggesting portal insufficiency (see later section), even in a patient with other competing liver diagnosis (e.g., fatty liver, autoimmune hepatitis etc.) and also in a patient without obvious portal hypertension. Figure 18.2 depicts a timeline of various terminologies used to describe NCIPH.[32-34]

EPIDEMIOLOGY

Prevalence of NCIPH remains underestimated in most resource-constrained scenarios. In a prospective study from southern India, spanning over a period of 1 year (2009–2010), 203 (35%) of

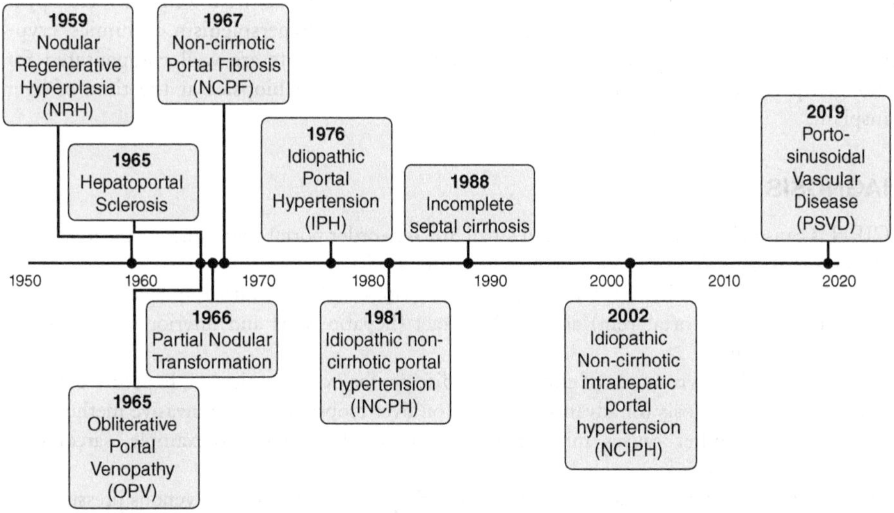

Figure 18.2 Timeline depicting changing nomenclature for idiopathic non-cirrhotic intrahepatic portal hypertension (NCIPH).

583 consecutive adult patients with portal hypertension were labeled as "cryptogenic cirrhosis" prior to biopsy. Only 39 of these 203 patients underwent liver biopsy, which revealed NCIPH in 16 (41%) patients.[35] In India, contribution of NCIPH to portal hypertension varies from 5% to 25% and depends on factors like modalities used to confirm diagnosis and stage of disease.[27,36,37] Improvement in socioeconomic status may lead to gradual decrease in prevalence of NCIPH, but it still continues to be an important cause of portal hypertension in India.[27] NCIPH is a rarity in the developed world. On the other hand, Schistosomiasis induced pre-sinusoidal portal hypertension, is a common cause of esophageal varices and variceal bleed in Africa.[38]

ETIOPATHOGENESIS

There are only isolated reports of familial NCIPH and it appears to be a complex disorder with interaction of both environmental factors and possible underlying genetic predilection.[27]

The increased prevalence of NCIPH in the resource-limited world and localization to small portal vein radicles points to active involvement of the gut and "poverty-linked thrombophilia" in the pathogenesis.[27] Endothelial-mesenchymal transition[39] and imbalance of vasoactive molecules (e.g., nitric oxide, endothelin) and imbalance of primary hemostasis (von-Willebrand factor and its cleaving protease)[40] have also been implicated.

Other associated factors that may hint at pathogenic mechanisms are immune-deficiency conditions (e.g., common variable immunodeficiency), immune-mediated diseases (e.g., rheumatoid arthritis, celiac disease, inflammatory bowel disease), toxins and drugs (e.g., arsenicosis, some anti-retroviral drugs/chemotherapeutic agents, azathioprine), or hematological conditions (e.g., hypovitaminosis B12, imbalance of primary hemostasis, myeloproliferative disease).[28,41,42]

It is possible that NCIPH develops as a consequence of environmental factors related to poor socio-economic conditions, like gut contamination secondary to poor sanitation. As access to clean water and sanitation improves, NCIPH may decline in incidence in these settings.

CLINICAL PRESENTATION

NCIPH typically presents in early adulthood (second/third decade) with well-tolerated upper gastrointestinal variceal bleeds or splenomegaly with/without hypersplenism. It mimics "cryptogenic cirrhosis" in all aspects and even though most patients are well compensated for prolonged period, few patients are diagnosed only on explant biopsies at the time of liver transplant.

DIAGNOSIS

NCIPH is caused by chronic occlusion of small 3rd/4th-order portal vein radicles. The diagnosis is currently based on fulfilling all the following criteria[27,28]

a. Presence of portal hypertension—usually via gastroesophageal varices or splenomegaly
b. Patent inflow (portal vein) and outflow tract (hepatic veins and inferior vena-cava) on Doppler scan
c. Absence of known causes of chronic liver disease, for example, alcohol, hepatitis B and C
d. Absence of cirrhosis (or advanced fibrosis) on liver biopsy or via noninvasive methods
e. Absence of other causes mimicking NCIPH on histology, for example, sarcoidosis, schistosomiasis

Hepatic venous pressure gradient (wedged hepatic pressure–free hepatic venous pressure) reflects sinusoidal pressure and it is usually normal in up to one-third of NCIPH patients and can serve to distinguish it from cirrhosis.[36]

Liver biopsy is the key to ruling out advanced fibrosis/cirrhosis, thereby confirming NCIPH. In addition, adequate liver biopsy (with at least six portal tracts) shows findings suggesting portal venous insufficiency, namely sclerosed/dilated portal vein radicles, sinusoidal dilation, multiplicity of portal vessels (equivalent to portal cavernoma at the level of portal triad), or parenchymal extinction.[44] These findings may often be subtle and require experienced hepato-pathologist for interpretation. It can also assess for other pre-sinusoidal causes of portal hypertension (e.g., schistosomiasis).

Thrombocytopenia, often noted in NCIPH, adds a layer of complexity to perform a liver biopsy with need for either a transjugular route or post biopsy use of foam gel sealant. Liver biopsy therefore is not commonly feasible in a resource-constrained setting, leading to these patients being mislabeled as having "cryptogenic cirrhosis."

Natural History

Most published studies show a good prognosis and overall survival in patients with NCIPH.[45] Goel et al.,[46] in a recent large retrospective cohort study from India ($n = 172$), showed an excellent 5-year transplant-free survival (97%) but a definite risk of decompensation (23%) and portal vein thrombosis (28%) on follow-up. Similarly, a follow-up study of Western patients (n = 62) demonstrated an overall survival of 100%, 78%, and 56% at 1, 5, and 10 years, respectively (Table 18.1).

Patients are prone to complications of portal hypertension (variceal bleed, ascites, encephalopathy in late stages), macrovascular involvement (e.g., portal vein thrombosis), and microvascular involvement (e.g., hepato-pulmonary syndrome, porto-pulmonary hypertension, glomerulonephritis). Some patients may need liver transplant secondary to worsening of liver dysfunction or portal hypertension and also due to development of hepatoma.

Although survival is decreased as compared to the general population, it appears to be much better than comparable clinical stages of cirrhosis. The usual predictors of mortality in cirrhosis (Baveno-VI staging, hepatic venous pressure gradient) may not accurately predict outcomes in these patients, requiring further research.

MANAGEMENT

Management strategies, including primary (nonselective beta blockers) and secondary (endoscopic variceal ligation) prophylaxis of variceal bleed, are similar to that of patients with cirrhosis.

TABLE 18.1 ■ **Short-and Medium-Term Transplant-Free Survival in 172 NCIPH Patients—Retrospective Cohort Study[45]**

Baveno-VI Clinical Stage	Description	Number of Patients	1-Year Survival	5-Year Survival
Stage 0	HVPG <10 mm Hg, no varices	2	100%*	-
Stage 1	HVPG >10 mm Hg, no varices	4	100%*	-
Stage 2	Non-bleeding varices	77	100%	100%
Stage 3	Bleeding varices	60	98%	98%
Stage 4	Development of ascites	29	96.6%	96.6%
Stage 5	Second decompensating event	0	-	-
Stage 6	Late decompensation	0	-	-
Total		172	-	97%

HVPG: hepatic venous pressure gradient.
*Alive with a median follow-up of 32 months (range: 16–217 months).

As NCIPH is a pure vasculopathy, hepatic decompensation is usually late in the course. Transjugular intrahepatic portosystemic shunt or surgical portosystemic shunt thus can be considered in cases of difficult-to-control variceal bleeds. Only occasionally is splenectomy necessary for symptomatic hypersplenism.[36]

The decompensating events, even though late in the course, are managed as per guidelines pertaining to cirrhosis. Some patients may eventually need liver transplant.

Active evaluation and adequate managing of the various coexistent conditions (e.g., celiac disease, arsenicosis) can be helpful in overall prognosis of these patients.[47]

References

1. Poddar U, Thapa BR, Rao KL, Singh K. Etiological spectrum of esophageal varices due to portal hypertension in Indian children: is it different from the West? *J Gastroenterol Hepatol.* 2008;23(9):1354-1357.
2. Yachha SK, Khanduri A, Sharma BC, Kumar M. Gastrointestinal bleeding in children. *J Gastroenterol Hepatol.* 1996;11(10):903-907.
3. Cox K, Ament ME. Upper gastrointestinal bleeding in children and adolescents. *Pediatrics.* 1979;63(3): 408-413.
4. Simon EG, Joseph AJ, George B, et al. Aetiology of paediatric portal hypertension: experience of a tertiary care centre in South India. *Trop Doct.* 2009;39(1):42-44.
5. Grama A, Pîrvan A, Sîrbe C, et al. Extrahepatic portal vein thrombosis, an important cause of portal hypertension in children. *J Clin Med.* 2021;10(12):2703.
6. Ferri PM, Ferreira AR, Fagundes ED, Liu SM, Roquete ML, Penna FJ. Portal vein thrombosis in children and adolescents: 20 years experience of a pediatric hepatology reference center. *Arq Gastroenterol.* 2012;49(1):69-76.
7. El-Karaksy HM, El-Koofy N, Mohsen N, Helmy H, Nabil N, El-Shabrawi M. Extrahepatic portal vein obstruction in Egyptian children. *J Pediatr Gastroenterol Nutr.* 2015;60(1):105-109.
8. Afaa TJ, Amegan-Aho KH, Richardson E, Goka B. Diagnosis and management of extrahepatic oesophageal variceal bleed in children in a low resourced setting. *Ghana Med J.* 2020;54(4):274-278.
9. Kim JH, Lee YS, Kim SH, Lee SK, Lim MK, Kim HS. Does umbilical vein catheterization lead to portal venous thrombosis? Prospective US evaluation in 100 neonates. *Radiology.* 2001;219(3):645-650.
10. Koshy A, Jeyakumari M. High FVIII level is associated with idiopathic portal vein thrombosis in South India. *Am J Med.* 2007;120(6):552.e9-11.
11. Koshy A, Jeyakumari M. Factor V Leiden is not commonly associated with idiopathic portal vein thrombosis in southern India. *Indian J Gastroenterol.* 2006;25(3):140-142.
12. Koshy A, Jeyakumari M. Prothrombin G20210A gene variant is not associated with idiopathic portal vein thrombosis in an area endemic for portal vein thrombosis. *Ann Hematol.* 2006;85(2):126-128
13. Sharma S, Kumar SI, Poddar U, Yachha SK, Aggarwal R. Factor V Leiden and prothrombin gene G20210A mutations are uncommon in portal vein thrombosis in India. *Indian J Gastroenterol.* 2006;25(5): 236-239.
14. Sarin SK, Bansal A, Sasan S, Nigam A. Portal-vein obstruction in children leads to growth retardation. *Hepatology.* 1992;15(2):229-233.
15. Mehrotra RN, Bhatia V, Dabadghao P, Yachha SK. Extrahepatic portal vein obstruction in children: anthropometry, growth hormone, and insulin-like growth factor I. *J Pediatr Gastroenterol Nutr.* 1997; 25(5):520-523.
16. Maksoud-Filho JG, Gonçalves ME, Cardoso SR, Gibelli NE, Tannuri U. Long-term follow-up of children with extrahepatic portal vein obstruction: impact of an endoscopic sclerotherapy program on bleeding episodes, hepatic function, hypersplenism, and mortality. *J Pediatr Surg.* 2009;44(10):1877-1883.
17. Thomas V, Jose T, Kumar S. Natural history of bleeding after esophageal variceal eradication in patients with extrahepatic portal venous obstruction; a 20-year follow-up. *Indian J Gastroenterol.* 2009;28(6): 206-211.
18. Sen Sarma M, Srivastava A, Yachha SK, Poddar U. Ascites in children with extrahepatic portal venous obstruction: etiology, risk factors and outcome. *Dig Liver Dis.* 2020;52(12):1480-1485.
19. Sarin SK, Sollano JD, Chawla YK, et al. Consensus on extra-hepatic portal vein obstruction. *Liver Int.* 2006;26(5):512-519.

20. Poddar U, Bhatnagar S, Yachha SK. Endoscopic band ligation followed by sclerotherapy: is it superior to sclerotherapy in children with extrahepatic portal venous obstruction? *J Gastroenterol Hepatol.* 2011;26(2): 255-259.
21. Lautz TB, Keys LA, Melvin JC, Ito J, Superina RA. Advantages of the meso-Rex bypass compared with portosystemic shunts in the management of extrahepatic portal vein obstruction in children. *J Am Coll Surg.* 2013;216(1):83-89.
22. Ateş O, Hakgüder G, Olguner M, Seçil M, Karaca I, Akgür FM. Mesenterico left portal bypass for variceal bleeding owing to extrahepatic portal hypertension caused by portal vein thrombosis. *J Pediatr Surg.* 2006;41(7):1259-1263.
23. Dhiman RK, Saraswat VA, Valla DC, et al. Portal cavernoma cholangiopathy: consensus statement of a working party of the Indian National Association for Study of the Liver. *J Clin Exp Hepatol.* 2014;4(suppl 1): S2-S14.
24. Shin SM, Kim S, Lee JW, et al. Biliary abnormalities associated with portal biliopathy: evaluation on MR cholangiography. *AJR Am J Roentgenol.* 2007;188(4):W341-W347.
25. Sharma M, Rameshbabu CS. Portal cavernoma cholangiopathy: an endoscopic ultrasound based imaging approach. *J Clin Exp Hepatol.* 2014;4(suppl 1):S53-S61.
26. Ravindranath A, Sen Sarma M, Yachha SK, et al. Outcome of portosystemic shunt surgery on pre-existing cholangiopathy in children with extrahepatic portal vein obstruction. *J Hepatobiliary Pancreat Sci.* 2020;27(3):141-148.
27. Goel A, Ramakrishna B, Zachariah U, et al. What makes non-cirrhotic portal hypertension a common disease in India? Analysis for environmental factors. *Indian J Med Res.* 2019;149(4):468-478.
28. Schouten JNL, Garcia-Pagan JC, Valla DC, Janssen HLA. Idiopathic noncirrhotic portal hypertension. *Hepatology.* 2011;54:1071-1081.
29. Sarin SK, Khanna R. Non-cirrhotic portal hypertension. *Clin Liver Dis.* 2014;18(2):451-476. doi:10.1016/j.cld.2014.01.009.
30. Goel A, Elias JE, Eapen CE, Ramakrishna B, Elias E. Idiopathic non-cirrhotic intrahepatic portal hypertension (NCIPH)-newer insights into pathogenesis and emerging newer treatment options. *J Clin Exp Hepatol.* 2014;4:247-256.
31. Goel A, Ramakrishna B, Madhu K, et al. Idiopathic noncirrhotic intrahepatic portal hypertension is an ongoing problem in India. *Hepatology.* 2011;54:2275-2276.
32. De Gottardi A, Rautou PE, Schouten J, et al. Porto-sinusoidal vascular disease: proposal and description of a novel entity. *Lancet Gastroenterol Hepatol.* 2019;4(5):399-411. doi:10.1016/S2468-1253(19)30047-0.
33. Kmeid M, Liu X, Ballentine S, Lee H. Idiopathic non-cirrhotic portal hypertension and porto-sinusoidal vascular disease: review of current data. *Gastroenterology Res.* 2021;14(2):49-65. doi:10.14740/gr1376.
34. Guido M, Sarcognato S, Sonzogni A, et al. Obliterative portal venopathy without portal hypertension: an underestimated condition. *Liver Int.* 2016;36(3):454-460. doi:10.1111/liv.12936.
35. Goel A, Madhu K, Zachariah U, et al. A study of aetiology of portal hypertension in adults (including the elderly) at a tertiary centre in southern India. *Indian J Med Res.* 2013;137:922-927.
36. Khanna R, Sarin SK. Non-cirrhotic portal hypertension: diagnosis and management. *J Hepatol.* 2014;60(2):421-441. doi:10.1016/j.jhep.2013.08.013.
37. Dhiman RK, Chawla Y, Vasishta RK, et al. Non-cirrhotic portal fibrosis (idiopathic portal hypertension): experience with 151 patients and a review of the literature. *J Gastroenterol Hepatol.* 2002;17:6-16.
38. Opio CK, Kazibwe F, Ocama P, Rejani L, Belousova EN, Ajal P. Profiling lifetime episodes of upper gastrointestinal bleeding among patients from rural Sub-Saharan Africa where schistosoma mansoni is endemic. *Pan Afr Med J.* 2016;24:296.
39. Sato Y, Nakanuma Y. Role of endothelial-mesenchymal transition in idiopathic portal hypertension. *Histol Histopathol.* 2013;28(2):145-154.
40. Goel A, Alagammai PL, Nair SC, et al. ADAMTS13 deficiency, despite well-compensated liver functions in patients with noncirrhotic portal hypertension. *Indian J Gastroenterol.* 2014;33:355-363.
41. Maiwall R, Goel A, Pulimood AB, et al. Investigation into celiac disease in Indian patients with portal hypertension. *Indian J Gastroenterol.* 2014;33:517-523.
42. Goel A, Christudoss P, George R, et al. Arsenicosis, possibly from contaminated groundwater, associated with noncirrhotic intrahepatic portal hypertension. *Indian J Gastroenterol.* 2016;35:207-215.
43. Goel A, Ramakrishna B, Muliyil J, et al. Use of serum vitamin B12 level as a marker to differentiate idiopathic noncirrhotic intrahepatic portal hypertension from cryptogenic cirrhosis. *Dig Dis Sci.* 2013;58:179-187.

44. Guido M, Alves VAF, Balabaud C, et al. Histology of portal vascular changes associated with idiopathic non-cirrhotic portal hypertension: nomenclature and definition. *Histopathology*. 2019;74(2):219-226. doi:10.1111/his.13738.
45. Siramolpiwat S, Seijo S, Miquel R, et al. Idiopathic portal hypertension: natural history and long-term outcome. *Hepatology*. 2013. Available at: http://dx.doi.org/10.1002/hep.26904.
46. Goel A, Zachariah U, Ramakrishna B, Elias E, Eapen CE. Baveno-VI clinical staging of cirrhosis underestimates 5-year survival after variceal bleed in cryptogenic chronic liver disease patients in India. *Eur J Gastroenterol Hepatol*. 2021;33(9):1232-1234.
47. Eapen CE, Nightingale P, Hubscher SG, et al. Non-cirrhotic intrahepatic portal hypertension: associated gut diseases and prognostic factors. *Dig Dis Sci*. 2011;56:227-235.

CHAPTER 19

Cirrhosis in the Tropics

Ângelo Zambam de Mattos

KEY POINTS

- Cirrhosis and chronic liver diseases rank 10th among the diseases with the highest mortality rate worldwide.
- Cirrhosis may present in a compensated stage (usually asymptomatic) or in a decompensated stage (manifested by ascites, variceal bleeding, hepatic encephalopathy, or jaundice).
- Ascites in cirrhosis is highly associated with a serum-ascites albumin gradient ≥1.1 g/dL and an ascitic total protein level <2.5 g/dL.
- Sodium restriction and diuretics (e.g., spironolactone and furosemide) are the mainstays of ascites treatment.
- Variceal bleeding should be treated with a vasoactive drug (i.e., terlipressin, octreotide, or somatostatin), antibiotic prophylaxis (norfloxacin or ceftriaxone), and endoscopic therapy (preferably variceal ligation).
- Hepatic encephalopathy is usually managed with lactulose. Rifaximin may be used if encephalopathy recurs despite the use of lactulose.
- Spontaneous bacterial peritonitis is characterized by a polymorphonuclear count $>250/mm^3$ in ascites and is treated with antibiotics combined with albumin infusion in certain cases.
- Hepatorenal syndrome should be treated with a vasoconstrictor (i.e., terlipressin or noradrenaline) associated with albumin.

Introduction

Cirrhosis is the final stage of chronic liver disease, especially chronic hepatitis B and C, alcohol-related liver disease, and nonalcoholic fatty liver disease. It is the consequence of a long-term wound-healing process in the liver, which leads to deposition of fibrotic tissue, formation of regenerative nodules, vascular rearrangement, and portal hypertension.[1]

Epidemiology

In 2019, it was estimated that 1.69 billion people had cirrhosis or chronic liver diseases (global prevalence of 20,710.1 per 100,000 persons), leading to 1.47 million deaths worldwide (mortality rate of 18 per 100,000 persons). Cirrhosis and chronic liver diseases are the conditions with the 10th highest mortality rate in the world. Mortality rate is particularly high in some tropical countries, such as Egypt, Cambodia, Myanmar, and Mexico (Figure 19.1).[1]

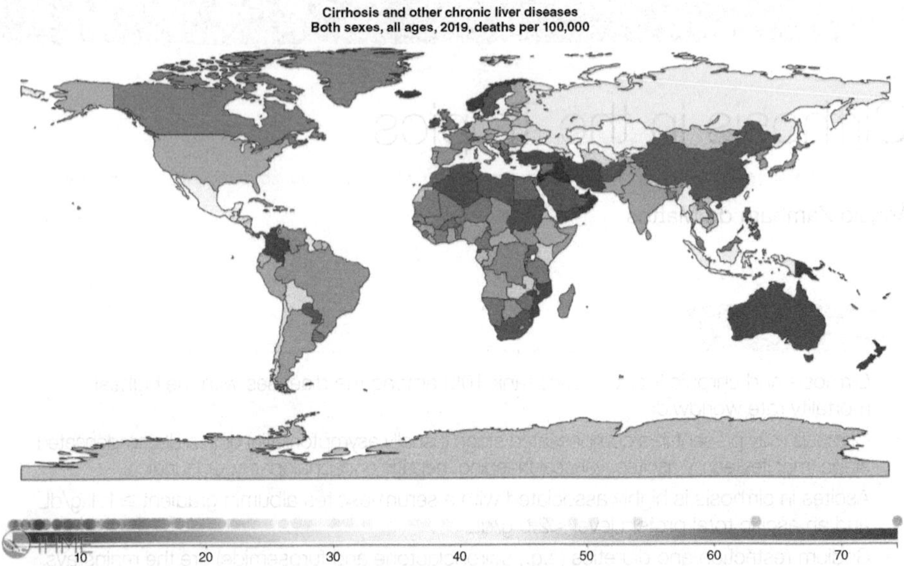

Figure 19.1 Worldwide mortality due to cirrhosis or other chronic liver diseases in 2019. (From Institute for Health Metrics Evaluation. Used with permission. All rights reserved.)

Presentation

Cirrhosis is traditionally classified as compensated and decompensated. Patients with compensated cirrhosis usually are asymptomatic and have a survival of approximately 12 years. Decompensated cirrhosis is associated with a survival of 2 to 4 years and is typically manifested by ascites, variceal bleeding, hepatic encephalopathy (HE), or jaundice. Decompensation may present in a nonacute manner, with a slowly progressive development of mild ascites, HE or jaundice (nonacute decompensation), or in an acute form, leading to hospital admission due to rapid development of moderate-large ascites, HE, digestive bleeding, or infection (acute decompensation).[2]

Acute-on-chronic liver failure (ACLF) is an extreme form of acute decompensation of cirrhosis, characterized by one or more organ failures developing in a short period of time with high mortality.[3] ACLF is diagnosed in nearly 35% of patients admitted with acute decompensation and carries a 90-day mortality of 58%. Mortality has been reported to be higher in South America (73%) and South Asia (68%).[4] There are different definitions and diagnostic criteria for ACLF, but the one proposed by the Chronic Liver Failure Consortium (CLIF-C)[3] seems to have the best performance for predicting mortality.[5] The prognosis of patients with ACLF diagnosed according to this definition can be estimated by the CLIF-C ACLF score,[6] which yields better results compared to other prognostic scores for this population and has been validated in tropical settings, such as Brazil.[7]

Acute decompensation may follow one of three different paths: stable decompensated cirrhosis (no readmissions nor development of ACLF in 90 days, 1-year mortality of 9.5%); unstable decompensated cirrhosis (further hospital admission in 90 days, without ACLF, 90-day and 1-year mortality rates of 21.0% and 35.6%, respectively); and pre-ACLF (development of ACLF in 90 days, 90-day and 1-year mortality rates of 53.7% and 67.4%, respectively).[8]

Diagnosis

Liver biopsy is the reference standard for the diagnosis of cirrhosis, although this is being replaced by noninvasive methods. More frequently the diagnosis is usually made through the analysis of clinical, laboratory, imaging, and endoscopic data: presence of chronic liver disease or risk factors for cirrhosis, stigmata of cirrhosis, ascites, jaundice, low platelet count, irregular liver surface, splenomegaly, esophageal varices, among others. Noninvasive methods (elastography, AST to platelet ratio index [APRI], Fibrosis-4 index [FIB-4], and others) could also aid in this diagnosis, but their cut-off points vary according to the cause of liver disease.[9] Among noninvasive methods, elastography seems to have a better performance for the detection of cirrhosis when compared to APRI, for instance, but serum markers might be more widely available in resource-limited countries.[10]

Management of Cirrhosis Complications

Hepatocellular carcinoma (HCC) will be approached in a specific chapter of this book, but it should be highlighted that patients with cirrhosis must be submitted to surveillance with ultrasound every 6 months[11-13] and that adding alpha-fetoprotein to the surveillance strategy could improve sensitivity.[14]

ASCITES

Ascites is the most common expression of decompensation of cirrhosis. Patients who develop ascites grades 2 or 3 for the first time must undergo diagnostic paracentesis, including polymorphonuclear (PMN) leukocyte count, culture, total protein concentration, and serum-ascites albumin gradient (SAAG). Ascites due to cirrhosis is highly associated with a SAAG $\geq$1.1 g/dL and an ascitic total protein $<$2.5 g/dL. Whenever a patient with cirrhosis and ascites develops a decompensation or is admitted to the hospital, a diagnostic paracentesis (including at least PMN count and culture of ascites) should be considered.[15,16]

Ascites should be initially managed through dietary sodium restriction (2g or 90 mmol/day) and diuretics, with the aim of a weight loss of 0.5 kg/day for patients without peripheral edema or 1 kg/day for those with edema. Aldosterone antagonists (e.g., spironolactone, which could be started at 100 mg/day and increased up to 400 mg/day in increments of 100 mg every 3–5 days) are the preferred diuretics for mobilizing ascites. The addition of loop diuretics (e.g., furosemide, which could be initiated at 40 mg/day and increased up to 160 mg/day) should be considered if the desired weight loss is not achieved.[15-17] In patients with recidivating ascites both classes of diuretics could be initiated simultaneously.[15,16,18] No specific treatment is formally recommended for ascites grade 1 (only detected by imaging methods).[15,16]

Patients with ascites grade 3 should be treated with large-volume paracentesis, with volume expansion with intravenous albumin 8 g per liter of ascites removed (6–8 g/L according to the American Association for the Study of Liver Diseases [AASLD]), especially for paracentesis $>$5 L.[15,16,19] For patients with ACLF, the benefits of albumin have been demonstrated even for modest-volume paracentesis.[20] After therapeutic paracentesis, diuretics could be started if no contraindications are present.[15,16] Ascites should be sent for analysis of PMN count and culture in every therapeutic paracentesis.[15]

Ascites is considered refractory when it cannot be mobilized with diuretics or recurs soon after large-volume paracentesis despite sodium restriction and diuretics. This condition is usually treated with large-volume paracentesis combined with albumin infusion,[15,16] but transjugular intrahepatic portosystemic shunt (TIPS) might be associated with improved survival, particularly when covered stents are used.[21,22] Given the poor prognosis associated with refractory ascites, such patients should be considered for liver transplantation when possible.[15,16]

Long-term albumin infusion is being studied for patients with cirrhosis and ascites.[23-25] However, evidence still is insufficient for a formal recommendation to be made.[15,26]

VARICEAL BLEEDING

Prophylaxis of First Variceal Bleeding or First Decompensation

Esophageal varices are present in 42% of patients with compensated cirrhosis and 72% of those with decompensated cirrhosis. Bleeding from esophageal varices occurs at a rate of 5% to 15% per year, with a mortality of approximately 20%. In order to avoid variceal bleeding, until recently, primary prophylaxis with a nonselective beta-blocker (NSBB—i.e., propranolol, nadolol, or carvedilol) or with endoscopic variceal ligation (EVL) was indicated for individuals with high-risk varices (medium- or large-sized varices or small varices in the presence of red marks or cirrhosis classified as Child-Pugh C).[16,27,28]

However, in 2021, the Baveno VII Consensus[26] proposed substantial changes in this regard, based on an RCT that has demonstrated improved prognosis in individuals with clinically significant portal hypertension (CSPH) who were treated with NSBBs, despite the absence of high-risk varices.[29] According to the Baveno VII Consensus, prophylaxis with NSBB against decompensation of cirrhosis (not only variceal bleeding) should be considered in all patients with compensated cirrhosis and CSPH (hepatic venous pressure gradient—HVPG ≥10 mm Hg). Individuals under prophylaxis with NSBB can spare variceal screening with esophagogastroduodenoscopy (EGD). On the other hand, patients with decompensated cirrhosis who are not under NSBB should be submitted to variceal screening with EGD.[26]

This consensus has also reinforced that CSPH is very unlikely in individuals with liver stiffness measurement (LSM) by transient elastography ≤15 kPa plus platelet count ≥150,000/mm^3, while LSM ≥25 kPa, LSM ≥20 kPa plus platelet count <150,000/mm^3, or LSM ≥15 kPa plus platelet count <110,000/mm^3 are associated with high risk of CSPH, indicating prophylaxis with NSBB.[26,30,31] Considering that HVPG measuring is an invasive procedure and that both HVPG measuring and elastography are not widely available in resource-limited settings, we understand that individuals with compensated cirrhosis and other signs suggestive of CSPH might also be considered for prophylaxis (esophageal varices of any grade, gastric varices, enlarged spleen, collateral circulation or enlarged portal vein on imaging exams, low platelet count, among others).

When indicated, propranolol should be started at doses of 20 to 40 mg twice daily and increased up to 320 mg/day if necessary (160 mg/day if ascites[28] and probably not over 80 mg/day if refractory ascites[16]). Ideally, the dose is titrated according to HVPG, but given the invasive character of its measurement, it is usually titrated in order to achieve a heart rate of 55 to 60 beats per minute, with a systolic blood pressure ≥90 mm Hg. Carvedilol should be started at 6.25 mg/day and increased to 12.5 mg/day if tolerated.[28] The Baveno VII Consensus gives preference to carvedilol over propranolol if available.[26] Nadolol is another potential option, when available. NSBBs should be avoided in individuals with systolic blood pressure <90 mm Hg, sodium <130 mmol/L, or acute kidney injury (AKI).[16]

Patients with compensated cirrhosis who have contraindications or intolerance to NSBB should undergo variceal screening with EGD if they have LSM ≥20 kPa or platelet count ≤150,000/mm^3 (LSM and platelet count should be repeated annually if not reaching these cutoffs). In the presence of high-risk varices and considering NSBB is potentially contraindicated, they should be evaluated for EVL.[26] EVL should be repeated every 2 to 8 weeks until variceal eradication, after which an EGD should be repeated once at 3 to 6 months, and every 6 to 12 months thereafter.[28]

Acute Variceal Bleeding

When digestive bleeding develops in a patient with cirrhosis, admission to the intensive care unit is strongly advised, and patients should receive careful volume expansion in order to achieve hemodynamic stability, as well as oxygen supplementation if necessary (including airway protection if neurological impairment or persistent hematemesis). However, blood transfusions should be restrictive and target a hemoglobin level of 7 to 8 g/dL as further expansion of the intravascular bed could worsen the bleed.[26,32] Removal of blood from the gut by the administration of lactulose (orally if the patient is safe to have intake, or by enemas) should be considered in order to prevent HE. Besides, abdominal imaging (contrast-enhanced imaging or, at least, ultrasound with Doppler studies, depending on renal function) is recommended for all patients with variceal bleeding in order to examine the splanchnic vascular system and to exclude HCC.[26]

A vasoactive drug that decreases portal pressure should be started as early as possible, preferably before EGD, and kept for 3 to 5 days. Alternatives are intravenous terlipressin 2 mg every 4 hours during the first 2 days and 1 mg every 4 hours thereafter; intravenous bolus of octreotide 50 μg, followed by 50 μg/hour; or intravenous bolus of somatostatin 250 μg, followed by 250 μg/hour.[16,26-28,33]

Digestive bleeding is a risk factor for infections in cirrhosis, and primary prophylaxis should be initiated as soon as possible (at the moment of admission) and maintained for 7 days. Norfloxacin 400 mg twice a day orally is usually prescribed, but ceftriaxone 1 g/day intravenously should be preferred in settings with high prevalence of multidrug-resistant (MDR) bacteria, for individuals already on prophylaxis with norfloxacin, or for those who present with ≥2 of the following criteria: ascites, HE, severe malnutrition, or bilirubin >3 mg/dL.[16,26-28,34]

EGD should be performed in the first 12 hours of the bleeding episode (in the absence of contraindications, intravenous erythromycin 250 mg 30 to 120 minutes before EGD may be useful). EVL is the endoscopic treatment of choice for esophageal varices, and sclerotherapy should be reserved for situations in which EVL is not technically feasible.[16,26-28,35] After endoscopic/pharmacological hemostasis, early pre-emptive covered TIPS (within 24–72 hours from the bleeding episode) could be considered to reduce the risk of rebleeding for patients classified as Child-Pugh B with active bleeding during EGD (particularly for those with a Child-Pugh score >7 points), Child-Pugh C (<14 points), or for individuals with HVPG >20 mm Hg at the time of hemorrhage.[16,26-28,36]

TIPS is also indicated as a rescue therapy for individuals with persistent bleeding or early rebleeding after 1 or 2 attempts of endoscopic and pharmacological treatment. Balloon tamponade or removable, covered, and self-expanding esophageal stents could be used as a bridge therapy.[16,26-28,36] Balloon tamponade provides temporary hemostasis in up to 80% of cases, but it is associated with a mortality rate near 20%. Ideally it should be used for a maximum of 24 hours, and it is advisable that the patient is intubated (to avoid aspiration pneumonia) and, if available, in the intensive care unit.[16,28]

Balloon tamponade should be reserved for hemodynamically unstable patients with massive refractory bleeding until a more definitive treatment can be provided. The three most commonly used devices are: the Linton-Nachlas tube, which has a single gastric balloon and usually has two ports (gastric balloon inflation port and gastric suction port); the Sengstaken-Blakemore tube, which has a gastric balloon and an esophageal balloon and usually has three ports (gastric balloon inflation port, esophageal balloon inflation port, and gastric suction port); and the Minnesota tube, which has a gastric balloon and an esophageal balloon, as well as four ports (gastric balloon inflation port, esophageal balloon inflation port, gastric suction port, and esophageal suction port). After the device is in place, the patient should be kept with the head of the bed elevated to 45°, continuous suction should be considered for the first 12 hours, and frequent assessments for bleeding, mucosal ulcerations, and balloon pressure are recommended.[37]

Secondary Prophylaxis

Secondary prophylaxis against variceal bleeding should be performed by combining EVL with NSBB (carvedilol or propranolol), which usually should be started on the sixth day after the bleeding episode.[16,26-28]

HEPATIC ENCEPHALOPATHY

HE is a neurological dysfunction associated with liver insufficiency and portosystemic shunts. According to the West Haven criteria, it can be classified as follows: grade I, presenting with shortened attention span, altered sleep rhythm, impairment of subtraction or addition, and anxiety, among other symptoms; grade II, presenting with lethargy, disorientation, confusion, inappropriate behavior, and asterixis, among other manifestations; grade III, characterized by semi-stupor and being responsive to stimuli; and grade IV, characterized by coma. Minimal encephalopathy is diagnosed through psychometric or neuropsychological tests. The main precipitating factors are infections, digestive bleeding, diuretics overdose, electrolyte disturbances, use of psychoactive drugs, and constipation. Aside from approaching the precipitating factor, the first line treatment is lactulose, which could be started at a dose of 25 mL orally twice a day and adjusted with the aim of achieving two to three soft bowel movements per day. Rifaximin 550 mg twice daily may be associated if HE recurs despite the use of lactulose. Other treatments, such as neomycin, metronidazole, or L-ornithine L-aspartate, might also be considered, but they represent suboptimal options.[38]

INFECTIONS

Spontaneous Bacterial Peritonitis

Spontaneous bacterial peritonitis (SBP) is a spontaneous infection of the ascitic fluid in the absence of another identifiable intra-abdominal source, likely caused by bacterial translocation. Diagnosis should be assumed when a PMN count >250/mm^3 is detected in ascites. Treatment combining antibiotics and albumin infusion (1.5 g/kg on the first day and 1 g/kg on the third day) reduces the risk of renal impairment and improves survival.[39] Despite international guidelines recommending that albumin at the abovementioned doses are administrated to all patients with SBP,[15,16] in settings where the availability of albumin is restricted, one might consider prioritizing patients with bilirubin ≥4 mg/dL or with creatinine ≥1 mg/dL, since they had worse prognosis in the original trial.[39] Moreover, there are authors who defend that lower doses of albumin might also be useful.[40]

There is an increasing prevalence of MDR bacteria in infections in cirrhosis worldwide, and some tropical countries are particularly affected. According to an international prospective cohort study, 34% of infections in patients with cirrhosis were caused by MDR bacteria, a prevalence that was greater in Asia, and especially in India, where MDR bacteria were detected in 73% of isolates.[41] In a Brazilian study MDR bacteria were detected in 37.5% of isolates of individuals with cirrhosis.[42] Therefore empirical antibiotic therapy should ideally be based on local resistance profiles. In the absence of local data a suggestion of broad-spectrum empirical antibiotic treatment is given in Table 19.1.[16,43] Antibiotics should be revised according to culture when it becomes available. If possible, a diagnostic paracentesis should be repeated 48 hours after the beginning of antibiotics to evaluate treatment response. In the absence of a decrease of at least 25% in PMN count, antibiotic spectrum should be broadened and the possibility of secondary peritonitis should be considered.[15]

Secondary prophylaxis should be implemented after the first episode of SBP and maintained for as long as the patient has ascites or until transplantation. Norfloxacin 400 mg once a day is the antibiotic of choice. Ciprofloxacin, rifaximin, and sulfamethoxazole/trimethoprim might be

TABLE 19.1 ■ **Empirical Antibiotic Therapy for the Most Common Infections in Cirrhosis**

	Community-Acquired Infections	Healthcare-Associated and Nosocomial Infections*
Spontaneous bacterial peritonitis	Third-generation cephalosporins or piperacillin-tazobactam	Carbapenems ± vancomycin, or daptomycin, or linezolid
Skin and soft tissue infections	Piperacillin-tazobactam or third-generation cephalosporins + oxacillin	Third-generation cephalosporins or meropenem + oxacillin, or glycopeptide, or daptomycin, or linezolid
Pneumonia	Piperacillin-tazobactam or ceftriaxone + macrolide	Ceftazidime or meropenem + levofloxacin ± glycopeptide or linezolid
Urinary tract infection	Uncomplicated—ciprofloxacin or sulfamethoxazole/trimethoprim	Uncomplicated—fosfomycin or nitrofurantoin
	Sepsis—third-generation cephalosporins or piperacillin-tazobactam	Sepsis—meropenem + glycopeptide

*Healthcare-associated infections in settings with low prevalence of multidrug-resistant bacteria could be treated as community-acquired infections, except if sepsis.
Based on recommendations from the European Association for the Study of the Liver.[16]

alternatives, but evidence supporting these options is still limited. Primary prophylaxis is indicated in the context of bleeding passing through the digestive tract (irrespective of the presence of ascites, as outlined in the Variceal Bleeding subsection) and when total protein level in ascites is <1.5 g/dL in patients with signs of advanced dysfunction of the liver (Child-Pugh ≥9 with bilirubin ≥3 mg/dL) or the kidneys (creatinine ≥1.2 mg/dL, blood urea nitrogen ≥25 mg/dL, or sodium ≤130 mmol/L), a situation in which long-term norfloxacin 400 mg daily improves survival.[44]

Extraperitoneal Infections

Patients with cirrhosis are immunocompromised, and infections are extremely common. However, their presentation may be subtle and high clinical suspicion is of the utmost importance in order for the treatment not to be delayed. The diagnostic criteria for extraperitoneal infections in patients with cirrhosis are usually similar to those used for patients without liver disease. Considering the high prevalence of infections caused by MDR bacteria in individuals with cirrhosis, a broad-spectrum empirical antibiotic therapy is recommended until culture results are available, and a suggestion for the most common infections is provided in Table 19.1.[16,43] Evidence does not support a general recommendation for albumin infusion in patients with cirrhosis and extraperitoneal infections at this time.[45]

ACUTE KIDNEY INJURY AND HEPATORENAL SYNDROME

AKI is present in almost 30% of patients hospitalized for acute decompensation of cirrhosis, although hepatorenal syndrome (HRS) is the culprit in less than half of AKI cases.[46] AKI is diagnosed in an individual with cirrhosis when there is an increase in serum creatinine ≥0.3 mg/dL in 48 hours or ≥50% from baseline assumed to have occurred in the previous 7 days. Mortality appears to increase substantially in patients with AKI stage ≥1b (increase in creatinine ≥1.5-fold to 2-fold compared to the baseline with maximum creatinine ≥1.5 mg/dL, increase in creatinine >2-fold, increase in creatinine ≥0.3 mg/dL to a value ≥4 mg/dL, or necessity of dialysis).[16,47-50]

Despite not being the most common cause of AKI in cirrhosis, HRS certainly carries some of the worst prognosis. HRS-AKI (formerly referred to as HRS type 1) is diagnosed in patients with cirrhosis and ascites who develop AKI, without improvement after 48 hours of suspension of diuretics and volume expansion with albumin 1 g/kg/day, as long as shock, use of nephrotoxic drugs, and parenchymal renal injury (evidenced by urinary protein ≥500 mg/24 hours, ≥50 red blood cells/high power field, abnormal findings on renal imaging) are ruled out.[15,16,47] In patients using a urinary catheter, a urinary output ≤0.5 mL/kg over ≥6 hours might be an alternative diagnostic parameter.[51] HRS-non-AKI (HRS-NAKI, previously called HRS type 2) can be divided in to the following: HRS-acute kidney disease (HRS-AKD), which is diagnosed in patients with cirrhosis and ascites who have an estimated glomerular filtration rate <60 mL/minute per 1.73 m^2 or who develop an increase in creatinine <50% from baseline for up to 3 months, without structural renal damage; and HRS-chronic kidney disease (HRS-CKD), which is diagnosed in patients with cirrhosis and ascites who have an estimated glomerular filtration rate <60 mL/minute per 1.73 m^2 for >3 months, without structural renal damage.[51]

AKI stage 1a should be managed by removing risk factors. AKI stage ≥1b should be managed with complete withdrawal of diuretics and volume expansion with albumin 1 g/kg/day for 48 hours. In the absence of improvement and if the patient meets the other diagnostic criteria for HRS (see above), treatment combining a vasoconstrictor and albumin (1 g/kg on the first day and 20–40 g/day thereafter) should be initiated and maintained for up to 14 days. Moreover, it is worth noting that HRS is a sign of end-stage liver disease and should prompt an evaluation for liver transplantation.[15,16]

Terlipressin is the vasoconstrictor supported by the most robust body of evidence and should be started at doses of 0.5 to 1.0 mg every 4 to 6 hours. If creatinine does not decrease by ≥25% in 2 days, doses can be doubled every 48 hours, up to 12 mg/day. Treatment can be suspended if creatinine does not decrease ≥50% after 7 days of the highest dose or if there is no improvement at all in 3 days.[16,52-58] Alternatively, noradrenaline (0.5–3.0 mg/hour, with the aim of increasing mean arterial pressure by ≥10 mm Hg) could be combined with albumin.[15,59-64] Both terlipressin and noradrenaline combined with albumin are superior to albumin alone or to the combination of midodrine, octreotide, and albumin in the treatment of HRS.[65]

Terlipressin is more expensive than noradrenaline, but the former can be administered in a regular ward, while the latter should be administered in an intensive care setting. Brazilian studies have demonstrated that a strategy with terlipressin is more economically feasible than noradrenaline.[66,67] Moreover, a recent RCT performed in patients with HRS and ACLF has demonstrated that terlipressin is superior to noradrenaline regarding HRS reversal and mortality reduction.[68]

In the absence of terlipressin and if an intensive care unit is not available, the combination of midodrine and octreotide (along with albumin at the previously mentioned doses) might be an option. Midodrine could be initiated at 7.5 mg orally every 8 hours, and octreotide at 100 μg subcutaneously every 8 hours. Doses could be progressively increased up to 12.5 mg and 200 μg every 8 hours, respectively, if creatinine fails to decrease by ≥25% from baseline. However, it must be highlighted that the combination of midodrine and octreotide is a suboptimal treatment and that an RCT comparing it with terlipressin had to be prematurely terminated due to the significant superiority of the latter (complete response in 4.8% of patients receiving midodrine and octreotide and in 55.5% of those receiving terlipressin, $p < 0.001$).[69]

References

1. GBD 2019 Diseases and Injuries Collaborators. Global burden of 369 diseases and injuries in 204 countries and territories, 1990–2019: a systematic analysis for the Global Burden of Disease Study 2019. *Lancet.* 2020;396(10258):1204-1222. doi:10.1016/S0140-6736(20)30925-9.

2. D'Amico G, Bernardi M, Angeli P. Towards a new definition of decompensated cirrhosis. *J Hepatol.* 2022;76(1):202-207. doi:10.1016/j.jhep.2021.06.018.
3. Moreau R, Jalan R, Gines P, et al. Acute-on-chronic liver failure is a distinct syndrome that develops in patients with acute decompensation of cirrhosis. *Gastroenterology.* 2013;144(7):1426-1437, 1437.e1-9. doi:10.1053/j.gastro.2013.02.042.
4. Mezzano G, Juanola A, Cardenas A, et al. Global burden of disease: acute-on-chronic liver failure, a systematic review and meta-analysis. *Gut.* 2022;71(1):148-155. doi:10.1136/gutjnl-2020-322161.
5. Leão GS, Lunardi FL, Picon RV, Tovo CV, de Mattos AA, de Mattos Â. Acute-on-chronic liver failure: a comparison of three different diagnostic criteria. *Ann Hepatol.* 2019;18(2):373-378. doi:10.1016/j.aohep.2019.01.001.
6. Jalan R, Saliba F, Pavesi M, et al. Development and validation of a prognostic score to predict mortality in patients with acute-on-chronic liver failure. *J Hepatol.* 2014;61(5):1038-1047. doi:10.1016/j.jhep.2014.06.012.
7. Picon RV, Bertol FS, Tovo CV, de Mattos Â. Chronic liver failure-consortium acute-on-chronic liver failure and acute decompensation scores predict mortality in Brazilian cirrhotic patients. *World J Gastroenterol.* 2017;23(28):5237-5245. doi:10.3748/wjg.v23.i28.5237.
8. Trebicka J, Fernandez J, Papp M, et al. The PREDICT study uncovers three clinical courses of acutely decompensated cirrhosis that have distinct pathophysiology. *J Hepatol.* 2020;73(4):842-854. doi:10.1016/j.jhep.2020.06.013.
9. European Association for the Study of the Liver. EASL Clinical Practice Guidelines on non-invasive tests for evaluation of liver disease severity and prognosis: 2021 update. *J Hepatol.* 2021;75(3):659-689. doi:10.1016/j.jhep.2021.05.025.
10. Mattos AZ, Mattos AA. Transient elastography vs. aspartate aminotransferase to platelet ratio index in hepatitis C: a meta-analysis. *Ann Hepatol.* 2017;16(3):349-357. doi:10.5604/16652681.1235477.
11. European Association for the Study of the Liver. EASL Clinical Practice Guidelines: management of hepatocellular carcinoma. *J Hepatol.* 2018;69(1):182-236. doi:10.1016/j.jhep.2018.03.019.
12. Heimbach JK, Kulik LM, Finn RS, et al. AASLD guidelines for the treatment of hepatocellular carcinoma. *Hepatology.* 2018;67(1):358-380. doi:10.1002/hep.29086.
13. Marrero JA, Kulik LM, Sirlin CB, et al. Diagnosis, staging, and management of hepatocellular carcinoma: 2018 Practice Guidance by the American Association for the Study of Liver Diseases. *Hepatology.* 2018;68(2):723-750. doi:10.1002/hep.29913.
14. Tzartzeva K, Obi J, Rich NE, et al. Surveillance imaging and alpha fetoprotein for early detection of hepatocellular carcinoma in patients with cirrhosis: a meta-analysis. *Gastroenterology.* 2018;154(6):1706-1718.e1. doi:10.1053/j.gastro.2018.01.064.
15. Biggins SW, Angeli P, Garcia-Tsao G, et al. Diagnosis, evaluation, and management of ascites, spontaneous bacterial peritonitis and hepatorenal syndrome: 2021 Practice Guidance by the American Association for the Study of Liver Diseases. *Hepatology.* 2021;74(2):1014-1048. doi:10.1002/hep.31884.
16. European Association for the Study of the Liver. EASL Clinical Practice Guidelines for the management of patients with decompensated cirrhosis. *J Hepatol.* 2018;69(2):406-460. doi:10.1016/j.jhep.2018.03.024.
17. Santos J, Planas R, Pardo A, et al. Spironolactone alone or in combination with furosemide in the treatment of moderate ascites in nonazotemic cirrhosis: a randomized comparative study of efficacy and safety. *J Hepatol.* 2003;39(2):187-192. doi:10.1016/s0168-8278(03)00188-0.
18. Angeli P, Fasolato S, Mazza E, et al. Combined versus sequential diuretic treatment of ascites in non-azotaemic patients with cirrhosis: results of an open randomised clinical trial. *Gut.* 2010;59(1):98-104. doi:10.1136/gut.2008.176495.
19. Ginès P, Titó L, Arroyo V, et al. Randomized comparative study of therapeutic paracentesis with and without intravenous albumin in cirrhosis. *Gastroenterology.* 1988;94(6):1493-1502. doi:10.1016/0016-5085(88)90691-9.
20. Arora V, Vijayaraghavan R, Maiwall R, et al. Paracentesis-induced circulatory dysfunction with modest-volume paracentesis is partly ameliorated by albumin infusion in acute-on-chronic liver failure. *Hepatology.* 2020;72(3):1043-1055. doi:10.1002/hep.31071.
21. Bai M, Qi XS, Yang ZP, Yang M, Fan DM, Han GH. TIPS improves liver transplantation-free survival in cirrhotic patients with refractory ascites: an updated meta-analysis. *World J Gastroenterol.* 2014;20(10):2704-2714. doi:10.3748/wjg.v20.i10.2704.

22. Bureau C, Thabut D, Oberti F, et al. Transjugular intrahepatic portosystemic shunts with covered stents increase transplant-free survival of patients with cirrhosis and recurrent ascites. *Gastroenterology.* 2017;152(1):157-163. doi:10.1053/j.gastro.2016.09.016.
23. Caraceni P, Riggio O, Angeli P, et al. Long-term albumin administration in decompensated cirrhosis (ANSWER): an open-label randomised trial. *Lancet.* 2018;391(10138):2417-2429. doi:10.1016/S0140-6736(18)30840-7.
24. Solà E, Solé C, Simón-Talero M, et al. Midodrine and albumin for prevention of complications in patients with cirrhosis awaiting liver transplantation: a randomized placebo-controlled trial. *J Hepatol.* 2018;69(6):1250-1259. doi:10.1016/j.jhep.2018.08.006.
25. Sandi BB, Leão GS, de Mattos AA, de Mattos Â. Long-term albumin administration in patients with cirrhosis and ascites: a meta-analysis of randomized controlled trials. *J Gastroenterol Hepatol.* 2021; 36(3):609-617. doi:10.1111/jgh.15253.
26. de Franchis R, Bosch J, Garcia-Tsao G, Reiberger T, Ripoll C, Faculty BV. Baveno VII: renewing consensus in portal hypertension. *J Hepatol.* 2022;76(4):959-974. doi:10.1016/j.jhep.2021.12.022.
27. de Franchis R, Faculty BV. Expanding consensus in portal hypertension: Report of the Baveno VI Consensus Workshop: stratifying risk and individualizing care for portal hypertension. *J Hepatol.* 2015;63(3):743-752. doi:10.1016/j.jhep.2015.05.022.
28. Garcia-Tsao G, Abraldes JG, Berzigotti A, Bosch J. Portal hypertensive bleeding in cirrhosis: risk stratification, diagnosis, and management: 2016 practice guidance by the American Association for the study of liver diseases. *Hepatology.* 2017;65(1):310-335. doi:10.1002/hep.28906.
29. Villanueva C, Albillos A, Genescà J, et al. β blockers to prevent decompensation of cirrhosis in patients with clinically significant portal hypertension (PREDESCI): a randomised, double-blind, placebo-controlled, multicentre trial. *Lancet.* 2019;393(10181):1597-1608. doi:10.1016/S0140-6736(18)31875-0.
30. Abraldes JG, Bureau C, Stefanescu H, et al. Noninvasive tools and risk of clinically significant portal hypertension and varices in compensated cirrhosis: the "Anticipate" study. *Hepatology.* 2016;64(6): 2173-2184. doi:10.1002/hep.28824.
31. Maurice JB, Brodkin E, Arnold F, et al. Validation of the Baveno VI criteria to identify low risk cirrhotic patients not requiring endoscopic surveillance for varices. *J Hepatol.* 2016;65(5):899-905. doi:10.1016/j.jhep.2016.06.021.
32. Villanueva C, Colomo A, Bosch A, et al. Transfusion strategies for acute upper gastrointestinal bleeding. *N Engl J Med.* 2013;368(1):11-21. doi:10.1056/NEJMoa1211801.
33. Seo YS, Park SY, Kim MY, et al. Lack of difference among terlipressin, somatostatin, and octreotide in the control of acute gastroesophageal variceal hemorrhage. *Hepatology.* 2014;60(3):954-963. doi:10.1002/hep.27006.
34. Fernández J, Ruiz del Arbol L, Gómez C, et al. Norfloxacin vs ceftriaxone in the prophylaxis of infections in patients with advanced cirrhosis and hemorrhage. *Gastroenterology.* 2006;131(4):1049-1056; quiz 1285. doi:10.1053/j.gastro.2006.07.010.
35. Lo GH, Lai KH, Cheng JS, et al. Emergency banding ligation versus sclerotherapy for the control of active bleeding from esophageal varices. *Hepatology.* 1997;25(5):1101-1104. doi:10.1002/hep.510250509.
36. Nicoară-Farcău O, Han G, Rudler M, et al. Effects of early placement of transjugular portosystemic shunts in patients with high-risk acute variceal bleeding: a meta-analysis of individual patient data. *Gastroenterology.* 2021;160(1):193-205.e10. doi:10.1053/j.gastro.2020.09.026.
37. Bridwell RE, Long B, Ramzy M, Gottlieb M. Balloon tamponade for the management of gastrointestinal bleeding. *J Emerg Med.* 2022;62(4):545-558. doi:10.1016/j.jemermed.2021.11.004.
38. American Association for the Study of Liver Diseases, European Association for the Study of the Liver. Hepatic encephalopathy in chronic liver disease: 2014 practice guideline by the European Association for the Study of the Liver and the American Association for the Study of Liver Diseases. *J Hepatol.* 2014;61(3):642-659. doi:10.1016/j.jhep.2014.05.042.
39. Sort P, Navasa M, Arroyo V, et al. Effect of intravenous albumin on renal impairment and mortality in patients with cirrhosis and spontaneous bacterial peritonitis. *N Engl J Med.* 1999;341(6):403-409. doi:10.1056/NEJM199908053410603.
40. de Araujo A, de Barros Lopes A, Rossi G, et al. Low-dose albumin in the treatment of spontaneous bacterial peritonitis: should we change the standard treatment? *Gut.* 2012;61(9):1371-1372. doi:10.1136/gutjnl-2011-301739.

41. Piano S, Singh V, Caraceni P, et al. Epidemiology and effects of bacterial infections in patients with cirrhosis worldwide. *Gastroenterology*. 2019;156(5):1368-1380.e10. doi:10.1053/j.gastro.2018.12.005.
42. Costabeber AM, Mattos AA, Sukiennik TC. Prevalence of bacterial resistance in hospitalized cirrhotic patients in Southern Brazil: a new challenge. *Rev Inst Med Trop Sao Paulo*. 2016;58:36. doi:10.1590/S1678-9946201658036.
43. Mattos AA, Wiltgen D, Jotz RF, Dornelles CMR, Fernandes MV, Mattos Â. Spontaneous bacterial peritonitis and extraperitoneal infections in patients with cirrhosis. *Ann Hepatol*. 2020;19(5):451-457. doi:10.1016/j.aohep.2020.04.010.
44. Fernández J, Navasa M, Planas R, et al. Primary prophylaxis of spontaneous bacterial peritonitis delays hepatorenal syndrome and improves survival in cirrhosis. *Gastroenterology*. 2007;133(3):818-824. doi:10.1053/j.gastro.2007.06.065.
45. Leão GS, John Neto G, Jotz RF, Mattos AA, Mattos Â. Albumin for cirrhotic patients with extraperitoneal infections: a meta-analysis. *J Gastroenterol Hepatol*. 2019;34(12):2071-2076. doi:10.1111/jgh.14791.
46. Desai AP, Knapp SM, Orman ES, et al. Changing epidemiology and outcomes of acute kidney injury in hospitalized patients with cirrhosis: a US population-based study. *J Hepatol*. 2020;73(5):1092-1099. doi:10.1016/j.jhep.2020.04.043.
47. Angeli P, Ginès P, Wong F, et al. Diagnosis and management of acute kidney injury in patients with cirrhosis: revised consensus recommendations of the International Club of Ascites. *J Hepatol*. 2015; 62(4):968-974. doi:10.1016/j.jhep.2014.12.029.
48. Fagundes C, Barreto R, Guevara M, et al. A modified acute kidney injury classification for diagnosis and risk stratification of impairment of kidney function in cirrhosis. *J Hepatol*. 2013;59(3):474-481. doi:10.1016/j.jhep.2013.04.036.
49. Schacher FC, Mattos AA, Mulazzani CM, et al. Impact of actue kidney injury staging on prognosis of patients wit cirrhosis. *Arq Gastroenterol*. 2020;57(3):244-248. doi:10.1590/S0004-2803.202000000-46.
50. Leão GS, de Mattos AA, Picon RV, et al. The prognostic impact of different stages of acute kidney injury in patients with decompensated cirrhosis: a prospective cohort study. *Eur J Gastroenterol Hepatol*. 2021;33(1S suppl 1):e407-e412. doi:10.1097/MEG.0000000000002120.
51. Angeli P, Garcia-Tsao G, Nadim MK, Parikh CR. News in pathophysiology, definition and classification of hepatorenal syndrome: a step beyond the International Club of Ascites (ICA) consensus document. *J Hepatol*. 2019;71(4):811-822. doi:10.1016/j.jhep.2019.07.002.
52. Salerno F, Gerbes A, Ginès P, Wong F, Arroyo V. Diagnosis, prevention and treatment of hepatorenal syndrome in cirrhosis. *Gut*. 2007;56(9):1310-1318. doi:10.1136/gut.2006.107789.
53. Solanki P, Chawla A, Garg R, Gupta R, Jain M, Sarin SK. Beneficial effects of terlipressin in hepatorenal syndrome: a prospective, randomized placebo-controlled clinical trial. *J Gastroenterol Hepatol*. 2003; 18(2):152-156.
54. Sanyal AJ, Boyer T, Garcia-Tsao G, et al. A randomized, prospective, double-blind, placebo-controlled trial of terlipressin for type 1 hepatorenal syndrome. *Gastroenterology*. 2008;134(5):1360-1368. doi:10.1053/j.gastro.2008.02.014.
55. Martín-Llahí M, Pépin MN, Guevara M, et al. Terlipressin and albumin vs albumin in patients with cirrhosis and hepatorenal syndrome: a randomized study. *Gastroenterology*. 2008;134(5):1352-1359. doi:10.1053/j.gastro.2008.02.024.
56. Neri S, Pulvirenti D, Malaguarnera M, et al. Terlipressin and albumin in patients with cirrhosis and type I hepatorenal syndrome. *Dig Dis Sci*. 2008;53(3):830-835. doi:10.1007/s10620-007-9919-9.
57. Boyer TD, Sanyal AJ, Wong F, et al. Terlipressin plus albumin is more effective than albumin alone in improving renal function in patients with cirrhosis and hepatorenal syndrome type 1. *Gastroenterology*. 2016;150(7):1579-1589.e2. doi:10.1053/j.gastro.2016.02.026.
58. Wong F, Pappas SC, Curry MP, et al. Terlipressin plus albumin for the treatment of type 1 hepatorenal syndrome. *N Engl J Med*. 2021;384(9):818-828. doi:10.1056/NEJMoa2008290.
59. Alessandria C, Ottobrelli A, Debernardi-Venon W, et al. Noradrenalin vs terlipressin in patients with hepatorenal syndrome: a prospective, randomized, unblinded, pilot study. *J Hepatol*. 2007;47(4):499-505. doi:10.1016/j.jhep.2007.04.010.
60. Sharma P, Kumar A, Shrama BC, Sarin SK. An open label, pilot, randomized controlled trial of noradrenaline versus terlipressin in the treatment of type 1 hepatorenal syndrome and predictors of response. *Am J Gastroenterol*. 2008;103(7):1689-1697. doi:10.1111/j.1572-0241.2008.01828.x.

61. Singh V, Ghosh S, Singh B, et al. Noradrenaline vs. terlipressin in the treatment of hepatorenal syndrome: a randomized study. *J Hepatol.* 2012;56(6):1293-1298. doi:10.1016/j.jhep.2012.01.012.
62. Ghosh S, Choudhary NS, Sharma AK, et al. Noradrenaline vs terlipressin in the treatment of type 2 hepatorenal syndrome: a randomized pilot study. *Liver Int.* 2013;33(8):1187-1193. doi:10.1111/liv.12179.
63. Goyal O, Sidhu S, Sehgal N, Puri S. Noradrenaline is as effective as terlipressin in hepatorenal syndrome type 1: a prospective, randomized trial. *J Assoc Physicians India.* 2016;64(9):30-35.
64. Saif RU, Dar HA, Sofi SM, Andrabi MS, Javid G, Zargar SA. Noradrenaline versus terlipressin in the management of type 1 hepatorenal syndrome: a randomized controlled study. *Indian J Gastroenterol.* 2018;37(5):424-429. doi:10.1007/s12664-018-0876-3.
65. Best LM, Freeman SC, Sutton AJ, et al. Treatment for hepatorenal syndrome in people with decompensated liver cirrhosis: a network meta-analysis. *Cochrane Database Syst Rev.* 2019;9:CD013103. doi:10.1002/14651858.CD013103.pub2.
66. Mattos ÂZ, Mattos AA, Ribeiro RA. Terlipressin versus noradrenaline in the treatment of hepatorenal syndrome: systematic review with meta-analysis and full economic evaluation. *Eur J Gastroenterol Hepatol.* 2016;28(3):345-351. doi:10.1097/MEG.0000000000000537.
67. Mattos ÂZ, Mattos AA, Ribeiro RA. Terlipressin versus noradrenaline for hepatorenal syndrome. Economic evaluation under the perspective of the Brazilian Public Health System. *Arq Gastroenterol.* 2016;53(2):123-126. doi:10.1590/S0004-28032016000200014.
68. Arora V, Maiwall R, Rajan V, et al. Terlipressin is superior to noradrenaline in the management of acute kidney injury in acute on chronic liver failure. *Hepatology.* 2020;71(2):600-610. doi:10.1002/hep.30208.
69. Cavallin M, Kamath PS, Merli M, et al. Terlipressin plus albumin versus midodrine and octreotide plus albumin in the treatment of hepatorenal syndrome: a randomized trial. *Hepatology.* 2015;62(2):567-574. doi:10.1002/hep.27709.

CHAPTER 20

Metabolic Dysfunction Associated Steatotic Liver Disease in Resource-Limited Settings

Mark W. Sonderup ■ Luis Antonio Diaz ■ Juan Pablo Arab ■ Marco Arrese

KEY POINTS

- Metabolic dysfunction associated steatotic liver (MASLD), previously known as nonalcoholic fatty liver disease (NAFLD), is currently a global epidemic burdening health systems worldwide
- MASLD is closely linked to obesity and type 2 diabetes (T2DM), which in turn are risk factors for disease severity.
- Despite being a potentially serious condition, MASLD is largely underappreciated and remains absent on national and global health agendas.
- Some low- and middle-income countries bear the highest burden of obesity and T2DM globally and predictably have high MASLD prevalence, although good-quality data is lacking.
- Identification of cases with advanced fibrosis or cirrhosis using simple, non-invasive tools is critical to reducing liver disease burden.
- MASLD management in resource-limited settings should emphasize prevention physician education and take advantage of existing infrastructure to attempt multi-disciplinary approaches.

Metabolic dysfunction associated steatotic liver (MASLD), previously known as nonalcoholic fatty liver disease (NAFLD), refers to a spectrum of liver conditions spanning from isolated steatosis to steatohepatitis that can lead to serious liver disease, including cirrhosis, cancer, and death.[1] The condition, which is intrinsically linked to obesity and type 2 diabetes mellitus (T2DM), is reaching epidemic proportions worldwide and is associated with significant morbidity and mortality resulting in substantial healthcare costs and economic losses.[2,3] MASLD is considered a "silent" disease because most affected people are asymptomatic for long periods until they develop advanced disease.[4,5] The nosology of the excessive lipid accumulation in the liver had changed recently. In 2019, an international panel of experts recommended renaming nonalcoholic fatty liver disease (NAFLD) to metabolic dysfunction–associated fatty liver disease (MAFLD)[6] and adopting a set of positive criteria to diagnose the diseases that are independent of alcohol intake or other liver diseases.[7] This change was welcomed by the international community, but there was some criticisms due to the effects of the new definition on biomarker development and ongoing clinical trials as well as because of the lack of proper thresholds for alcohol intake.[8] For that reason, a multinational effort led by the American Association for the Study of Liver Diseases, the European Association for the Study of the Liver, the Latin American Association for the Study of the Liver, as well as other societies and organizations aimed to readdress the issue of the nomenclature and classification of hepatic steatosis. In the new proposal, excessive fat accumulation in the liver is referred to as steatotic liver disease (SLD), which serves as an overarching term to encompass the various etiologies of excessive lipid accumulation in the liver. This overarching term includes steatosis due to metabolic dysfunction, now termed MASLD, steatosis in the context of alcohol-related liver disease (ALD), steatosis in the context of MASLD and increased alcohol intake (named Met-ALD), and other aetiologies.[9] The more aggressive form of MASLD is called metabolic dysfunction associated steatohepatitis (MASH). Initial analyses suggest that MASLD/MASH overlaps with NAFLD in 99% of the cases and they can be used interchangeably.[10]

Epidemiological data related to MASLD suggest a global prevalence of 30% in the general population in 2019.[11] However, MASLD prevalence estimates for many countries are imperfect because primary data from some regions are scarce. That said, epidemiological projections based on available data on obesity and T2DM in most regions are worrisome.[3] In this setting countries with low-resource or resource-limited health systems face many challenges and obstacles to providing care for MASLD patients including the implementation of appropriate risk stratification and referral pathways from primary care.

MASLD Epidemiology in Latin America (LATAM) and Sub-Saharan Africa (SSA)

MASLD IN LATIN AMERICA

Epidemiological data on liver diseases in this region is limited or absent for some countries. As in other parts of the world, noncommunicable diseases are the leading cause of mortality in the area, ranging from 62% in Costa Rica to 84% in Chile.[12] Regarding MASLD, this condition has an estimated prevalence of 30% in the Latin American population.[13] However, primary data from Latin American countries is scarce, with only few published studies reporting the MASLD prevalence from Brazil (35.2%), Chile (23%), Mexico (17%), and Colombia (26.6%).[14] It should be noted that most of the studies were performed more than a decade ago, and therefore it is likely that the current MASLD prevalence in the region is higher.[15] Of note, examination of epidemiological figures for obesity and T2DM as indirect estimates of MASLD prevalence in the region suggests that MASLD prevalence likely increased in the last decade.[15,13] Importantly, some data points to the fact that the prevalence of MASH as a cause of cirrhosis had increased more than any other etiology in the region, with 8% to 11% of deaths due to cirrhosis being related to MASH in 2016.[12]

Currently, the prevalence of obesity in LATAM is among the highest globally.[16] In recent years the prevalence of this condition in LATAM has been increasing faster than in the rest of the world, being more critical in people of low socioeconomic status.[17] Indeed, the increasing prevalence of obesity and overweight in LATAM poses a major public health challenge to the region.[18] The situation is more complex in children and adolescents, as one in five is overweight or obese. The transition from a predominantly underweight population to one that is overweight and obesity has been remarkably rapid in Latin America; this has been associated with changes in food systems and living environments characterized by greater availability, accessibility, and affordability of ultra-processed foods, as well as an increase in sedentary lifestyle.[19] The countries with the highest prevalence of obesity are Mexico (20.6% in men, 32.7% in women), Chile (22% in men, 30.3% in women), Costa Rica (15.4% in men, 28.8% in women), and Uruguay (23.3% in men, 25.4% in women).[16] Metabolic syndrome is another relevant risk factor for liver diseases that exhibit high prevalence rates (between 25% and 37%) in LATAM.[20,21] The recent Cardiovascular Risk Factor Multiple Evaluation in LATAM (CARMELA) study found a global prevalence of metabolic syndrome of 21%. The most affected cities were Mexico City (27%),

Barquisimeto (26%), Santiago (21%), and Bogota (20%), and the cities with the lowest prevalence were Lima (18%), Buenos Aires (17%), and Quito (14%).[22] Physical inactivity plays a fundamental role as a contributor to obesity and overweight and is highly prevalent in the region. LATAM corresponds to the area with the highest sedentary lifestyles globally, with a prevalence rate of insufficient physical activity of 32%.[23] This situation is also problematic in teenagers, since only 15% of adolescents are physically active.[24]

MASLD IN SUB-SAHARAN AFRICA

The SSA region includes 47 countries, most having low- or middle-income economic status, with 40.6% of the population urbanized. The per-capita gross national income is <1,657 USD and the per-capita health spend is 83 USD.[25] Data supporting MASLD as a growing cofactor in patients with viral hepatitis in sub-Saharan Africa is emerging. Equally, the metabolic risk factors underlying MASLD are prevalent and concerningly increasing, suggesting an environment where the population at risk for MASLD is burgeoning. The 2019 T2DM burden was estimated at 19 million but is projected to increase to 41 million by 2045, with a concerning 45 million sub-Saharan Africans having impaired glucose tolerance.[26] The metabolic syndrome components commonly associated with MASLD are prevalent and increasing in SSA. This is occurring within an environment of rapid urbanization (41% in 2019) and accompanying MASLD-enhancing dietary and lifestyle changes, including sedentary activities. Compounding this is food insecurity, driving a shift to lower nutritional value and more calorically loaded options.[27]

A 2016 meta-analysis of MASLD prevalence suggested a 13.5% (95% CI 5.67–28.7) MASLD prevalence in SSA. Even so, accurate data about MASLD in Africa is lacking, with published data often not based on a histological assessment of the liver. What is, however, apparent is that a transition in SSA is occurring from the health burden of communicable diseases such as HIV, tuberculosis, and malaria to the noncommunicable diseases that are often related to MASLD. Between 1990 and 2017, the disability-adjusted life years (DALY) due to noncommunicable diseases increased by 67%.[28] Furthermore, the median age of Africans with noncommunicable diseases is comparatively 10 years younger, suggesting a proportionally greater increase in prevalence.

As is observed globally, the obesity epidemic has not spared sub-Saharan Africa. The age-standardized body mass index (BMI) increased from 21 to 23 kg/m^2 and 21.9 to 24.9 kg/m^2 in men and women, respectively, between 1980 and 2014.[29] Concerningly, the trend is similarly observed in children with the obesity transition occurring in younger ages in those of school-going age. The transition is greater in females who are urban living and of greater socioeconomic status.[30]

Expectedly, the rise in obesity mirrors the growing prevalence of T2DM in SSA. MASLD prevalence, based mostly on radiological assessment in four studies of patients with T2DM, was 30.4%.[31] An astounding 156% T2DM increase in prevalence by 2045 is anticipated, with the number of adult with diabetes surging to 41 million.[26] A regional variation of undiagnosed T2DM prevalence is observed, with an overall pooled prevalence of 3.9% ranging from 1.46% in Southern Africa to 4.27% in Northern, 4.43% in Eastern, and 4.72% in Western Africa.[32]

Abnormal lipid profiles are prevalent in MASLD and present in up to 70% in those with simple steatosis and 72% in NASH. As a major risk factor for cardiovascular disease, a large systematic review determined an almost 26% prevalence of hyperlipidemia in the general African population.[33]

A global burden of disease study provides estimates of MASLD prevalence change from 1990 to 2017.[34] For the various regions of SSA, the trends have been as follows: in the Southern region it is estimated that MASLD cases per million have increased from 3.7 to 8.1, with age-standardized prevalence increasing from 9.3% to 11.4%; in the Central region from 2.3 to 6.2 MASLD cases per million, with age-standardized prevalence increasing from 6.5% to 7.5%; in the Eastern region from 7.1 to 18 MASLD cases per million, with an age-standardized prevalence increasing from 6% to 7%; and in the Western region from 8.4 to 23.2 MASLD cases per million, with the age-standardized prevalence increasing from 6.5% to 8%. Some additional data is provided below.

SOUTHERN SUB-SAHARAN AFRICA

T2DM is a surrogate marker for type 2 diabetes and has increased across all countries in the Southern region. Between 1980 and 2014, type 2 diabetes prevalence in men and women, respectively, in South Africa increased from 4.8% and 7.7% to 9.7% and 12.6%, while in Botswana the increase was from 2% and 3.8% to 7.6% and 9.5%, respectively.[35] Rates of obesity in the region are the highest in SSA, with rates in men and women being 11.7% and 37%, respectively. A liver biopsy–based study from South Africa of at-risk patients for MASLD yielded a prevalence of MASLD, simple steatosis, MASH, and advanced liver fibrosis of 87%, 51%, 36%, and 17%, respectively.[36] A major compounding factor is HIV prevalence and the consequences of massively upscaled antiretroviral therapy and the potential longer metabolic consequences of therapy. A prospective study of 301 HIV-positive patients undergoing a liver biopsy found 19.3% with MASLD, of whom 27.6% had steatohepatitis.[37]

CENTRAL SUB-SAHARAN AFRICA

Obesity is less prevalent in this region, with the proportion of those with a BMI of >30 (obese) ranging from 5.4% in Burundi to 17.5% in Equatorial Guinea. There is an apparent socioeconomic trend in these rates, with more affluent trending toward higher BMI rates.

EASTERN SUB-SAHARAN AFRICA

In 2017, Ethiopia estimated its prevalence of type 2 diabetes in adults (>35 years) at 5.1% and 2.1% for urban and rural dwellers, respectively. The pooled prevalence in a systematic review in 2020 for adult Ethiopians, either overweight or obese, was 19% and 5.4%, respectively.[38] Sudanese data demonstrated a MASLD prevalence of 50.3% in type 2 diabetics. Type 2 diabetes prevalence in north Sudan has been shown to be 19.1%.

WESTERN SUB-SAHARAN AFRICA

Obesity in Ghana has increased from 5.5% to 25.4% since 2010, with MASLD observed in 40% of a female cohort of peri- and post-menopausal women in 2020.[39] MASLD prevalence in Nigeria is observed in 9.5% to 16.7% of those with type 2 diabetes.

Unique Aspects of MASLD in SSA

STEATOSIS AND STEATOHEPATITIS IN AFRICANS

A puzzling aspect is that while steatosis has been commonly observed in Africans, data to support MASH are lacking, but where assessed, it seems to occur at a frequency less than in other ethnicities. Genetic factors play a role in ethnic variation and a host of candidate genes have been associated with MASLD including *PNPLA3* (patatin-like phospholipase domain-containing protein 3), *MBOAT7,* and *TM6SF2* (transmembrane 6 superfamily member 2) genes.[40] The rs738409[G] SNP of *PNPLA3* is independently associated with MASLD and HCC risk in patients with cirrhosis. The SNP has varying ethnic prevalence and has lowest expression in African Americans, who are more likely to have the protective rs6006460[T] *PNPLA3* allele. Subcutaneous fat stores may have a protective effect, as evidenced in a southern African study where African black women, despite having higher total body fat, subcutaneous body fat, BMI, and waist circumference, had a lower liver fat content on CT scan compared to Asians and Whites.[41]

PRO-MASLD DIETARY CHANGES

A nutritional transition is occurring in sub-Saharan Africa with a move from a traditional high-fiber, low-fat diet to a high-calorie one with increased intake of fast foods, sugar-sweetened drinks, and high fat consumption.[42] While these are factors not unique to sub-Saharan Africa, they are occurring in the context of a simultaneous rapid rise in other metabolic syndrome risk factors. Data from South Africa supports the elevated intake of sugar-sweetened drinks. This is coupled with a marked reduction in leisure-time physical activity. This confluence of factors may well lead to a significant increase in MASLD risk. Finally, infection with the human immunodeficiency virus (HIV) plays an important role in MASLD in SSA. This is discussed in the HIV chapter in this book.

Current Challenges in Addressing the Public Health Problem of MASLD in LATAM and SSA as Examples of Low-Resource Healthcare Settings

The constantly increasing MASLD figures in limited-resource settings such as LATAM and SSA imply many challenges.[18] Obesity and T2DM burden in LATAM and the liver disease burden related to the endemicity of hepatitis B in addition to hepatitis C, alcohol, and aflatoxin in SSA make the potential added burden of MASLD very concerning. However, it equally presents an opportunity to consider integrating health opportunities. In fact, health system fragmentation is a barrier to tackling MASLD and building on existing efforts of integration of care around metabolic diseases may be a way to better manage MASLD. Importantly, design and implementation of efficient and effective models of care for patients with MASLD are crucial.[43]

Other challenges around MASLD in resource-limited regions are lack of disease awareness, limited educational opportunities for healthcare providers, and lack of effective strategies for the prevention and treatment of the condition and its common comorbidities. In fact, in most of the current guidance documents for the management of T2DM, hypertension, and dyslipidemia, MASLD is barely mentioned.

Regarding public policies addressing MASLD, a recent modeling study suggests that the establishment of public health policies on MASLD-related conditions could result in lower burden of disease and resulting complications.[44] Some examples of public policies to address MASLD include fiscal measures such as using judicious taxes and subsidies to promote healthier diet, policies for the procurement and provision of healthy food, particularly in schools, and measures for promoting healthy diet and physical activity through mass media campaigns and holistic planning of non-communicable disease management.

From the clinical standpoint, a key issue in MASLD management refers to the identification of cases with advanced fibrosis or cirrhosis and use of proper referral pathways to liver specialists.[45,46] Most guidelines suggest the use of two-step assessment of fibrosis using, first, simple noninvasive tools such as FIB-4 score, followed by evaluation of liver stiffness with transient elastography (TE).[45] Unfortunately, availability of TE is limited in low-resource settings, which determine difficulties in applying currently recommended algorithms (Figure 20.1).

CLINICAL APPROACH TO MASLD

Diagnosis: Most patients with MASLD are asymptomatic. Hepatomegaly is a common finding, secondary to fat infiltration of the liver. Mild elevations of ALT and AST are usually present (but their normality does not exclude MASLD), usually two to three times the upper limit of normal, and with ALT slightly higher than AST. Alkaline phosphatase and ferritin can also be slightly elevated.[47] The diagnosis of MASLD is mainly of exclusion and requires (1) presence of fat in the

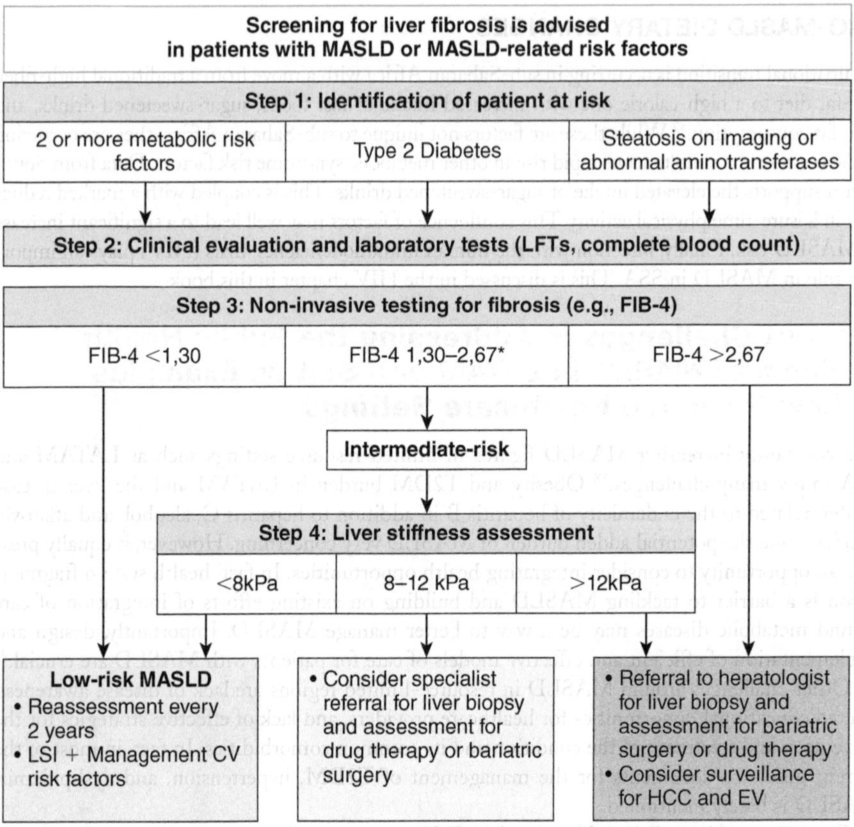

Figure 20.1 Suggested algorithm for evaluation of liver fibrosis in patients with MASLD or MASLD-related risk factors. Fibrosis evaluation with noninvasive scores (Fibrosis 4 [FIB-4] as preferred tool) should be carried out as triaging test. If abnormal, evaluation is followed by liver stiffness assessment using vibration-controlled transient elastography (VCTE) to evaluate liver fibrosis and hepatology consultation. (Adapted from ref. 45. CV: cardiovascular, EV: esophageal varices, HCC: hepatocellular carcinoma, LSI: lifestyle interventions.)

liver (detected by imaging or biopsy), (2) lack of significant alcohol consumption, and (3) exclusion of other causes of liver disease (i.e., viral hepatitis, autoimmune, drug-induced liver injury, etc.).

Management: The management of the patient with MASLD is mainly focused on prevention. However, important aspects of lifestyle modifications should be taken into account. These include the following: decrease or abstinence of alcohol consumption, as well as other MASLD-inducing beverages like sugar drinks; intake of Mediterranean-type diet (low in carbohydrates and processed foods); weight loss (recommended 7–10% of body weight); exercise implementation (150–200 minutes of moderate-intensity exercise per week); immunization against viral hepatitis; and proper control of comorbidities (including T2DM, obesity, hypertension and dyslipidemia).[48,49] Finally, it should be noted that cardiovascular disease is the number-one cause of death in these patients, and therefore maximization of cardiovascular prevention is a must (dyslipidemia, blood pressure control, etc.). Currently, there are no specific drugs recommended for the treatment of MASLD/MASH.[50] Some medications like vitamin E addressing oxidative stress, metformin and pioglitazone for T2DM control, or semaglutide for weight control have been studied (some with better results than others) but no strong recommendation for either is currently present.[51]

LOOKING TO THE FUTURE

Coordinated efforts are needed to address MASLD in low-resources regions.[52] Existing programs designed to manage both communicable and non-communicable diseases may incorporate assessment of NAFLD to attempt and use proper referral pathways to identify patients with advanced fibrosis and cirrhosis and reduce liver disease burden. This also would favor multidisciplinary approaches.[53] Also, disease prevention should be emphasized through wide promotion of healthy lifestyles.

Institutional strengthening allowing to conduct impactful research is important to promote awareness and good practices around MASLD. In that regard, collaboration with high income countries where MASLD has been researched for a long time (e.g., the United States and parts of western Europe) may help to create international networks as well as may contribute to more relevant participation of resource-limited countries in large international clinical trials improving MASLD research in these areas. Building large biobanks from well characterized patient populations integrating clinical, genetic, biomarkers and OMICs information is also key to this end. Scientific societies devoted to the study of the liver and all those that group physicians and health professionals caring for patients with poor metabolic health may have a pivotal role in improving the situation by joining both political and scientific efforts. Extensive collaboration between these societies with governments, non-governmental organizations, pharmaceutical industry, and other stakeholders is urgently needed to advance the MASLD public health policies agenda that allows us to address this disease in resource-limited settings with a whole of society approach.

References

1. Younossi Z, Tacke F, Arrese M, et al. Global perspectives on nonalcoholic fatty liver disease and nonalcoholic steatohepatitis. *Hepatology*. 2019;69:2672-2682.
2. Younossi ZM. Non-alcoholic fatty liver disease: a global public health perspective. *J Hepatol*. 2019;70: 531-544.
3. Estes C, Chan HLY, Chien RN, et al. Modelling NAFLD disease burden in four Asian regions: 2019–2030. *Aliment Pharmacol Ther*. 2020;51:801-811.
4. Bugianesi E. Fatty liver disease: putting the spotlight on a silent menace for young adults. *Lancet Gastroenterol Hepatol*. 2020;5:236-238.
5. Lindenmeyer CC, McCullough AJ. The natural history of nonalcoholic fatty liver disease: an evolving view. *Clin Liver Dis*. 2018;22:11-21.
6. Eslam M, Sanyal AJ, George J, International Consensus Panel. MAFLD: a consensus-driven proposed nomenclature for metabolic associated fatty liver disease. *Gastroenterology*. 2020;158:1999-2014.e1.
7. Eslam M, Newsome PN, Sarin SK, et al. A new definition for metabolic dysfunction-associated fatty liver disease: an international expert consensus statement. *J Hepatol*. 2020;73(1):202-209. doi:10.1016/j.jhep.2020.03.039.
8. Younossi ZM, Rinella ME, Sanyal AJ, et al. From NAFLD to MAFLD: implications of a premature change in terminology. *Hepatology*. 2021;73(3):1194-1198. doi:10.1002/hep.31420.
9. Rinella ME, Lazarus JV, Ratziu V, et al. NAFLD Nomenclature Consensus Group. A multi-society Delphi consensus statement on new fatty liver disease nomenclature. *Hepatology*. 2023. doi:10.1097/HEP.0000000000000520.
10. Hagström H, Vessby J, Ekstedt M, Shang Y. 99% of patients with NAFLD meet MASLD criteria and natural history is therefore identical. *J Hepatol*. 2023. doi:10.1016/j.jhep.2023.08.026.
11. Younossi ZM, Golabi P, Paik JM, Henry A, Van Dongen C, Henry L. The global epidemiology of nonalcoholic fatty liver disease (NAFLD) and nonalcoholic steatohepatitis (NASH): a systematic review. *Hepatology*. 2023;77(4):1335-1347. doi:10.1097/HEP.0000000000000004.
12. GBD 2017 Cirrhosis Collaborators. The global, regional, and national burden of cirrhosis by cause in 195 countries and territories, 1990–2017: a systematic analysis for the Global Burden of Disease Study 2017. *Lancet Gastroenterol Hepatol*. 2020;5:245-266.

13. Rojas YAO, Cuellar CLV, Barron KMA, Verdugo JPA, Miranda AL. Non-alcoholic fatty liver disease prevalence in Latin America: a systematic review and meta-analysis. *Ann Hepatol.* 2022;18(3):528-535. doi:10.1016/j.aohep.2019.04.005.
14. Pinto Marques Souza de Oliveira C, Pinchemel Cotrim H, Arrese M. Nonalcoholic fatty liver disease risk factors in Latin American populations: current scenario and perspectives. *Clin Liver Dis (Hoboken).* 2019;13:39-42.
15. Lopez-Velazquez JA, Silva-Vidal KV, Ponciano-Rodriguez G, et al. The prevalence of nonalcoholic fatty liver disease in the Americas. *Ann Hepatol.* 2014;13:166-178.
16. Ng M, Fleming T, Robinson M, et al. Global, regional, and national prevalence of overweight and obesity in children and adults during 1980–2013: a systematic analysis for the Global Burden of Disease Study 2013. *Lancet.* 2014;384:766-781.
17. Halpern B, Louzada M, Aschner P, et al. Obesity and COVID-19 in Latin America: a tragedy of two pandemics: official document of the Latin American Federation of Obesity Societies. *Obes Rev.* 2021;22:e13165.
18. Arab JP, Diaz LA, Dirchwolf M, et al. NAFLD: challenges and opportunities to address the public health challenge in Latin America. *Ann Hepatol.* 2021;24:100359.
19. Cominato L, Di Biagio GF, Lellis D, Franco RR, Mancini MC, de Melo ME. Obesity prevention: strategies and challenges in Latin America. *Curr Obes Rep.* 2018;7:97-104.
20. Cuevas A, Alvarez V, Carrasco F. Epidemic of metabolic syndrome in Latin America. *Curr Opin Endocrinol Diabetes Obes.* 2011;18:134-138.
21. Marquez-Sandoval F, Macedo-Ojeda G, Viramontes-Horner D, Fernandez Ballart JD, Salas Salvado J, Vizmanos B. The prevalence of metabolic syndrome in Latin America: a systematic review. *Public Health Nutr.* 2011;14:1702-1713.
22. Escobedo J, Schargrodsky H, Champagne B, et al. Prevalence of the metabolic syndrome in Latin America and its association with sub-clinical carotid atherosclerosis: the CARMELA cross sectional study. *Cardiovasc Diabetol.* 2009;8:52.
23. Guthold R, Stevens GA, Riley LM, Bull FC. Worldwide trends in insufficient physical activity from 2001 to 2016: a pooled analysis of 358 population-based surveys with 1.9 million participants. *Lancet Glob Health.* 2018;6:e1077-e1086.
24. Aguilar-Farias N, Martino-Fuentealba P, Carcamo-Oyarzun J, et al. A regional vision of physical activity, sedentary behaviour and physical education in adolescents from Latin America and the Caribbean: results from 26 countries. *Int J Epidemiol.* 2018;47:976-986.
25. Spearman CW, Sonderup MW. Health disparities in liver disease in sub-Saharan Africa. *Liver Int.* 2015; 35:2063-2071.
26. International Diabetes Federation. IDF Diabetes Atlas, 10th ed. Brussels, Belgium: IDF; 2021. Available at: https://www.diabetesatlas.org.
27. Nettle D, Andrews C, Bateson M. Food insecurity as a driver of obesity in humans: the insurance hypothesis. *Behav Brain Sci.* 2017;40:e105.
28. Gouda HN, Charlson F, Sorsdahl K, et al. Burden of non-communicable diseases in sub-Saharan Africa, 1990–2017: results from the Global Burden of Disease Study 2017. *Lancet Glob Health.* 2019;7:e1375-e1387.
29. NCD Risk Factor Collaboration (NCD-RisC) – Africa Working Group. Trends in obesity and diabetes across Africa from 1980 to 2014: an analysis of pooled population-based studies. *Int J Epidemiol.* 2017;46:1421-1432.
30. Muthuri SK, Francis CE, Wachira LJ, et al. Evidence of an overweight/obesity transition among school-aged children and youth in Sub-Saharan Africa: a systematic review. *PLoS One.* 2014;9:e92846.
31. Younossi ZM, Golabi P, de Avila L, et al. The global epidemiology of NAFLD and NASH in patients with type 2 diabetes: a systematic review and meta-analysis. *J Hepatol.* 2019;71:793-801.
32. Dessie G, Mulugeta H, Amare D, et al. A systematic analysis on prevalence and sub-regional distribution of undiagnosed diabetes mellitus among adults in African countries. *J Diabetes Metab Disord.* 2020; 19:1931-1941.
33. Noubiap JJ, Bigna JJ, Nansseu JR, et al. Prevalence of dyslipidaemia among adults in Africa: a systematic review and meta-analysis. *Lancet Glob Health.* 2018;6:e998-e1007.
34. Ge X, Zheng L, Wang M, Du Y, Jiang J. Prevalence trends in non-alcoholic fatty liver disease at the global, regional and national levels, 1990–2017: a population-based observational study. *BMJ Open.* 2020;10:e036663.
35. NCD Risk Factor Collaboration (NCD-RisC). Worldwide trends in diabetes since 1980: a pooled analysis of 751 population-based studies with 4.4 million participants. *Lancet.* 2016;387:1513-1530.

36. Kruger FC, Daniels C, Kidd M, et al. Non-alcoholic fatty liver disease (NAFLD) in the Western Cape: a descriptive analysis. *S Afr Med J.* 2010;100:168-171.
37. Sonderup MW, Wainwright H, Hall P, Hairwadzi H, Spearman CW. A clinicopathological cohort study of liver pathology in 301 patients with human immunodeficiency virus/acquired immune deficiency syndrome. *Hepatology.* 2015;61:1721-1729.
38. Kassie AM, Abate BB, Kassaw MW. Prevalence of overweight/obesity among the adult population in Ethiopia: a systematic review and meta-analysis. *BMJ Open.* 2020;10:e039200.
39. Setroame AM, Kormla Affrim P, Abaka-Yawson A, et al. Prevalence of metabolic syndrome and nonalcoholic fatty liver disease among premenopausal and postmenopausal women in Ho Municipality: a cross-sectional study. *Biomed Res Int.* 2020;2020:2168381.
40. Trépo E, Valenti L. Update on NAFLD genetics: from new variants to the clinic. *J Hepatol.* 2020;72:1196-1209.
41. Naran NH, Haagensen M, Crowther NJ. Steatosis in South African women: how much and why? *PLoS One.* 2018;13:e0191388.
42. Steyn NP, McHiza ZJ. Obesity and the nutrition transition in Sub-Saharan Africa. *Ann N Y Acad Sci.* 2014;1311:88-101.
43. Lazarus JV, Mark HE, Anstee QM, et al. Advancing the global public health agenda for NAFLD: a consensus statement. *Nat Rev Gastroenterol Hepatol.* 2022;19:60-78.
44. Diaz LA, Fuentes-Lopez E, Ayares G, et al. The establishment of public health policies and the burden of non-alcoholic fatty liver disease in the Americas. *Lancet Gastroenterol Hepatol.* 2022;7(6):552-559. doi:10.1016/S2468-1253(22)00008-5.
45. Kanwal F, Shubrook JH, Adams LA, et al. Clinical care pathway for the risk stratification and management of patients with nonalcoholic fatty liver disease. *Gastroenterology.* 2021;161:1657-1669.
46. Armstrong MJ, Marchesini G. Referral pathways for NAFLD fibrosis in primary care: no longer a "needle in a haystack". *J Hepatol.* 2019;71:246-248.
47. Rinella ME, Neuschwander-Tetri BA, Siddiqui MS, et al. AASLD Practice Guidance on the clinical assessment and management of nonalcoholic fatty liver disease. *Hepatology.* 2023;77(5):1797-1835. doi:10.1097/HEP.0000000000000323.
48. Younossi ZM, Zelber-Sagi S, Henry L, Gerber LH. Lifestyle interventions in nonalcoholic fatty liver disease. *Nat Rev Gastroenterol Hepatol.* 2023. doi:10.1038/s41575-023-00800-4.
49. Manikat R, Nguyen MH. Nonalcoholic fatty liver disease and non-liver comorbidities. *Clin Mol Hepatol.* 2023;29(suppl):s86-s102. doi:10.3350/cmh.2022.0442.
50. Tilg H, Byrne CD, Targher G. NASH drug treatment development: challenges and lessons. *Lancet Gastroenterol Hepatol.* 2023;8(10):943-954. doi:10.1016/S2468-1253(23)00159-0.
51. Rinella ME, Neuschwander-Tetri BA, Siddiqui MS, et al. AASLD Practice Guidance on the clinical assessment and management of nonalcoholic fatty liver disease. *Hepatology.* 2023;77(5):1797-1835. doi:10.1097/HEP.0000000000000323.
52. Diaz LA, Ayares G, Arnold J, et al. Liver Diseases in Latin America: current status, unmet needs, and opportunities for improvement. *Curr Treat Options Gastroenterol.* 2022;20(3):261-278. doi:10.1007/s11938-022-00382-1.
53. Lazarus JV, Anstee QM, Hagstrom H, et al. Defining comprehensive models of care for NAFLD. *Nat Rev Gastroenterol Hepatol.* 2021;18:717-729.

CHAPTER 21

Aflatoxins in Liver Disease

Mirghani A. Yousif

KEY POINTS

- Aflatoxins (AFs) are structurally related mycotoxins produced as food-borne metabolites by different strains of *Aspergillus flavus* and *Aspergillus parasiticus*.
- Sub-Saharan Africa is one of the areas that experience the highest exposure risk to AFs, with approximately 40% of aflatoxin-induced liver cancers.
- AFB1 affects many human organs; however, the liver is the most importantly affected one, as it causes hepatocellular carcinoma (HCC) upon chronic exposure.
- Different degrees of liver injury in animals and humans have been attributed to high intake of AF-contaminated food, and many studies have suggested an association between liver cirrhosis and AF exposure.
- Aflatoxicosis has no specific antidote. Treatment is supportive.
- Measures exist for pre- and post-harvest treatment of grains to decrease aflatoxin exposure.

Introduction

Aflatoxins (AFs) are structurally related mycotoxins produced as food-borne metabolites by different strains of *Aspergillus flavus* and *Aspergillus parasiticus* in a temperate and humid environment. Tropical and subtropical zones are prone to their growth.[1] The most suitable range of growth temperature is 12°C to 40°C, and the required moisture range is 3% to 18%.[1] These fungi are predominantly growing on farm-to-table cereals and nuts foodstuffs in tropical climates, namely Southeast Asia and sub-Saharan Africa.[3-5] AFs are produced on cereal grains during growth, harvest, storage, or transportation.[6] About 18 different types of AFs are globally distributed; however, the dominant ones are AFB1, AFB2, AFG1, AFG2, AFM1, and AFM2.[7] Out of these, AFB1 is named by the International Agency for Research on Cancer (IARC) as a class one carcinogen and it is the most prevalent and toxic type of AF.[8]

Aflatoxins Biological Effects

AFB1 affects many human organs; however, the liver is the most importantly affected, as AFB1 causes hepatocellular carcinoma (HCC) upon chronic exposure.[9,10] By the action of family microsomal CYP450 enzymes, AFB1 is converted to a more toxic epoxide, AFB1-8,9-epoxide (AFBO).[11] The majority of AFB1 tissue toxicity is attributed to the highly reactive epoxide AFBO due to its binding capacity to macromolecules as proteins and DNA.[10] AFBO is fully detoxified by glutathione transferases (GSH) when it crosses mitochondrial membrane and goes through phase II metabolism.[11] Thus mitochondria play a critical role in AFB1 metabolism and detoxification, which is important in the pathogenesis of aflatoxicosis and therefore needs detailed investigation. Studies have shown that AFB1 impairs mitochondrial functions such as permeability.[12,13] Moreover, AFB1 induces oxidative stress and disruption of lipid metabolism.[14]

EPIDEMIOLOGY

Environmental exposure to AFs and its effects on the liver have recently gained public interest, as high consumption of AF-contaminated foodstuff increases endemicity of regional liver diseases.[15] Global epidemiology of liver diseases varies from one region to another. Many risk factors, such as heavy consumption of alcohol,[16] pesticides, and chemicals,[17] were observed to have an influence on AF effects on the liver. AF exposure risk is estimated to affect around 4 billion people worldwide.[18,19] Sub-Saharan Africa is one of the areas that experience the highest exposure risk to AFs, and approximately 40% of AF-induced liver cancer occurs in the region.[20] In Tanzania, the nationwide overall risk for AF-induced liver cancer was estimated to be 2.95 per 100,000 people.[21] In Nigeria and Mali, overall median risks AF-induced liver cancer were, respectively, 1.4 and 2.7 per 100,000.[22]

Aflatoxins Effects on the Liver

The hepatotoxic effects of AFs were fully established decades ago.[23,24] Mycotoxins showed adverse effects on humans and animals that lead to illnesses and economic losses.[25] It is known that AFs have hepatotoxic, hepatocarcinogenic, teratogenic, mutagenic, and immunosuppressive effects.[26] Animals are not equally affected by AF. Factors such as sex, age, and breed play a significant role in toxicity, as some animals are more resistant while others are more susceptible.[27] In all animals the liver is the target organ of the toxin. AFs toxicity and the type of diseases depend on the volume and time pattern of exposure. High doses of AFs cause severe hepatocellular necrosis, while prolonged low doses lead to enlargement of the liver.[28]

Acute aflatoxicosis is less common than chronic disease, although it often leads to death, as reported in Kenya and Tanzania.[29-31] Indeed, acute aflatoxicosis is characterized by hemorrhagic necrosis of the liver, bile duct proliferation, edema, and lethargy.[18] In addition, occurrence of acute symptoms and signs of jaundice, vomiting, abdominal pain, and diarrhea were attributed to ingestion of home grain maize contaminated with high levels of AFs.[31] Chronic exposure to AFs results in immune suppression, cancer, and other pathological conditions.[32]

Different degrees of liver injury in animals and humans have been attributed to high intake of AF-contaminated food, and many studies have suggested an association between liver cirrhosis and AF exposure.[33,34] Although this point is still controversial, cryptogenic cases of cirrhosis have been associated with high AF exposure in sub-Saharan African countries, and a meta-analysis has suggested that AF could be a risk factor for cirrhosis development.[35]

In sub-Saharan African countries, high consumption of AF-contaminated foods is known as an etiologic factor for HCC.[36] Approximately 28% of new cases of liver cancer are linked to AF exposure worldwide, and due to climatic and poor storage conditions.[37,38] Two main risk factors influence the risk of liver cancer induced by AF, namely hepatitis B virus infection and high level of AF exposure.[39] Unfortunately, both of these factors are common in Africa, which helps explain why nearly 40% of global AF-induced liver cancer occurs in that region.[20] The main mechanism to explain AF-induced HCC is associated with AF-driven mutational activity.[40]

In regions with high frequency of hepatitis B virus carriers and AF exposure, the mean age of presentation of HCC is often decreased to as young as 33 years.[41] The risk of HCC increases in individuals with hepatitis B virus infection who are potentially exposed to AFs. Indeed, chronic exposure to AFs in individuals with hepatitis B leads to a mutation in the TP53 gene (Codon 249), which has been extensively described to lead to early HCC.[42] In addition, aflatoxins exert various health conditions. These include malnutrition, delayed physical and mental maturity, reproduction, and nervous system diseases.[18,43,44] Exposure to AF during pregnancy can affect embryo and leads to infant teratogenicity.[45]

AFLATOXICOSIS DIAGNOSIS

Aflatoxicosis detection in humans is difficult due to the variations in clinical signs and to the immune suppression caused by infectious diseases. Measurement of a breakdown product in urine within 24 hours after exposure is the most often used diagnostic procedure.[68]

Aflatoxicosis can be diagnosed by a wide range of signs and symptoms that include vomiting, abdominal pain and hemorrhaging, pulmonary edema, acute liver damage, loss of digestive tract function, convulsions, cerebral edema, and coma.[47] AFs in body fluids and tissues can be best determined in urine via a screening qualitative test.[48] Mycotoxins can also be detected using immunology tests such as ELISA and immunoabsorbent (ELISA).[49,50] Although ELISA has proven to be easily used and to detect low levels of AF, it needs well-equipped laboratories, trained personnel, and it takes hours.[51]

AF EXPOSURE PREVENTION MEASURES

AF contamination of commodities is increasing worldwide, especially in sub-Saharan Africa and other tropical regions. Ground nuts and maize constitute the two essential diet crops in these areas. Due to improper storage and transportation, these crops are prone to contamination by aflatoxigenic fungi. Reduction of contamination levels could be achieved by controlling factors that enhance mycotoxin formation, namely temperature, moisture, and physical damage to seeds during transportation or due to infestation of insects and pests. The prevention processes should be initiated early, prior to fungal infestation and hence mycotoxins production. These processes include selection of plant varieties resistant to AF-producing fungi[52] and control of moisture, insect, and rodent during storage.[53]

AF PRE- AND POST-HARVEST REDUCTION

A wide range of pre- and post-harvest AF reduction measures can reduce AF contamination in food. Biological control is specifically applied in pre-harvest stage, while other chemical and physical measures are used in post-harvest settings.[54] Biologically non-toxigenic strains of *A. flavus* have been used as field crop control protection.[55] Physical sorting technology is also used to select out the substandard quality of crops through physical properties differentiation of size, color, shape, and visible detection of fungal growth.[56] Other methods include electromagnetic[57] and ozone fumigation.[58] Interestingly, esterified glucomannan (EG) has been preferred in poultry animals due to its high AF binding ability,[59] and it seems to ameliorate the adverse effects of AF in the liver aflatoxicosis.[60] More attention is needed also by stakeholders involved in the supply chain to prevent and reduce mycotoxins production in dairy animal feed reduce AFM1 residues in milk.[1]

AF TREATMENT

Aflatoxicosis has no specific antidote. Treatment against AFs has been attempted with the use of a number of pharmacological compounds that either enhance detoxification processes in animals or prevent the epoxide production that leads to chromosomal damage.[62,63] Oltipraz and chlorophyll are able to decrease the biologically effective dose but are understudied.[64] Supportive treatment is important, and steroids as well as N-acetyl cysteine have been tried in animals, with no studies performed in humans.[65]

References

1. Verma R. Aflatoxin cause DNA damage. *Int J Hum Genet.* 2004;4:231-236.
2. Duncan HE, Hagler M. *Aflatoxins and other mycotoxins. Oklahoma Cooperative Extension, Fact Sheet (CR-2105 - 1203).* Oklahoma, USA; 2008.
3. Gong YY, Watson S, Routledge MN. Aflatoxin exposure and associated human health effects, a review of epidemiological studies. *Food Saf (Tokyo).* 2016;4:14-27.
4. Mutegi C, Cotty, P, Bandyopadhyay R. Prevalence and mitigation of aflatoxins in Kenya (1960-to date). *World Mycotoxin J.* 2018;11:341.
5. Opoku N, Achaglinkame MA, Amagloh FK. Aflatoxin content in cereal-legume blends on the Ghanaian market far exceeds the permissible limit. *Food Secur.* 2018;10:1539-1545.
6. Salem M, Kamel K, Yousef M, Hassan G, El-Nouty F. Protective role of ascorbic acid to enhance semen quality of rabbits treated with sublethal doses of aflatoxin B1. *Toxicology.* 2001;62:209-218.
7. Luo Y, Liu X, Li J. Updating techniques on controlling mycotoxins: a review. *Food Control.* 2018; 89:123-132.
8. Ostry V, Malir F, Toman J, Grosse Y. Mycotoxins as human carcinogens: the IARC Monographs classification. *Mycotoxin Res.* 2017;33:65-73.
9. Wogan GN, Kensler TW, Groopman JD. Present and future directions of translational research on aflatoxin and hepatocellular carcinoma: a review. *Food Addit Contam Part A Chem Anal Control Expo Risk Assess.* 2012;29:249-257.
10. Rushing BR, Selim MI. Aflatoxin B1: a review on metabolism, toxicity, occurrence in food, occupational exposure, and detoxification methods. *Food Chem Toxicol.* 2019;124:81-100.
11. Deng J, Zhao L, Zhang NY, et al. Aflatoxin B1 metabolism: regulation by phase I and II metabolizing enzymes and chemoprotective agents. *Mutat Res Rev Mutat Res.* 2018;778:79-89.
12. Liu Y, Wang W. Aflatoxin B1 impairs mitochondrial functions, activates ROS generation, induces apoptosis and involves Nrf2 signal pathway in primary broiler hepatocytes. *Anim Sci J.* 2016;87:1490-1500.
13. Wang WJ, Xu ZL, Yu C, Xu XH. Effects of aflatoxin B1 on mitochondrial respiration, ROS generation and apoptosis in broiler cardiomyocytes. *Anim Sci J.* 2017;88:1561-1568.
14. Rotimi OA, Rotimi SO, Goodrich JM, Adelani IB, Agbonihale E, Talabi G. Time-course effects of acute aflatoxin B1 exposure on hepatic mitochondrial lipids and oxidative stress in rats. *Front Pharmacol.* 2019;10:467.
15. Melaram R. Environmental risk factors implicated in liver disease: a mini-review. *Front Public Health.* 2021;9:738.
16. Pimpin L, Cortez-Pinto H, Negro F, et al. Burden of liver disease in Europe: epidemiology and analysis of risk factors to identify prevention policies. *J Hepatol.* 2018;69:718-735.
17. Blair A, Ritz B, Wesseling C, Freeman LB. Pesticides and human health. *Occup Environ Med.* 2015;72(2):81-82. doi:10.1136/oemed-2014-102454.
18. Williams JH, Phillips TD, Jolly PE, Stiles JK, Jolly CM, Aggarwal D. Human aflatoxicosis in developing countries: a review of toxicology, exposure, potential health consequences, and interventions. *Am J Clin Nutr.* 2004;80(5):1106-1122. doi:10.1093/ajcn/80.5.1106.
19. Dhakal A, Sbar E. Aflatoxin Toxicity. In: *StatPearls [Internet].* Treasure Island, FL: StatPearls Publishing; 2022.
20. Liu Y, Wu F. Global burden of aflatoxin-induced hepatocellular carcinoma: a risk assessment. *Environ Health Perspect.* 2010;118:818-824.
21. Kimanya ME, Routledge MN, Mpolya E, et al. Estimating the risk of aflatoxin-induced liver cancer in Tanzania based on biomarker data. *PLoS One.* 2021;6:e0247281.
22. Ingenbleek L, Verger P, Gimou MM, et al. Human dietary exposure to chemicals in sub-Saharan Africa: safety assessment through a total diet study. *Lancet Planet Health.* 2020;4:e292-e300.
23. Newberne PM, Butler WH. Acute and chronic effects of aflatoxin on the liver of domestic and laboratory animals: a review. *Cancer Res.* 1969;29:236-250.

24. Zuckerman A, Rees K, Inman D, Petts V. Site of action of aflatoxin on human liver cells in culture. *Nature.* 1967;214:814-815.
25. Hussein HS, Brasel JM. Toxicity, metabolism, and impact of mycotoxins on humans and animals. *Toxicology.* 2001;67:101-134.
26. Oguz H, Hadimli H, Kurtoglu V, Erganis O. Evaluation of humoral immunity of broilers during chronic aflatoxin (50 and 100 ppb) and clinoptilolite exposure. *Revue de Médecine Vétérinaire.* 2003;154:483-486.
27. Richard JL. Discovery of aflatoxins and significant historical features. *Toxin Rev.* 2008;27:171-201.
28. Lakkawar AW, Chattopadhyay SK, Johri TS. Experimental aflatoxin B1 toxicosis in young rabbits-a clinical and patho-anatomical study. *Slov Vet Res.* 2004;41:73-81.
29. Ngindu A, Kenya P, Ocheng D, et al. Outbreak of acute hepatitis caused by aflatoxin poisoning in Kenya. *Lancet.* 1982;319:1346-1348.
30. Azziz-Baumgartner E, Lindblade K, Gieseker K, et al. Case–control study of an acute aflatoxicosis outbreak, Kenya, 2004. *Environ Health Perspect.* 2005;113:1779-1783.
31. Kamala A, Shirima C, Jani B, et al. Outbreak of an acute aflatoxicosis in Tanzania during 2016. *World Mycotoxin J.* 2018;11:311-320.
32. Hsieh D. Potential human health hazards of mycotoxins. In: Natori S, Hashimoto K, Ueno Y, eds. *Mycotoxins and Phytotoxins.* Third Joint Food and Agriculture Organization/W.H.O./United Nations Environment Program International Conference of Mycotoxins. Amsterdam, The Netherlands: Elsevier; 1988:69-80.
33. Saad-Hussein A, Shahy EM, Shaheen W, et al. Comparative hepatotoxicity of Aflatoxin B1 among workers exposed to different organic dust with emphasis on polymorphism role of glutathione S-Transferase gene. *Open Access Maced J Med Sci.* 2016;4:312.
34. Wouters ATB, Casagrande RA, Wouters F, et al. An outbreak of aflatoxin poisoning in dogs associated with aflatoxin B1–contaminated maize products. *J Vet Diagn Invest.* 2013;25:282-287.
35. Mekuria AN, Routledge MN, Gong YY, Sisay M. Aflatoxins as a risk factor for liver cirrhosis: a systematic review and meta-analysis. *BMC Pharmacol Toxicol.* 2020;21:1-8.
36. Huţanaşu C, Sfarti C, Trifan A, Huţanaşu M, Stanciu C. Contaminarea cu aflatoxine a alimentelor–factor suplimentar de risc pentru patologia hepatică cronică [Aflatoxin contamination of food: additional risk factor for chronic liver diseases]. *Rev Med Chir Soc Med Nat Iasi.* 2009;113(4):1061-1065.
37. Amuzie C, Bandyopadhyay R, Bhat RV, et al. Mycotoxin control in low- and middle-income countries. In: Wild CP, Miller JD, Groopman JD, eds. 2016.
38. Bandyopadhyay R, Ortega-Beltran A, Akande A, et al. Biological control of aflatoxins in Africa: current status and potential challenges in the face of climate change. *World Mycotoxin J.* 2016;9(5):771-789. https://doi.org/10.3920/WMJ2016.2130.
39. Joint F. *Evaluations of the Joint FAO/WHO Expert Committee on Food Additives. CADMIUM.* 2020. Available at: http://appswhoint/food-additives-contaminants-jecfa-database/chemicalaspx.
40. Wild CP, Gong YY. Mycotoxins and human disease: a largely ignored global health issue. *Carcinogenesis.* 2010;31:71-82.
41. Chang MH, Chen CJ, Lai MS, et al. Universal hepatitis B vaccination in Taiwan and the incidence of hepatocellular carcinoma in children. Taiwan Childhood Hepatoma Study Group. *N Engl J Med.* 1997;336:1855-1859.
42. Ozturk M. p53 mutation in hepatocellular carcinoma after aflatoxin exposure. *Lancet.* 1991;338(8779):1356-1359. doi:10.1016/0140-6736(91)92236-u.
43. El Khoury D, Fayjaloun S, Nassar M, Sahakian J, Aad YP. Updates on the effect of mycotoxins on male reproductive efficiency in mammals. *Toxins (Basel).* 2019;11:515.
44. Alsayyah A, ElMazoudy R, Al-Namshan M, Al-Jafary M, Alaqeel N. Chronic neurodegeneration by aflatoxin B1 depends on alterations of brain enzyme activity and immunoexpression of astrocyte in male rats. *Ecotoxicol Environ Saf.* 2019;182:109407.
45. Smith LE, Prendergast AJ, Turner PC , Humphrey JH, Stoltzfus RJ. Aflatoxin exposure during pregnancy, maternal anemia, and adverse birth outcomes. *Am J Trop Med Hyg.* 2017;96(4):770-776. doi:10.4269/ajtmh.16-0730.
46. World Health Organization (WHO). *Food Safety Digest: Aflatoxins.* Geneva: Department of Food Safety and Zoonoses, World Health Organization; 2018.

47. Dohlman E. *Mycotoxin Hazards and Regulations: Impacts on Food and Animal Feed Crop Trade*. International Trade and Food Safety, AER-828; 2008:97-108. Retrieved from November 11, 2011. USDA Economic Research Service.
48. Hooper DG, Bolton VE, Guilford FT, Straus DC. Mycotoxin detection in human samples from patients exposed to environmental molds. *Int J Mol Sci*. 2009;10(4):1465-1475. doi:10.3390/ijms10041465.
49. Scott PM, Trucksess MW. Application of immunoaffinity columns to mycotoxin analysis. *J AOAC Int*. 1997;80:941-949. Int. J. Mol. Sci. 2009, 10.
50. Yike I, Distler AM, Ziady AG, Dearborn DG. Mycotoxin adducts on human serum albumin: biomarkers of exposure to *Stachybotrys chartarum*. *Environ Health Perspect*. 2006;114:1221-1226.
51. Dallasta C, Ingletto G, Corradini R, Galaverna G, Marchelli R. Fluorescence enhancement of aflatoxins using native and substituted cyclodextrins. *J Incl Phenom Macrocycl Chem*. 2003;45(3):257-263.
52. Bruns HA. Controlling aflatoxin and fumonisin in maize by crop management. *Toxin Rev*. 2003;22: 153-173. doi:10.1081/TXR-120024090.
53. Magnussen A, Parsi MA. Aflatoxins, hepatocellular carcinoma and public health. *World J Gastroenterol*. 2013;19(10):1508-1512. doi:10.3748/wjg.v19.i10.1508.
54. Udomkun P, Wiredu AN, Nagle M, Müller J, Vanlauwe B, Bandyopadhyay R. Innovative technologies to manage aflatoxins in foods and feeds and the profitability of application: a review. *Food Control*. 2017;76:127-138. doi:10.1016/j.foodcont.2017.01.008.
55. Cotty PJ. Biocompetitive exclusion of toxigenic fungi. In: Barug D, Bhatnagar D, van Egdmond HP, van der Kamp JW, van Osenbruggen WA, Visconti A, eds. *The mycotoxin Factbook*. Wageningen Academic Publishers: 2006:179-197.
56. Fandohan P, Zoumenou D, Hounhouigan DJ, Marasas WFO, Wingfield MJ, Hell K. Fate of aflatoxins and fumonisins during the processing of maize into food products in Benin. *Int J Food Microbiol*. 2005;98(3):249-269.
57. Herzallah S, Alshawabkeh K, Al Fataftah A. Aflatoxin decontamination of artificially contaminated feeds by sunlight, γ-radiation, and microwave heating. *J Appl Poult Res*. 2008;17:515-521.
58. Inan F, Pala M, Doymaz I. Use of ozone in detoxification of aflatoxin B_1 in red pepper. *J Stored Prod Res*. 2007;43:425-429.
59. Basmacioglu H, Oguz H, Ergul M, Col R, Birdane Y. Effect of dietary esterified glucomannan on performance, serum biochemistry and haematology in broilers exposed to aflatoxin. *Czech J Anim Sci*. 2005; 50:31-39.
60. Colakoglu F, Donmez HH. Effects of aflatoxin on liver and protective effectiveness of esterified glucomannan in merino rams. *ScientificWorldJournal*. 2012;2012:462925.
61. Milićević DR, Milešević J, Gurinović M, et al. Dietary exposure and risk assessment of aflatoxin M1 for children aged 1 to 9 years old in Serbia. *Nutrients*. 2021;13:4450. doi:10.3390/nu13124450.
62. Kensler TW, Davis EF, Bolton MG. Strategies for chemoprotection against aflatoxin-induced liver cancer. In: Eaton D, Groopman JD, eds. *The toxicology of aflatoxins: Human Health, Veterinary, and Agricultural Significance*. London: Academic Press; 1993:281-306.
63. Hayes JD, Pulford DJ, Ellis EM, et al. Regulation of rat glutathione S-transferase A5 by cancer chemopreventive agents: mechanisms of inducible resistance to aflatoxin B1. *Chem Biol Interact*. 1998; 111-112:51-67.
64. Wang JS, Shen X, He X, et al. Protective alterations in phase 1 and 2 metabolism of aflatoxin B1 by oltipraz in residents of Qidong, People's Republic of China. *J Natl Cancer Inst*. 1999;91:347-354.
65. Tras B, Faki HE, Kutahya ZO, Bahcivan E, Dik B, Uney K. The effects of dexamethasone and minocycline alone and combined with N-acetylcysteine and vitamin E on serum matrix metalloproteinase-9 and coenzyme Q10 levels in aflatoxin B1 administered rats. *Pol J Vet Sci*. 2022;25:419-427.

CHAPTER 22

Tropical Herb-Induced Liver Injury by Pyrrolizidine Alkaloids

Rolf Teschke ■ Xingshun Qi ■ Tran Dang Xuan ■ Axel Eickhoff

KEY POINTS

- In tropical and subtropical regions disease clusters of life-threatening HSOS (hepatic sinusoidal obstruction syndrome) may be observed, causally related to the ingestion of plant products containing 1,2-unsaturated pyrrolizidine alkaloids (PAs).
- The early diagnosis of PA-related HSOS is difficult to be established because symptoms are unspecific and liver tests are normal or only marginally increased, but in suspected later stages the use of blood pyrrole-protein adducts and the updated Roussel Uclaf Causality Assessment Method (RUCAM) may be helpful.
- Unsaturated PAs target preferentially hepatic sinusoids leading to their obstruction and in the late stage of the disease to ascites as key clinical features that should be differentiated from ascites caused by a variety of chronic liver diseases.
- Treatment options must ensure stopping the ingestion of PAs, should focus on ascites by using diuretic drugs and reducing fluid intake, and will require anticoagulation therapy as early therapeutic intervention.

Introduction

Pyrrolizidine alkaloids (PAs) are found in variable amounts as ingredients of worldwide growing plants,[1-5] but only some have a potential role in the etiology of pulmonary hypertension, congenital anomalies,[6] and hepatotoxicity.[1,6,7] The PA-related herb-induced liver injury (HILI), commonly known as hepatic sinusoidal obstruction syndrome (HSOS), occurs wherever plants containing 1,2-unsaturated PAs grow and are consumed,[1,7] including tropical and subtropical regions[8-12] like Afghanistan,[8,9] India,[10,11] and Tadjistan.[12] In analogy to humans[1,7-17] animals such as cattle may suffer from HSOS after consumption of plants containing PAs[2] in a similar way as rats[5] and mice,[2] allowing for studies on mechanistic steps leading to HSOS.[2,5]

Pathogenesis

PAs are synthesized by roots of plants and represent heterocyclic organic chemicals that consist of a necine base esterified with a necic acid.[1,3] The necine base typically includes pyrrolizidine, a bicyclic aliphatic hydrocarbon consisting of two fused five-membered rings with a nitrogen at the bridgehead.[3] PAs *per se* are not toxic unless the saturated ring is transferred to their 1,2-unsaturated structure, shown for retronecine with its double bond between C1 and C2 (Figure 22.1). The conversion to unsaturated PAs with its 1,2-unsaturated necine base occurs in the plant

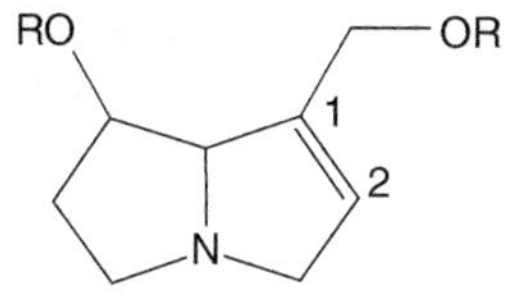

Figure 22.1 Basic structure of a toxic 1,2-unsaturated pyrrolizidine alkaloid. The toxicity of a PA is caused by the double bond between C1 and C2. R illustrates the position of different necic acids. Of note, the chemical structure of non-toxic PAs is similar to the structure shown above except that the double bond between C1 and C2 is missing.[1]

through dehydrogenation. After uptake by humans or animals, toxification of 1,2-unsaturated PAs proceeds preferentially via the microsomal cytochrome P450 (CYP) isoforms CYP 3A4 and CYP 2C19 in the hepatocytes.[1,3]

The 1,2-unsaturated PAs are injurious to hepatocytes and the liver sinusoidal endothelial cells (LSECs).[1,2,5,18-20] Hepatocellular injury is common for the hepatocytes, with focus on mitochondrial damage, overproduction of reactive oxygen species, and depletion of intracellular glutathione. Unsaturated PAs passing the liver cell membranes typically cause HSOS as evidenced by detachment of endothelial cells in small sinusoidal hepatic and interlobular veins, leading to toxicity characterized by edema, necrosis, intrahepatic congestion, portal hypertension, and liver impairment.[20]

Epidemiology

PA-containing plants were identified in many tropical and subtropical regions but research on HSOS cases is limited, shown also for Ghana, where PAs were found in herbal products and honey.[21] On the contrary, reports on HSOS from other countries classified large-scale intoxications by PAs correctly as outbreaks or clusters and less correctly as epidemics or endemics, occurring when food like bread was consumed, prepared from grain contaminated with PAs derived from co-harvested plants.[8-12,22] HSOS cases presenting recent outbreaks were reported from Afghanistan,[8,9,22] India,[10,11] Tadjistan,[12] Ethiopia,[23-26] and Iraq.[27]

In Afghanistan, a first HSOS outbreak was published in 1976,[8] confirmed in 1978,[22] with a second outbreak reported in 2010.[9] The first outbreak occurred following a 2-year period of severe drought and affected many patients with massive ascites and emaciation.[8] Clinical and pathological studies revealed typical cases of HSOS. The outbreak was caused by bread made from wheat contaminated with PAs from seeds of *Heliotropium* plants. Examination of 7,200 inhabitants showed evidence of liver disease in 22.6%. Clinical improvement was observed in 13 cases after 3 to 9 months, and in three cases liver biopsies showed almost complete disappearance of initial abnormalities.[8] Further studies revealed heliotrine as the main PA causing HSOS.[22] Characteristic morphological findings of the liver showed centrilobular hemorrhagic necrosis, followed by occlusive changes in the hepatic veins, finally resulting in non-portal cirrhosis. The sequence of changes suggested primary parenchymal injury and secondary obstructive lesions at the sinusoidal level.[22]

In India a minor HSOS outbreak of 25 patients with rapidly developing ascites due to portal hypertension was reported in 1976.[10] Illness started with mild pain in the epigastrium and the right upper abdominal quadrant, followed by a drop of urinary output and rapidly filling ascites in all patients in the absence of jaundice.[10] Liver histology was similar to the report from Afghanistan.[22] In the cohort of India 11 patients died, out of 25 patients retrieved from a population of 350 people.[10] HSOS was probably caused by cereals mixed with seeds of the plant *Crotalaria* sp. containing PAs.[11]

In Tadjistan an HSOS outbreak in 1992/1993 included 3,906 patients and was ascribed to the use of bread from wheat contaminated with PAs derived from *Heliotropium lasiocarpum* and their seeds collected with the wheat.[12] Clinical features included abdominal pain, nausea or vomiting, and asthenia (stage I); hepatomegaly combined with stage I (stage II); ascites plus features of stages I and II (stage III); and alteration of consciousness (stage IV).

In Ethiopia an outbreak of fatal liver disease of unidentified cause led to a case-control epidemiological study collecting information from the affected (case) area and a non-affected adjacent area (control) using a structured questionnaire,[23] showing that residents of the affected sites relied more on unprotected or protected well as a source of drinking water while most of the non-affected depended on fresh water from river or unprotected spring. This suggested that the problem of the case area could be linked to the special water source.[23] Subsequent clinical, laboratory, toxicological, and histopathologic studies classified the fatal liver disease as HSOS due to PAs[24] contaminating water from the unprotected well,[25] in which the PA-containing plant *Ageratum* sp. abundantly thrived.[26] In addition, PAs were found in Tela, an Ethiopian culture drink similar to beer. Overall, these conditions describe the challenges of finding HSOS and searching for the origin of PAs.

In Iraq a small HSOS outbreak of 14 patients was reported, in those who consumed wheat accidentally contaminated with *Senecio* seeds containing PAs.[27] Clinical presentation of this cohort included ascites (100%), abdominal pain (100%), hepatomegaly (57%), vomiting (50%), jaundice (43%), and splenomegaly (36%). Liver tests were slightly increased: bilirubin 4.6 mg (normal 0.2–1.0), alanine aminotransferase (ALT) 51.9 U/L (5-20), and aspartate aminotransferase (AST) 37.4 U/L (5-20). Children were at higher risk. Among the 14 patients, the overall fatality rate was 14.3%, resulting from liver failure and bleeding esophageal varices.[27]

Considering countries reporting clusters of PA-based HSOS, causes were tentatively ascribed to the consumption of food made from contaminated grain[8-12,22,27] or to drinks and drinking water.[23-26] With respect to grain, PAs may contaminate the grain via PA-containing plants co-harvested with the grain, or theoretically also through pre-harvest PA uptake by the grain from the soil contaminated with PAs. Indeed, to elucidate the origin of the widespread contaminations of plant-derived commodities with PAs, co-cultures of PA-containing Senecio jacobaea plants were used with various PA-free acceptor plants.[28] Plants grown in the vicinity of the Senecio donor plants contained significant amounts of the PAs, which previously had been synthesized in the Senecio plants. These findings illustrate that typical phytochemicals like PAs are commonly transferred and exchanged between living plants. As opposed to the broad spectrum of PAs in Senecio, in the acceptor plants nearly exclusively jacobine is accumulated. This indicates that this alkaloid is exuded specifically by the Senecio roots.[28] These conditions that may be applicable, for instance, to the *Senecio*-dependent HSOS of the cohort from Iraq,[27] resembling heavy metal uptake from contaminated soil by vegetables.[29]

Diagnostic Approaches

Clinical Presentation

Sporadic cases of HSOS by PAs occurring in tropical and subtropical regions remain mostly undetected, because clinical features are unspecific and found with many other diseases.[10] However, conditions are better if clusters of HSOS cases emerge facilitating early suspicion. Medical history regarding consumption of products potentially contaminated with plants containing PAs is primarily justified, although rarely expedient. Initial symptoms such as minor abdominal pains, vomiting or nausea, and asthenia are vague and of little diagnostic value.[12] With disease progression, key features include severe abdominal pains and rapidly developing ascites[8,12,27] while jaundice may be present[27] or not.[10,27] Despite loss of appetite and low caloric intake, patients with PA-induced HSOS suffer from concomitant weight increase due to fluid accumulation as edema and ascites.

Routine Laboratory Assessment

Serum activities of ALT or AST are slightly increased or within the normal range, thereby not helpful to suspect the diagnosis of a liver injury. Similarly, serum bilirubin may be normal or slightly increased.[27]

Pyrrole-protein Adducts

When available, highly appreciated are diagnostic biomarkers of blood pyrrole-protein adducts (PPAs), which help diagnose HSOS by PAs.[6,13-17,30,31] These biomarkers are mechanism based, resulting from reactive metabolites generated during degradation of unsaturated PAs and due to covalent binding to DNA, albumin, and other proteins. The formed PPAs leave the injured hepatocytes and enter the systemic circulation.

Causality Assessment Using Rucam

As for other HILI cases,[32] to validly exclude potential differential diagnoses, a formal causality assessment using RUCAM (Roussel Uclaf Causality Assessment Method) is proposed and was reported in 28 PA HSOS cases,[14,15] but recommended is now the updated RUCAM.[33] HSOS is also known after cytoreductive therapy prior to hematopoietic stem cell transplantation, chemotherapeutic regimes,[34,35] and PA-containing herbal remedies.[2,7,13-17,36,37]

Imaging Data

Diagnostic options include Doppler ultrasound looking for intrahepatic vessel changes, to be confirmed by computed tomography, magnetic resonance imaging, or digital subtraction angiography, if needed.[14]

Treatment

Apart from cessation of PA exposure, symptomatic treatment is important to manage ascites by restriction of water and sodium intake, use of diuretics such as furosemide and spironolactone, infusion of albumin, or serial paracentesis if drug therapy is ineffective.[38] In addition, early anticoagulant therapy should be initiated with low molecular weight heparin (100 IU/kg every 12 hours by subcutaneous injection as the anticoagulant of choice), either combined with or followed by oral use of warfarin.[38] Rarely done due to high costs, other therapeutic options may include transjugular intrahepatic portosystemic shunt (TIPS) and liver transplantation.[38]

References

1. Teschke R, Vongdala N, Quan NV, Quy TN, Xuan TD. Toxifying 1,2-unsaturated pyrrolizidine alkaloids causing human hepatic sinusoidal obstruction syndrome. *Int J Mol Sci.* SI: Molecular Toxicology. 2021;22:10419. doi:10.3390/ijms221910419.
2. Neuman MG, Cohen L, Opris M, Nanau RM, Hyunjin J. Hepatotoxicity of pyrrolizidine alkaloids. *J Pharm Pharm Sci.* 2015;18:825-843. doi:10.18433/j3bg7j.
3. Schramm S, Köhler N, Rozhon W. Pyrrolizidine alkaloids: Biosynthesis, biological activities and occurrence in crop plants. *Molecules.* 2019;24(3):498. doi:10.3390/molecules24030498.
4. Steinhoff B. Pyrrolizidine alkaloid contamination in herbal medicinal products: limits and occurrence. *Food Chem Toxicol.* 2019;130:262-266. doi:10.1016/j.fct.2019.05.026.
5. EMA (European Medicines Agency). *Public Statement on the Use of Herbal Medicinal Products Containing Toxic,* Unsaturated Pyrrolizidine Alkaloids *(PAs) Including Recommendations Regarding Contamination of Herbal Medicinal Products with Pyrrolizidine Alkaloids.* 2020. Last updated 8 July 2020. Available at: https://www.ema.europa.eu/en/documents/public-statement/public-statement-use-herbal-medicinal-products-containing-toxic-unsaturated-pyrrolizidine-alkaloids_en.pdf.

6. Edgar JA, Molyneux RJ, Colegate SM. Pyrrolizidine alkaloids: potential role in the etiology of cancers, pulmonary hypertension, congenital anomalies, and liver disease. *Chem Res Toxicol.* 2015;28:4-20.
7. Teschke R, Eickhoff A. Herbal hepatotoxicity in traditional and modern medicine: actual key issues and new encouraging steps. *Front Pharmacol.* 2015;6:72. doi:10.3389/fphar.2015.00072.
8. Mohabbat O, Younos MS, Merzad AA, Srivastava RN, Sediq GG, Aram GN. An outbreak of hepatic veno-occlusive disease in north-western Afghanistan. *Lancet.* 1976;308:269-271. doi:10.1016/s0140-6736(76)90726-1.
9. Kakar F, Akbarian Z, Leslie T, et al. An outbreak of hepatic veno-occlusive disease in western Afghanistan associated with exposure to wheat flour contaminated with pyrrolizidine alkaloids. *J Toxicol.* 2010;2010:313280. doi:10.1155/2010/313280.
10. Tandon RK, Tandon BN, Tandon HD. Study of an epidemic of venoocclusive disease in India. *Gut.* 1976;17:849-855.
11. Tandon BN, Tandon HD, Tandon RK, Narndranathan M, Joshi YK. An epidemic of veno-occlusive disease of the liver in central India. *Lancet.* 1976;308:271-272. doi:10.1016/S0140-6736(76)90727-3.
12. Chauvin P, Dillon JC, Moren A. Épidémie d'intoxication alimentaire á l'héliotrope, tadjikistan, Novembre 1992–Mars 1993. *Cahiers d'Études et de Recherches Francophones/Santé.* 1994;4:263-268.
13. Ruan J, Gao H, Li N, Xue J, Chen J, Ke C, et al. Blood pyrrole-protein adducts—A biomarker of pyrrolizidine alkaloid-induced liver injury in humans. *J Environ Sci Health C Environ Carcinog Ecotoxicol Rev.* 2015;33:404-421. doi:10.1080/10590501.2015.1096882.
14. Gao H, Li N, Wang JY, Zhang SC, Lin G. Definitive diagnosis of hepatic sinusoidal obstruction syndrome induced by pyrrolizidine alkaloids. *J Dig Dis.* 2012;13:33-39. doi:10.1111/j.1751-2980.2011.00552.x.
15. Gao H, Ruan JQ, Chen J, et al. Blood pyrrole-protein adducts as a diagnostic and prognostic index in pyrrolizidine alkaloid-hepatic sinusoidal obstruction syndrome. *Drug Des Devel Ther.* 2015;9:4861-4868. doi:10.2147/DDDT.S87858.
16. Frenzel C, Teschke R. Herbal hepatotoxicity: clinical characteristics and listing compilation. *Int J Mol Sci.* 2016;17:588. doi:10.3390/ijms17050588.
17. Teschke R, Larrey D, Melchart D, Danan G. Traditional Chinese Medicine (TCM) and herbal hepatotoxicity: RUCAM and the role of novel diagnostic biomarkers such as microRNAs. *Medicines.* 2016:3:18. doi:10.3390/medicines3030018.
18. Moreira R, Pereira DM, Valentão P, Andrade PB. Pyrrolizidine alkaloids: chemistry, pharmacology, toxicology and food safety. *Int J Mol Sci.* 2018;19:1668. doi:10.3390/ijms19061668.
19. Ghallab A. Pyrrolizidine alkaloids act by toxicity to sinusoidal endothelial cells of the liver. *Arch Toxicol.* 2019;93:3639-3640. doi:10.1007/s00204-019-02610-7.
20. Xu J, Wang W, Yang X, Xiong A, Yang L, Wang Z. Pyrrolizidine alkaloids: an update on their metabolism and hepatotoxicity mechanism. *Liver Res.* 2019;3:176-184.
21. Letsyo E, Jerz G, Winterhalter P, Beuerle T. Toxic pyrrolizidine alkaloids in herbal medicines commonly used in Ghana. *J Ethnopharmacol.* 2017;202:154-161. doi:10.1016/j.jep.2017.03.008.
22. Tandon HD, Tandon BN, Mattocks AR. An epidemic of veno-occlusive disease of the liver in Afghanistan pathologic features. *Am J Gastroenterol.* 1978;70(6):607-613.
23. Abebe D, Debella A, Tekabe F, et al. An outbreak of liver disease in Tahtay Koraro Woreda, Tigray region of Ethiopia: a case-control study for the identification of the etiologic agent. *Ethiop Med J.* 2012;50(suppl 2): 17-25.
24. Bane A, Seboxa T, Mesfin G, et al. An outbreak of veno-occlusive liver disease in northern Ethiopia, clinical findings. *Ethiop Med J.* 2012;50(suppl 2):9-16.
25. Debella A, Abebe D, Tekabe F, et al. Toxicity study and evaluation of biochemical markers towards the identification of the causative agent for an outbreak of liver disease in Tahtay Koraro Woreda, Tigray. *Ethiop Med J.* 2012;50(suppl 2):27-35.
26. Debella A, Abebe D, Tekabe F, et al. Physico-chemical investigation of consumables and environmental samples to determine the causative agent of liver disease outbreak in Tahitay Koraro Woreda, Tiray. *Ethiop Med J.* 2012;50(suppl 2):37-45.
27. Altaee MY. An outbreak of veno-occlusive disease of the liver in northern Iraq. *East Mediterr Health J.* 1998;4(1):142-148. Available at: https://apps.who.int/iris/handle/10665/117894.
28. Selmar D, Wittke C, Beck-von Wolffersdorff I, et al. Transfer of pyrrolizidine alkaloids between living plants: a disregarded source of contaminations. *Environ Pollut.* 2019;248:456-461. doi:10.1016/j.envpol.2019.02.026.

29. Vongdala N, Tran HD, Xuan TD, Teschke R, Khanh TD. Heavy metal accumulation in water, soil, and plants of municipal solid waste landfill in Vientiane, Laos. *Int J Environ Res Pub Health.* 2019;16(1):22. doi:10.3390/ijerph16010022.
30. Meunier L, Larrey D. DILI: biomarkers, requirements, candidates and validation. *Front Pharmacol.* 2019;10:1482.
31. Teschke R, Eickhoff A, Brown AC, Neuman MG, Schulze J. Diagnostic biomarkers in liver injury by drugs, herbs, and alcohol: tricky dilemma after EMA correctly and officially retracted Letter of Support. *Int J Mol Sci.* 2020;21:212.
32. Wang R, Qi X, Yoshida EM, et al. Clinical characteristics and outcomes of traditional Chinese medicine-induced liver injury: a systematic review. *Exp Rev Gastroenterol Hepatol.* 2018;12(4):425-434. doi:10.1080/17474124.2018.1427581.
33. Danan G, Teschke R. RUCAM in drug and herb induced liver injury: the update. In: Special Issue "Drug, Herb, and Dietary Supplement Hepatotoxicity," guest editors Rolf Teschke & Raúl J. *Andrade. Int J Mol Sci.* 2016;17(1):14. doi:10.3390/ijms17010014.
34. Fan CQ, Crawford JM. Sinusoidal obstruction syndrome (hepatic veno-occlusive disease). *J Clin Exp Hepatol.* 2014;4(4):332-346. doi:10.1016/j.jceh.2014.10.002.
35. DeLeve LD, Wang X, Wang L. VEGF-sdf1 recruitment of CXCR7+ bone marrow progenitors of liver sinusoidal endothelial cells promotes rat liver regeneration. *Am J Physiol Gastrointest Liver Physiol.* 2016;310(9):G739-G746. doi:10.1152/ajpgi.00056.2016.
36. Quan NV, Xuan TD, Teschke R. Potential hepatotoxins found in herbal medicinal products: a systematic review. *Int J Mol Sci.* 2020;21:5011. doi:10.3390/ijms21145011.
37. Wang X, Qi X, Guo X. Tusanqi-related sinusoidal obstruction syndrome in China: a systematic review of the literatures. *Medicine (Baltimore).* 2015;94(23):e942. doi:10.1097/MD.0000000000000942.
38. Yang XQ, Ye J, Li X, Li Q, Song YH. Pyrrolizidine alkaloids-induced hepatic sinusoidal obstruction syndrome: pathogenesis, clinical manifestations, diagnosis, treatment, and outcomes. *World J Gastroenterol.* 2019;25(28):3753-3763. doi:10.3748/wjg.v25.i28.3753.

CHAPTER 23

Alcohol-Related Liver Disease

Francisco Idalsoaga ■ Ashwani K. Singal ■ Marco Arrese ■ Juan P. Arab

KEY POINTS

- Alcohol-related liver disease (ALD) represents a spectrum of diseases caused by excessive alcohol consumption, including hepatic steatosis, steatohepatitis, different degrees of fibrosis, cirrhosis, and alcohol-related hepatitis.
- Clinical manifestations are observed in advanced stages, where it is possible to identify constitutional symptoms, jaundice, pain in the right hypochondrium, and stigmata of cirrhosis.
- For the diagnosis, it is essential to suspect and identify heavy alcohol consumption and demonstrate hepatocellular damage (by laboratory, imaging, and/or liver biopsy).
- The cornerstone of treatment is abstinence, which must be accompanied by support measures such as nutritional supplementation and management of alcohol withdrawal syndrome.
- In severe alcohol-related hepatitis with Maddrey's discriminant function ≥32 or MELD ≥20, corticosteroids should be used. Patients with MELD between 25 and 39 seem to benefit the most.
- The prognosis of ALD depends on the stage of the disease; in early stages survival is similar to that of the general population, while severe alcohol-related hepatitis has a mortality of 30% to 50% at 90 days.

Introduction

Alcohol-related liver disease (ALD) is one of the main causes of chronic liver disease worldwide and comprises a clinical-histologic spectrum including steatosis, steatohepatitis, different degrees of fibrosis, cirrhosis, and alcohol-related hepatitis (AH).[1] ALD is characterized by hepatocellular damage secondary to excessive alcohol consumption and it is associated with high morbidity and mortality. The natural history of ALD depends on whether one achieves alcohol abstinence or not. Hepatic steatosis is seen in approximately 90% to 95% of heavy drinkers, of which 10% will develop significant fibrosis, and of those, 5% to 10% will develop cirrhosis.[2,3] The most severe acute form of the disease is AH. This entity corresponds to a necro-inflammatory process that is commonly observed in patients with chronic hepatocellular damage. AH presents with rapid onset of jaundice and in severe cases may transition to acute-on-chronic liver failure. AH is associated with a high mortality rate of up to 30% to 50% at 3 months. Although most patients with AH already have cirrhosis, in those who have not, AH can also evolve into cirrhosis in 20% of cases.[4] Indeed, patients with AH are at increased risk of accelerated progression of fibrosis.[2]

Epidemiology

Alcohol consumption is an essential determinant of disease burden, with a significant social and economic impact worldwide.[5] Figure 23.1 depicts global alcohol consumption patterns. The World Health Organization (WHO) and the Institute for Health and Metrics Evaluation estimate that 3.3 million deaths globally are related to alcohol consumption each year.[6] Hazardous alcohol intake produces a catastrophic impact on social and work life, decreasing job performance, increasing labor absenteeism, road traffic injuries, domestic violence, suicide, and homicide.[7,8] Additionally, alcohol accounts for 10% of disability-adjusted life years (DALYs) in men.[9]

Alcohol use disorder (AUD) is one of the leading risk factors for disability and death worldwide[5] and constitutes the seventh leading risk factor for premature death and disability.[10] Although excessive alcohol consumption is frequent, AUD is usually underdiagnosed. Globally, a total of 5.1% of adults have AUD, affecting 8.6% of men and 1.7% of women.[6] Alcohol consumption also contributes to health inequalities, with alcohol-associated conditions being higher and more underreported in lower socioeconomic status (SES).[11-15] Indeed, while in high-income countries unrecorded alcohol corresponds to 11.4%, in low-middle-income countries unrecorded alcohol intake accounts for 40% of all alcohol consumed (45.4% in the South-East Asia Region, 70.5% in the Eastern Mediterranean Region).[6] In some tropical countries the consumption of homemade alcohol is very frequent. For example, in the Seychelles Islands the home brews ("Kalou" or palm toddy made of fermented palm sap, "Baka" of sugar-cane juice, and "Lapire" of fermented juice of various vegetables or fruit) are consumed by 52% of regular drinkers and they are more frequently consumed than products like beer or spirits.[16] Additionally, the consumption of home brews is associated strongly with low SES. In Ethiopia the most frequently consumed alcohol-associated beverages are the traditionally prepared "Areki," "Teje," and "Tella," which have high percentages of alcohol content.[17,18]

Many risk factors that influence the development of ALD have been identified[19-25]:

1. *Magnitude and duration of alcohol consumption:* The amount and duration of alcohol consumption constitute the most important risk factor for the development of chronic liver disease. The risk of cirrhosis increases by 30% in men who drink more than 40 g/day of alcohol and in women who drink more than 20 to 30 g/day. Of subjects with excessive and continuous alcohol consumption for more than 20 years, up to 50% will develop cirrhosis.
2. *Sex.* Women have a higher risk of disease (up to two times compared to men), with less alcohol consumption. The body composition, changes in absorption, and lower levels of the enzyme alcohol dehydrogenase (ADH) in the gastric mucosa have been described to play a role in the higher risk in women.
3. *Consumption pattern.* There is controversy regarding the risk of the pattern of excessive episodic consumption (defined as the consumption of more than 60 g of alcohol on one occasion) and the so-called "binge drinking" (defined as the consumption of ≥4 drinks in women or ≥5 drinks in men in 2 hours at least once a month). However, studies have shown that there is a risk of developing cirrhosis with both daily consumption and excessive episodic consumption.
4. *Individual susceptibility:* Multiple individual determinants increase susceptibility to alcohol-induced liver injury. Approximately 15% of heavy drinkers develop liver disease. Genetic polymorphisms (such as *PNPLA3*) and ethnicity (Hispanic and African-American) have been associated with an increased risk of cirrhosis related to alcohol consumption.
5. *Comorbidities.* Nutritional variations (obesity, malnourishment, and metabolic syndrome), other liver diseases (chronic viral hepatitis, nonalcohol-associated fatty liver disease, and hemochromatosis), and HIV infection all increase the risk of liver disease.

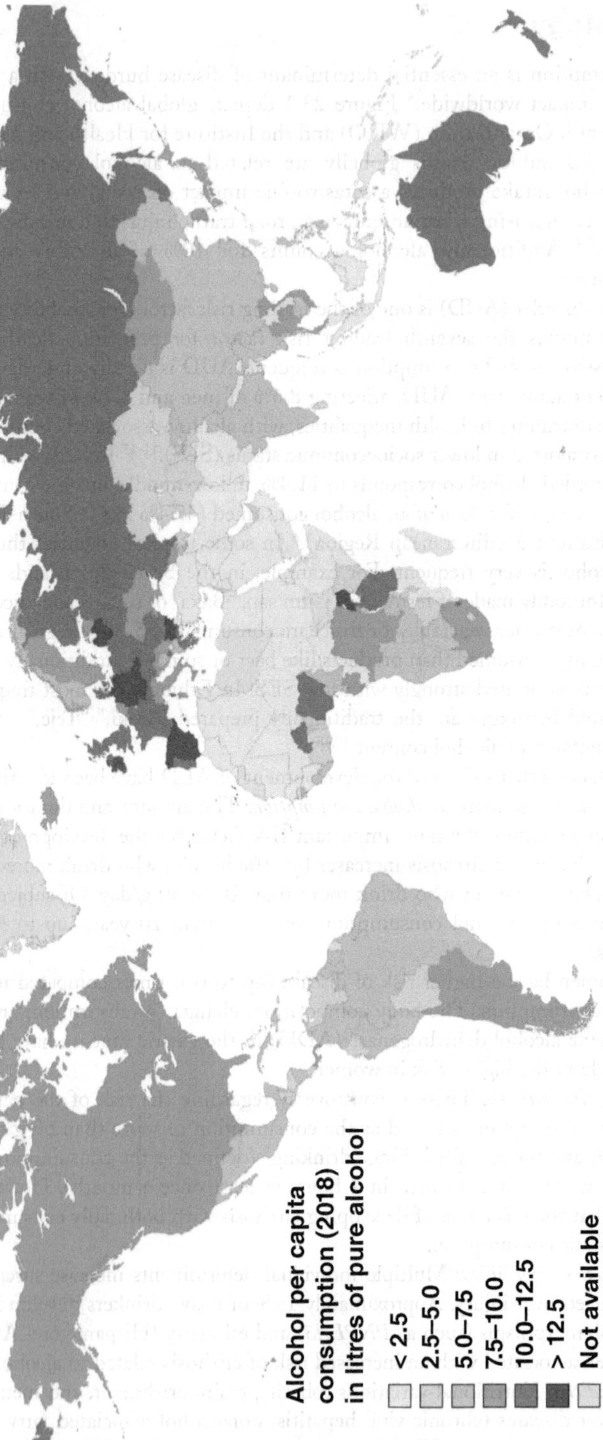

Figure 23.1 Total alcohol per capita consumption in liters of pure alcohol (2018).[6]

Pathogenesis

Alcohol is a substance that is toxic to the liver *per se*; thus the pathogenesis of ALD is mainly due to the consequences of its hepatic metabolization, activation of immunity, and an imbalance of cellular functions. The metabolism of alcohol in the liver (production of acetaldehyde and free radicals), activation of Kupffer cells (production of free radicals and hypoxia), and activation of hepatic stellate cells (fibrogenesis) are the main factors involved in the pathogenesis of ALD.[26,27] These processes lead to direct structural damage, oxidative damage, immune reactions, hypoxia, and peroxidation of fatty acids in the membranes, progressively constituting necrosis, inflammation, and fibrosis.[26-29]

The histological manifestations observed in ALD are steatosis, steatohepatitis, and fibrosis/cirrhosis, which generally coexist in various combinations (Figure 23.2). In steatosis a macrovesicular type of intracellular neutral fat deposition is observed displacing the nuclei of the hepatocytes, mainly in the centrilobular zone (acinus zone 3) and, in more severe cases, the entire parenchyma. Cirrhosis due to alcohol is histologically similar to cirrhosis due to other causes. AH is histologically characterized by hepatocyte damage, steatosis, increased cell volume (ballooning), Mallory-Denk hyaline bodies, presence of megamitochondria, bilirubinostasis, central perivenular inflammation, lobule neutrophil infiltration, pericellular and sinusoidal fibrosis, and confluent necrosis of hepatocytes in the most peripheral area of the acinus.[4,30]

Presentation

The symptoms and signs of ALD have a wide spectrum, ranging from asymptomatic patients with a normal physical examination to patients with multiple symptoms of decompensation

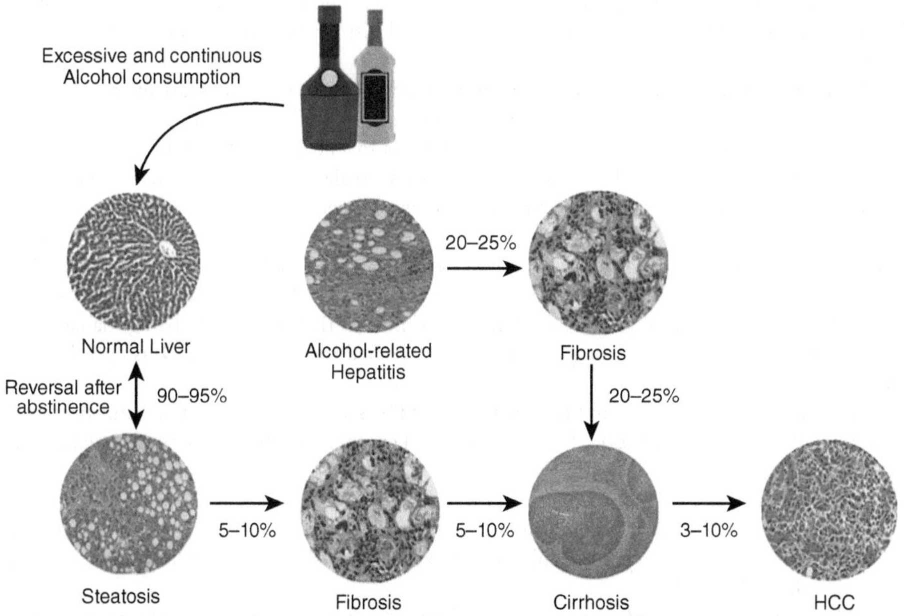

Figure 23.2 Spectrum of alcohol-related liver disease. In patients with excessive alcohol consumption, 90% to 95% develop steatosis. Of these patients, between 5% and 10% will develop fibrosis, and then between 5% and 10% will present with cirrhosis. Between 3% and 10% of those with cirrhosis will have HCC. In patients with AH between 20% and 25% will develop fibrosis, and of these, between 20% and 25% will have cirrhosis.[2,35]

and stigmata of chronic liver disease. More than 90% of individuals with ALD are asymptomatic or have non-specific symptoms. In those patients diagnosis is suspected upon observing abnormal laboratory or incidental abdominal ultrasound findings. Clinical manifestations are observed in advanced stages and are commonly represented by constitutional symptoms, jaundice, pain in the right upper quadrant, and stigmata of cirrhosis. Of note, AH can be seen at any stage of the disease. In patients with advanced chronic liver disease it is possible to find symptoms and signs secondary to cirrhosis or its complications. The most suggestive signs of alcohol-related cirrhosis are parotid hypertrophy, Dupuytren's contracture, and signs of feminization.[30,31]

AH has a wide spectrum of presentation, from mild symptoms to liver failure. The cardinal symptom/sign is rapid-onset jaundice. Additionally, among the most frequent manifestations are asthenia, anorexia, adynamia, fever, pain in the epigastrium or right hypochondrium, which can be very severe, and abdominal distension (secondary to ascites). On physical examination, patients may present with jaundice, hepatomegaly, ascites (due to decompensation of cirrhosis or temporary obstruction of the portal vein due to liver inflammation), hepatic encephalopathy, and eventually stigmata of cirrhosis.[32,33]

There are also extrahepatic manifestations of alcohol injury, such as neuropsychiatric disorders, hypovitaminosis (vitamin B12 and thiamine), cardiomyopathy, gastritis, pancreatitis, hypogonadism, polyneuritis, myopathy, hypoglycemia, and hyperglycemia, hypertriglyceridemia, macrocytic anemia, and thrombocytopenia.[34]

Diagnosis

It is essential to suspect and identify heavy alcohol consumption and demonstrate hepatocellular damage (by laboratory, imaging, and/or liver biopsy). No single laboratory marker can establish the diagnosis of ALD; thus the combination of medical history, laboratory, and clinical findings should be used.

Medical history and examination must be performed in a guilt-free environment and complement the information by interviewing relatives or close friends. To support the identification of patients with alcohol misuse, the Alcohol Use Disorders Inventory Test (AUDIT) is a validated tool to screen for patients with AUD. The AUDIT-C scale is an abbreviated adaptation of the AUDIT scale which has also been validated. This corresponds to a three-question scale on consumer habits.[35-37]

Patients with heavy alcohol use (>3 drinks per day in men and >2 drinks in women for >5 years) should always be counseled, highlighting the fact that they are at an increased risk for liver disease. Current clinical practice guidelines recommend that all patients being managed at primary care or admitted to the hospital should be screened routinely for AUD using validated questionnaires.[38]

In general, patients with harmful alcohol use should be screened with liver biochemistries and abdominal ultrasound examination. Furthermore, markers that are helpful in clinical practice are given as follows:

- *Markers suggestive of chronic heavy alcohol consumption:* Macrocytosis (mean corpuscular volume [MCV] >100), high gamma-glutamyl transferase (GGT), hypertriglyceridemia and increased HDL, hyperuricemia, decarboxylated transferrin, ethyl glucuronide (EtG), and ethyl sulfate.[2,31]
- *Markers suggestive of alcohol-associated liver disease:* Macrocytic anemia with thrombocytopenia, mild elevation of aminotransferases (may be normal), hyperbilirubinemia, hypoalbuminemia, and prolongation of prothrombin time (PT). An aspartate aminotransferase (AST or GOT)/alanine aminotransferase (ALT or GPT) ratio >2 (and particularly if >3) is suggestive of ALD but not of cirrhosis.

- *Markers suggestive of alcohol-related hepatitis:* rapid development or worsening of jaundice and liver-related complications, with serum total bilirubin >3 mg/dL; ALT (GPT) and AST (GOT) elevated >1.5 times the upper limit of normal but <400 U/L with the AST/ALT (GOT/GPT) ratio >1.5; elevation of GGT; and leukocytosis, predominantly neutrophilic and prolongation of PT.[2]

The stage of fibrosis is associated with long-term outcomes and should be evaluated with non-invasive radiologic methods and serum biomarkers.[39,40] The Enhanced Liver Fibrosis score and FibroTest, which are calculated by combining laboratory parameters and age, can rule out advanced fibrosis and have high negative predictive values (94% and 90%, respectively). The Fibrosis-4 score also may be used to exclude advanced fibrosis or cirrhosis. Transient elastography is a useful radiologic tool to evaluate fibrosis, with sensitivity and specificity of 86% and 94%, respectively, for diagnosing advanced fibrosis or cirrhosis.[39-43]

Imaging tests can aid in the diagnosis, supporting evidence of liver disease and excluding other causes of laboratory abnormalities. Fatty infiltration of the liver, fibrosis, hepatomegaly, splenomegaly, nodularity of the liver, and signs of portal hypertension can be seen. On computed tomography (CT) scan and magnetic resonance imaging (MRI), signs suggestive of cirrhosis due to ALD can be observed: an increase in the volume of the caudate lobe, visualization of the right posterior hepatic notch, and a smaller size of regenerative nodules (compared to cirrhosis due to viral hepatitis). Liver biopsy is also useful as a diagnostic and prognostic tool. However, its use should be evaluated on a case-by-case basis according to the risks and benefits of the procedure.

Management

Compared with other causes of cirrhosis (i.e., viral hepatitis), almost no pharmacological advances have been made in the management of patients with ALD in the past decades. The cornerstone of treatment is abstinence, which should be associated with measures such as nutritional supplementation and the management of alcohol withdrawal syndrome.[31] In addition, in cases of AH, severity should be stratified and corticosteroids could be used in cases with severe disease.[44] Additionally, patients with obesity or chronic HCV infection should be advised to avoid alcohol consumption.[31]

General management: Although abstinence does not guarantee a complete recovery from the disease, it is currently the mainstay of the treatment of ALD. The main drugs currently used to prevent relapse are acamprosate, naltrexone, nalmefene, topiramate, gabapentin, and baclofen.[45] However, naltrexone and acamprosate (despite being FDA-approved drugs for AUD) have not specifically been tested in ALD patients. Disulfiram, a frequently used drug, can cause severe hepatotoxicity and is contraindicated in this group of patients. One of the most commonly used drugs is baclofen, a γ-amino butyric acid-B receptor agonist. This drug is safe in patients with ALD and cirrhosis and is effective in increasing abstinence rates.[46] It is usually started at a dose of 5 mg three times a day (TID), and the dose can be increased at a 3- to 5-day interval based on patient tolerance (maximum dose is 15 mg TID). Acamprosate is usually used at a dose of 666 mg TID, and naltrexone can be used at doses of 50 mg QD per oral or 380 mg monthly intramuscular.

In patients with chronic alcohol consumption it is important to suspect and prevent alcohol withdrawal syndrome and to perform a timely psychiatric evaluation.

Management of cirrhosis: The management of cirrhosis from alcohol is the same as for cirrhosis from any other cause. The stage of the disease should be evaluated, and complications actively sought. In patients with advanced cirrhosis due to alcohol (MELD ≥15) who have discontinued consumption or have a favorable psychosocial profile, liver transplantation should be considered.

Treatment of AH: For the initial management of AH, the disease severity and the risk of complications should be evaluated. Severe AH is defined as a Maddrey's discriminant function score ≥ 32, MELD > 20, or encephalopathy.[44] Low-risk patients can improve only with abstinence from alcohol, nutritional support, and general measures. In contrast, patients with severe disease have a worse prognosis and additional treatment measures should be evaluated.

Abstinence is always the first measure and alcohol withdrawal syndrome should be suspected and avoided. Supportive measures include moderate hydration (overhydration can increase the risk of ascites and increased portal pressure) and nutritional therapy (malnutrition is a poor prognostic element, so it is essential to ensure consumption of 35–40 kcal/kg/day and protein 1 g/kg/day) as well as supplementation of vitamins (B complex vitamins, folic acid, and vitamin K) and minerals (magnesium, phosphorus, and zinc).

For severe AH, corticosteroids could be used. Corticosteroids, although controversial, are the first-line treatment for severe AH, since they reduce mortality in the short term.[4,30,31] The usual dose is prednisolone 40 mg/day for 1 month. Corticosteroids should not be used in patients with active infection, hepatitis B, or gastrointestinal bleeding. The response to corticosteroid treatment can be predicted using the Lille Model (based on age, albumin, bilirubin, creatinine, and PT), with a value ≥ 0.45 at 1 week predicting failure to corticosteroid treatment; corticosteroids should be discontinued in this group of patients.[47,48] Additionally, it has been recently described as an optimal therapeutic window for the use of steroids between MELD of 25 and 39, where the maximum benefit is achieved.[49]

Systemic inflammatory response syndrome (SIRS) at admission predisposes to acute kidney injury and multi-organ failure, which are associated with a poor prognosis. It is critical to take appropriate measures to prevent renal injury. Avoidance of nephrotoxic drugs, judicious use of diuretics, and low threshold for expanding circulating blood volume with albumin or saline infusions are recommended.[31]

It is important to remember that patients with severe AH have high mortality, and liver transplantation could be considered in the appropriate setting. Numerous studies have shown that early liver transplantation improves survival in patients with severe AH who have not responded to medical treatment. A comprehensive and individual evaluation of the patient should be carried out that includes many factors, including alcohol abstinence of approximately 6 months (although this varies per center).[31,50-52] Other therapies that act on the inflammation, fibrogenesis, oxidative stress, and immune activation pathways have been studied, such as pentoxifylline and TNF-alpha antagonists (infliximab and etanercept), but none have been shown to be useful.

The prognosis of ALD depends on the stage of the disease; on the one hand, patients with steatosis have a survival rate similar to that of the general population. On the other hand, patients with AH have a mortality of up to 50% at 3 months. Thus early liver transplantation is currently recommended for selected patients. In this sense the most important post-transplant prognostic factor is abstinence, and it should be pursued in all patients.

References

1. Gao B, Bataller R. Alcoholic liver disease: pathogenesis and new therapeutic targets. *Gastroenterology.* 2011;141:1572-1585.
2. Singal AK, Mathurin P. Diagnosis and treatment of alcohol-associated liver disease: a review. *JAMA.* 2021;326:165-176.
3. Mathurin P, Bataller R. Trends in the management and burden of alcoholic liver disease. *J Hepatol.* 2015;62:S38-S46.
4. Lucey MR, Mathurin P, Morgan TR. Alcoholic hepatitis. *N Engl J Med.* 2009;360:2758-2769.
5. Lopez AD, Williams TN, Levin A, et al. Remembering the forgotten non-communicable diseases. *BMC Med.* 2014;12:200.

6. World Health Organization. *Global Status Report on Alcohol and Health 2018*. Geneva, Switzerland: World Health Organization; 2019.
7. Cargiulo T. Understanding the health impact of alcohol dependence. *Am J Health Syst Pharm*. 2007;64:S5-S11.
8. Hadland SE, Xuan Z, Sarda V, et al. Alcohol policies and alcohol-related motor vehicle crash fatalities among young people in the US. *Pediatrics*. 2017;139:e20163037. doi:10.1542/peds.2016-3037.
9. Williams R, Aspinall R, Bellis M, et al. Addressing liver disease in the UK: a blueprint for attaining excellence in health care and reducing premature mortality from lifestyle issues of excess consumption of alcohol, obesity, and viral hepatitis. *Lancet*. 2014;384:1953-1997.
10. Griswold MG, Fullman N, Hawley C, et al. Alcohol use and burden for 195 countries and territories, 1990–2016: a systematic analysis for the Global Burden of Disease Study 2016. *Lancet*. 2018;392:1015-1035.
11. Rehm J, Mathers C, Popova S, Thavorncharoensap M, Teerawattananon Y, Patra J. Global burden of disease and injury and economic cost attributable to alcohol use and alcohol-use disorders. *Lancet*. 2009;373:2223-2233.
12. Probst C, Roerecke M, Behrendt S, Rehm J. Socioeconomic differences in alcohol-attributable mortality compared with all-cause mortality: a systematic review and meta-analysis. *Int J Epidemiol*. 2014;43:1314-1327.
13. Probst C, Roerecke M, Behrendt S, Rehm J. Gender differences in socioeconomic inequality of alcohol-attributable mortality: a systematic review and meta-analysis. *Drug Alcohol Rev*. 2015;34:267-277.
14. Harrison L, Gardiner E. Do the rich really die young? Alcohol-related mortality and social class in Great Britain, 1988–94. *Addiction*. 1999;94:1871-1880.
15. Díaz LA, Idalsoaga F, Fuentes-López E, et al. Impact of public health policies on alcohol-associated liver disease in Latin America: an ecological multinational study. *Hepatology*. 2021;74:2478-2490.
16. Perdrix J, Bovet P, Larue D, Yersin B, Burnand B, Paccaud F. Patterns of alcohol consumption in the Seychelles Islands (Indian Ocean). *Alcohol Alcohol*. 1999;34:773-785.
17. Bitew MS, Zewde MF, Wubetu M, Alemu AA. Consumption of alcohol and binge drinking among pregnant women in Addis Ababa, Ethiopia: prevalence and determinant factors. *PLoS One*. 2020;15:e0243784.
18. Wedajo Lemi B. Microbiology of Ethiopian traditionally fermented beverages and condiments. *Int J Microbiol*. 2020;2020:1478536.
19. Stein E, Cruz-Lemini M, Altamirano J, et al. Heavy daily alcohol intake at the population level predicts the weight of alcohol in cirrhosis burden worldwide. *J Hepatol*. 2016;65:998-1005.
20. Stickel F, Datz C, Hampe J, Bataller R. Pathophysiology and management of alcoholic liver disease: update 2016. *Gut Liver*. 2017;11:173-188.
21. Askgaard G, Grønbæk M, Kjær MS, Tjønneland A, Tolstrup JS. Alcohol drinking pattern and risk of alcoholic liver cirrhosis: a prospective cohort study. *J Hepatol*. 2015;62:1061-1067.
22. Sookoian S, Pirola CJ. How Safe is moderate alcohol consumption in overweight and obese individuals? *Gastroenterology*. 2016;150:1698-1703.e2.
23. Levy RE, Catana AM, Durbin-Johnson B, Halsted CH, Medici V. Ethnic differences in presentation and severity of alcoholic liver disease. *Alcohol Clin Exp Res*. 2015;39:566-574.
24. Stickel F, Buch S, Lau K, et al. Genetic variation in the PNPLA3 gene is associated with alcoholic liver injury in Caucasians. *Hepatology*. 2011;53:86-95.
25. Altamirano J, Higuera-de laTijera F, Duarte-Rojo A, et al. The amount of alcohol consumption negatively impacts short-term mortality in Mexican patients with alcoholic hepatitis. *Am J Gastroenterol*. 2011;106:1472-1480.
26. Kaplowitz N, Than TA, Shinohara M, Ji C. Endoplasmic reticulum stress and liver injury. *Semin Liver Dis*. 2007;27:367-377.
27. Lieber CS. Biochemical factors in alcoholic liver disease. *Semin Liver Dis*. 1993;13:136-153.
28. Szabo G, Petrasek J, Bala S. Innate immunity and alcoholic liver disease. *Dig Dis*. 2012;30(suppl 1):55-60.
29. Li S, Tan H-Y, Wang N, Feng Y, Wang X, Feng Y. Recent insights into the role of immune cells in alcoholic liver disease. *Front Immunol*. 2019;10:1328.
30. Arab JP, Roblero JP, Altamirano J, et al. Alcohol-related liver disease: clinical practice guidelines by the Latin American Association for the Study of the Liver (ALEH). *Ann Hepatol*. 2019;18:518-535.

31. Singal AK, Bataller R, Ahn J, Kamath PS, Shah VH. ACG Clinical Guideline: alcoholic liver disease. *Am J Gastroenterol.* 2018;113:175-194.
32. Mendenhall CL. Alcoholic hepatitis. *Clin Gastroenterol.* 1981;10:417-441.
33. Lischner MW, Alexander JF, Galambos JT. Natural history of alcoholic hepatitis. I. The acute disease. *Am J Dig Dis.* 1971;16:481-494.
34. Fernández-Solà J. Management of extrahepatic manifestations in alcoholic liver disease. *Clin Liver Dis.* 2013;2:89-91.
35. Bush K, Kivlahan DR, McDonell MB, Fihn SD, Bradley KA. The AUDIT Alcohol Consumption Questions (AUDIT-C): an effective brief screening test for problem drinking. Ambulatory Care Quality Improvement Project (ACQUIP). *Arch Intern Med.* 1998;158:1789-1795.
36. Bradley KA, DeBenedetti AF, Volk RJ, Williams EC, Frank D, Kivlahan DR. AUDIT-C as a brief screen for alcohol misuse in primary care. *Alcohol Clin Exp Res.* 2007;31:1208-1217.
37. Frank D, DeBenedetti AF, Volk RJ, Williams EC, Kivlahan DR, Bradley KA. Effectiveness of the AUDIT-C as a screening test for alcohol misuse in three race/ethnic groups. *J Gen Intern Med.* 2008; 23:781-787.
38. Crabb DW, Im GY, Szabo G, Mellinger JL, Lucey MR. Diagnosis and treatment of alcohol-associated liver diseases: 2019 practice guidance from the American Association for the Study of Liver Diseases. *Hepatology.* 2020;71:306-333.
39. de Franchis R, Baveno VI Faculty. Expanding consensus in portal hypertension: Report of the Baveno VI Consensus Workshop: stratifying risk and individualizing care for portal hypertension. *J Hepatol.* 2015;63:743-752.
40. Moreno C, Mueller S, Szabo G. Non-invasive diagnosis and biomarkers in alcohol-related liver disease. *J Hepatol.* 2019;70:273-283.
41. Thiele M, Madsen BS, Hansen JF, Detlefsen S, Antonsen S, Krag A. Accuracy of the Enhanced Liver Fibrosis Test vs FibroTest, elastography, and indirect markers in detection of advanced fibrosis in patients with alcoholic liver disease. *Gastroenterology.* 2018;154:1369-1379.
42. Bensamoun SF, Leclerc GE, Debernard L, et al. Cutoff values for alcoholic liver fibrosis using magnetic resonance elastography technique. *Alcohol Clin Exp Res.* 2013;37:811-817.
43. de Franchis R, Bosch J, Garcia-Tsao G, Reiberger T, Ripoll C, Baveno VII Faculty. Baveno VII—Renewing consensus in portal hypertension. *J Hepatol.* 2022;76:959-974.
44. Maddrey WC, Boitnott JK, Bedine MS, Weber Jr FL, Mezey E, White Jr RI. Corticosteroid therapy of alcoholic hepatitis. *Gastroenterology.* 1978;75:193-199.
45. Jonas DE, Amick HR, Feltner C, et al. Pharmacotherapy for adults with alcohol use disorders in outpatient settings: a systematic review and meta-analysis. *JAMA.* 2014;311:1889-1900.
46. Addolorato G, Leggio L, Ferrulli A, et al. Effectiveness and safety of baclofen for maintenance of alcohol abstinence in alcohol-dependent patients with liver cirrhosis: randomised, double-blind controlled study. *Lancet.* 2007;370:1915-1922.
47. Louvet A, Naveau S, Abdelnour M, et al. The Lille model: a new tool for therapeutic strategy in patients with severe alcoholic hepatitis treated with steroids. *Hepatology.* 2007;45:1348-1354.
48. Forrest EH, Atkinson SR, Richardson P, et al. Application of prognostic scores in the STOPAH trial: discriminant function is no longer the optimal scoring system in alcoholic hepatitis. *J Hepatol.* 2018; 68:511-518.
49. Arab JP, Díaz LA, Baeza N, et al. Identification of optimal therapeutic window for steroid use in severe alcohol-associated hepatitis: a worldwide study. *J Hepatol.* 2021;75:1026-1033.
50. Gonzalez A, Valero-Breton M, Huerta-Salgado C, Achiardi O, Simon F, Cabello-Verrugio C. Impact of exercise training on the sarcopenia criteria in non-alcoholic fatty liver disease: a systematic review and meta-analysis. *Eur J Transl Myol.* 2021;31:9630. doi:10.4081/ejtm.2021.9630.
51. Lucey MR, Im GY, Mellinger JL, Szabo G, Crabb DW. Introducing the 2019 American association for the study of liver diseases guidance on alcohol-associated liver disease. *Liver Transpl.* 2020;26:14-16.
52. Mathurin P, Moreno C, Samuel D, et al. Early liver transplantation for severe alcoholic hepatitis. *N Engl J Med.* 2011;365:1790-1800.

CHAPTER 24

Drug-Induced Liver Injury in Tropical Settings

Mark Sonderup

KEY POINTS

- DILI is likely underestimated in tropical settings
- The many diagnostic investigations required may not be readily available in resource-limited settings
- Clinical suspicion remains key to diagnosis given many DILI phenotypes
- Anti-TB, antiretroviral drugs, antibiotics, as well as herbal and dietary supplements are key causes of DILI
- Online tools like a RUCAM calculator can aid in the diagnosis, and stopping the offending drug is paramount in the treatment of DILI

Introduction

Drug-induced liver injuries (DILIs) are uncommon but potentially severe adverse drug reactions following exposure to a hepatotoxic drug. As most drug injuries are idiosyncratic, DILI should always be part of a differential diagnosis in patients presenting with an abnormal liver profile, either acutely or in a chronic setting. Abnormal liver profiles are a sensitive indicator of liver injury, but they are neither specific nor able to predict a subsequent clinical course in DILI. Key to DILI diagnosis remains vigilance and consideration to the possibility of DILI. A common characterization of DILI is to separate it into being either intrinsic or idiosyncratic, with idiosyncratic DILI being significantly more frequent. Intrinsic DILI is predictable and often dose dependent, as is observed in cases such as paracetamol/acetaminophen overdose. Mounting data suggests that the two characterizations are less distinct, but they remain good conceptual paradigms.[1] DILI incidence in low- and middle-income countries (LMIC) is poorly characterized, but it is likely high given the significant burden of disease. Few studies exist on an accurate incidence of DILI in certain LMIC regions such as sub-Saharan Africa. A clinicopathological study of 301 liver biopsies in HIV-positive patients in South Africa noted DILI in 42% of patients.[2] The leading drugs associated with DILI included cotrimoxazole, antiretroviral (ART) therapy, anti-tuberculosis (TB), and herbal or traditional remedies. In sub-Saharan Africa traditional medicine use is frequent, while in Asia a range of remedies, including ayurvedic and other herbals, are commonly used and implicated in drug- or toxin-induced liver injury.[3] The Latin America DILI Network (LATINDILIN) set up in 2011 has provided valuable insights into DILI in the region. The leading implicated drugs in the first 5 years of the registry included amoxicillin-clavulanate (AC), diclofenac, nimesulide, nitrofurantoin, cyproterone acetate, ibuprofen, anti-TB drugs, carbamazepine, phenytoin, and methimazole.[4] It is thus evident that in tropical regions DILI is an

TABLE 24.1 ■ **Leading Drugs Causing DILI in the South American DILI Network (LATINDILIN) Compared to Spain, the United States, and India**[5]

Drug	LATINDILIN (*n* = 311)	Spanish DILI Registry (*n* = 878)	DILIN (*n* = 899)	India (*n* = 313)
Amoxicillin-clavulanate	41	202	91	3
Nitrofurantoin	19	2	42	-
Diclofenac	18	16	12	1
Anti-TB drugs	12	28	-	181
Nimesulide$	12	9	-	2
Ibuprofen	9	27	1	2
Cyproterone	9	3	-	-
Carbamazepine	8	8	4	9
Methyldopa	6	0	11	0
Atorvastatin	5	18	8	5

$—not available in the United States.

important consideration in patients presenting with an unexplained abnormal liver profile. Table 24.1 compares the relative frequencies of leading causes of DILI in various regions compared to LATIDILIN.

Challenges in DILI Presentation and Diagnosis

DILI remains a diagnosis of exclusion based on a detailed history and extensive investigations including blood tests, hepatobiliary imaging, and possible liver biopsy. Causality scores such as the Roussel-UCLAF Causality Assessment Method (RUCAM) are useful (and easily found online) and intended to confirm or exclude the suspicion of DILI, but the diagnosis hinges on a complete diagnostic workup.[6] In LMIC viral infections are frequent and warrant exclusion, such as hepatitis A, B, C, D (in those with chronic hepatitis B infection), and E. Data from the DILI network in the United States (DILIN) demonstrated that almost 3% of patients with suspected DILI had positive anti-hepatitis E virus (HEV) IgM serology, suggesting that HEV should be part of DILI causality testing.[7] An Egyptian study found a much higher rate of almost 15% seropositivity. Of those with positive HEV IgM antibodies, 58% were HEV PCR positive.[8] Several countries in sub-Saharan Africa, including Namibia and Uganda, have experienced almost endemic outbreaks of hepatitis E, thus making it an important investigation to consider. Hepatitis E has been noted in several South American studies, although rates seem to be low, with cases of acute liver failure rarely observed.[9] Hepatitis E testing via anti-HEV antibodies is, in theory, relatively simple; however, the reliability of the currently available tests is poor, they are not readily available and none is WHO prequalified (further information on HEV is present in a chapter in the book).[10] Testing for hepatitis D is also not routinely available in many countries, adding to the challenge of excluding this as a co-factor or diagnosis.[11] Radiological assessment should exclude obvious pathologies such as Budd-Chiari syndrome, malignancy, or choledocholithiasis. Ultrasound, often more readily available, is ideal for this, but more advanced imaging may be warranted. Autoantibodies (antinuclear antibody and anti-smooth muscle antibody) and serum total IgG levels should be routinely obtained, as part of an autoimmune hepatitis evaluation. Low titers of autoantibodies, typically ≤1:80, are not infrequent and do not imply autoimmune hepatitis.[12] Liver biopsy, although not mandatory, can be a valuable adjunct in DILI assessment, although histological patterns may suggest a drug injury but are not diagnostic. Where DILI is suggested and polypharmacy is involved, it is difficult to ascertain on biopsy which drug is most likely implicated, unless a pathognomonic injury pattern is evident, for example, amiodarone and steatohepatitis. Biopsy is very useful to exclude other possible diagnoses, such as autoimmune hepatitis or an unusual drug injury pattern, for example, nodular regenerative hyperplasia (NRH).[1] In cholestatic injuries liver biopsy does allow for the evaluation of the severity of the bile duct injury and any features suggesting the development of ductopenia or the "vanishing bile duct syndrome." Although few data exist, biopsy may also guide whether adjunctive steroids may be helpful in managing a patient with DILI where, for example, an immune-allergic pattern is observed with a marked inflammatory component.[1] If possible, a portion of the biopsy should be sent for culture or for viral PCR testing, when required. This is especially useful in immunocompromised patients, for example, individuals with human immunodeficiency virus (HIV)/acquired immunodeficiency syndrome (AIDS), where fungal and TB culture of liver tissue is diagnostically useful. Other infections, e.g. malaria, should also be considered and appropriately excluded.[13]

Specific Drug Patterns of Injury

Drug-induced liver disease can be simply designated into three patterns of injury: hepatocellular, cholestatic, and mixed hepatocellular-cholestatic based on the biochemical pattern of serum liver enzyme elevations. Although drug-specific patterns of injury are not uniform, certain drugs tend to typically produce defined biochemical and histological patterns of injury. For example, cholestatic injury associated with AC, flucloxacillin, or terbinafine or hepatocellular injury associated with statins or nevirapine is typical. Given the burden of disease in tropical settings or LMIC, particularly HIV/AIDS and TB, certain drugs or drug classes are associated with DILI more frequently.[14]

Anti-Tuberculosis Drugs

The hepatotoxicity potential of first-line anti-TB drugs, as well as those used in managing multidrug-resistant (MDR)/extensively drug-resistant (XDR) TB, is well described. Anti-TB DILI is reported in 2% to 33% of patients depending on various DILI definitions and study populations.[15,16] Rifampicin, isoniazid, and pyrazinamide typically produce a hepatocellular type of liver injury days to weeks after initiating anti-TB therapy. Rifampicin can elicit a transient dose-dependent interference of bilirubin metabolism, producing an unconjugated hyperbilirubinemia without actual hepatocellular injury. More frequently, a hepatocellular injury can occur. Pyrazinamide can produce a range of both dose-dependent or idiosyncratic hepatotoxic injuries with an occasional immune-allergic hypersensitivity reaction with eosinophilia and liver injury or even granulomatous hepatitis. Isoniazid is primarily hepatically metabolized via acetylation by N-acetyltransferase-2. A metabolite is mono-acetyl hydrazine (MAH) with hepatotoxicity mediated via free radical generation, and, unlike classic hypersensitivity reactions, isoniazid rechallenge does not always evoke a rapid recurrence of hepatotoxicity. Acetylator status may play a role in isoniazid DILI, where in fast acetylators more than 90% of the drug is excreted as acetyl-isoniazid, whereas in slow acetylators, 67% is excreted as acetyl-isoniazid and a greater percentage of isoniazid is excreted as unchanged in urine. Acetylation status and DILI risk are not entirely clear as early data suggested fast acetylators generated acetyl-isoniazid, and thus toxic intermediates more rapidly; however, they clear MAH more rapidly. It is thus slow acetylators that accumulate more MAH over time and thus have overall greater exposure. They tend to develop higher ALT levels and are more likely to fail drug rechallenge.[17] Risk factors for DILI in patients receiving anti-TB treatment are well described in the literature. The most important risk factors include age >35 years, female gender, hepatitis B or C, alcohol use, slow acetylator status, abnormal baseline ALT, malnutrition, and HIV co-infection.[18]

As a combination of drugs are used in TB treatment, the likely offending drug is not always apparent. In patients on anti-TB therapy an elevation in the transaminases above three to five times the upper limit of normal (ULN) or any elevation in a symptomatic or jaundiced patient should prompt the immediate cessation of therapy. Rechallenge of TB drugs should ideally only be attempted once alanine aminotransferase (ALT) is <100 IU/L and jaundice has resolved. Rechallenge in patients in which DILI resulted in acute liver failure (jaundice with encephalopathy and/or coagulopathy) should not be attempted. Rechallenge of TB drugs is mostly safe and effective in 60% to 90% of patients, but frequent ALT monitoring during rechallenge is essential, with at least ALT monitoring three times weekly during rechallenge and weekly for 1 month following successful rechallenge.[19]

After allowing liver enzymes to improve, standard practice is to initiate a stepwise drug rechallenge using appropriate weight-based dosing of the individual drugs. Older data suggest that pyrazinamide is not rechallenged, although more recent data have suggested that pyrazinamide could be used as part of a drug rechallenge, albeit in selected patients and with due caution. It can be considered in those with TB meningitis, miliary TB, or where rifampicin or isoniazid rechallenge fails.[19]

Strategies to enhance recovery after anti-TB DILI have been looked at. A recent randomized controlled trial of administering intravenous N-acetyl cysteine to patients with confirmed anti-TB DILI demonstrated that it did not shorten the time to achieve an ALT <100 U/L but significantly reduced length of hospital stay.[20] In patients with HIV who develop TB after initiating ART therapy and are commenced on anti-TB treatment and who then develop jaundice, a diagnostic complicating factor is the clinical entity of TB immune reconstitution inflammatory syndrome (TB-IRIS), which becomes a differential diagnosis. Differentiating factors include the rapid development of systemic symptoms, jaundice, hepatomegaly, and possible ascites. The liver profile tends to demonstrate a more predominant cholestatic component, as opposed to the hepatocellular nature of anti-TB DILI.[21]

Antiretroviral Therapy

The burden of HIV/AIDS in LMIC, particularly sub-Saharan Africa, is enormous, with almost 75% of the global HIV/AIDS burden residing in this region.[22] Massive upscaling of ART programs has contributed to the decline in HIV mortality and morbidity; however, concomitant increased rates of DILI are also observed as a consequence of increasing numbers of people on ART.

NUCLEOSIDE REVERSE TRANSCRIPTASE INHIBITORS

Early data with first-generation nucleoside reverse transcriptase inhibitors (NRTIs) reported hepatotoxicity rates ranging from 7% with zidovudine, 9% to 13% with stavudine, to 16% with didanosine.[23] The newer and later-generation NRTI such as lamivudine, emtricitabine, tenofovir, and abacavir are associated with a significantly lower risk of liver injury. Hepatotoxicity is mediated through an infrequent but distinctive DILI pattern causing acute liver failure preceded by a tender mild hepatomegaly (due to macro- and microsteatosis) and lactic acidosis. The injury is mediated through NRTIs inhibiting mitochondrial gamma-polymerase, normally required for the maintenance of mitochondrial mass and function, thus impairing hepatic mitochondrial function.[24] Unlike the other NRTIs, abacavir toxicity or DILI potential is predictable in those with HLA-B*5701 phenotype. Finally, an uncommon didanosine-related liver injury produces portal fibrosis with NRH. Another rare variant is didanosine-related non-cirrhotic portal hypertension secondary to NRH and obliterative portal venopathy, where patients clinically manifest with portal hypertension features, including ascites and variceal hemorrhage.[25] Jaundice is infrequent and liver enzymes are modestly elevated. Mechanisms are thought to relate to didanosine damaging endothelial cells and producing thrombotic occlusion with secondary nodular hyperplasia. For their toxicity potential, older NRTIs, such as stavudine and didanosine, are mostly not used anymore.

NON-NUCLEOSIDE REVERSE TRANSCRIPTASE INHIBITORS

Nevirapine

In 17 randomized trials 10% of patients developed ALT/aspartate transaminase (AST) more than five times the ULN, and 6.3% were symptomatic.[25] Risk factors included hepatitis B or C coinfection, female gender, a CD4 greater than 250/mm^3 or where nevirapine was used as part of postexposure prophylaxis.[26] Overall, the 1% frequency of nevirapine DILI is significant, with an approximate 0.1% mortality. There are two patterns of nevirapine DILI—an early-onset drug hypersensitivity reaction/immune-mediated pattern within the first 6 to 8 weeks of therapy with abdominal pain, fever, rash, and jaundice, collectively a DRESS-type phenomenon (drug reaction with eosinophilia and systemic symptoms). The rash can be severe and be a toxic epidermal necrosis or Stevens-Johnson syndrome. The second hepatotoxicity mechanism is delayed onset and occurs 4 to 5 months after initiation. It is not immune-allergic/hypersensitivity in nature.

Efavirenz

Efavirenz, an NNRTI FDA-approved in 1998, is like nevirapine in its mechanism of action but has no molecular structural similarity. Elevations of ALT and AST greater than five times have been reported in 1% to 8% of patients, with higher elevations observed in hepatitis C coinfection. Occurrences of DRESS syndrome are less common than with nevirapine. Single nucleotide polymorphisms of cytochrome P450 2B6 producing slow metabolizer phenotypes are associated with efavirenz hepatotoxicity risk.[27] Efavirenz has demonstrated mitochondrial dysfunction with abnormal morphology and increased mitochondrial mass evoking apoptosis.[28] Efavirenz DILI has been reported noting three histologic patterns of injury: a nonspecific hepatitis with mild elevation of serum transaminases; a mixed cholestatic-hepatitis with mild to moderate jaundice and moderate elevation of transaminases, alkaline phosphatase (ALP), and gamma-glutamyl transferase (GGT); and a severe immuno-allergic DILI demonstrating submassive necrosis with markedly elevated transaminases, jaundice, and coagulopathy.[29] Affected patients are mainly women, younger than 30 years, many pregnant at time of initiating efavirenz-based ART.[29]

More recently, a prospective natural history study of 50 patients with efavirenz DILI was reported. Risk factors for the severe submissive necrosis pattern of injury remain similar, with a 14% mortality.[30] Prednisone was used as adjunctive therapy to aid resolution; however, full resolution of the severe injury took 6 to 12 months. Rilpivirine, a newer NNRTI, has demonstrated a twofold lower incidence of grade 2 to 4 liver adverse events compared with efavirenz.[31]

PROTEASE INHIBITORS

Protease inhibitors (PIs) have in general lower rates of hepatotoxicity with ALT/AST elevations >5 times the ULN reported in up to 15%. This is more frequent in those with hepatitis C coinfection. When used with ritonavir, as a dose-lowering "booster," the frequency and severity of ALT/AST elevation decreases. Atazanavir and indinavir increase serum unconjugated bilirubin due to the inhibition of *UDP glucuronyl-transferase*, producing a Gilbert syndrome–like effect. Here jaundice is not indicative of hepatic injury. Factors contributing to PI-induced hepatotoxicity include age, CD4 count, viral hepatitis coinfection, alcohol, and drug-drug interactions, for example, with anti-TB drugs.[32]

INTEGRASE INHIBITORS, FUSION INHIBITORS, AND CCR5 ANTAGONISTS

In 2005, the development of aplaviroc, a CCR5 antagonist, was halted because of severe hepatotoxicity. In contrast, maraviroc and vicriviroc have safer hepatotoxicity profiles. Case reports of maraviroc DILI have been issued, although, given the extensive range of other drugs used, causality is doubtful. Enfuvirtide, a fusion inhibitor, has demonstrated a consistent safety record. Integrase inhibitors, notably dolutegravir, have slowly been upscaled in LMIC as first-line therapy given better resistance and toxicity profiles.[33] A case report of a 28-year-old African woman developing acute liver failure and ultimately needing liver transplant has been published.[34]

Miscellaneous Drugs

Amoxicillin-Clavulanate

Several global DILI registries, including DILIN in the United States and LATINDILIN in South America, report AC-induced cholestatic or mixed cholestatic-hepatitis as a leading cause of DILI.[35] A 2011 genome-wide association study from 201 White European and US cases of AC-DILI demonstrated class I and II HLA genotypes affecting susceptibility to AC-DILI. Particular single nucleotide polymorphisms in HLA, HLA-A*02:01, and HLA-DRB1*15:01, strongly associated with AC-DILI susceptibility. Interestingly, an autoimmune gene, *PTPN22*, was also associated.[36] Although this study did not include patients from tropical or LMIC countries, a 2019 GWAS study did, and it confirmed the association with *PTPN22*, supporting an immune-mediated component to AC-DILI and many other drug injuries.[37]

Cotrimoxazole

Trimethoprim-sulfamethoxazole or cotrimoxazole is used in the prevention and treatment of *Pneumocystis jirovecii* pneumonia in HIV-infected or immunocompromised patients. It is implicated in causing a characteristic drug allergy or hypersensitivity with a DRESS phenomenon and an associated liver injury. An idiosyncratic hepatocellular injury is also described that can result in acute liver failure. A mixed-cholestatic or more predominant cholestatic pattern can emerge days or weeks into treatment with progressive jaundice. Histologically severe cholestasis can be demonstrated, with the development of a ductopenic or vanishing bile duct syndrome.[38] Given its widespread use, especially in HIV-positive patients, it should always be considered a causative factor when these patients present with abnormal liver enzymes.

Antifungals

Antifungals include the imidazoles, such as ketoconazole, fluconazole, and itraconazole, as well as terbinafine. Patterns of injury typically include mixed cholestatic-hepatocellular or pure cholestatic liver injuries. Vanishing bile duct syndrome has been linked to terbinafine, and cases of acute liver failure linked to ketoconazole are well described.[39,40]

Herbal and Dietary Supplement DILI

Herbal and dietary supplements (HDSs) as a cause of acute liver injury are increasing. This has been observed in registries, rising 7% to 9% in the 2004–2007 to 20% in the 2010–2014 period in DILIN.[41] Equally in LATINDILIN, initially 10% of cases were attributable to HDS.[4] Here a range of products were observed including anabolic steroids, Herbalife, and hydroxy-cut. The challenge is that HDS products may contain 5 to 20 ingredients, in uncertain concentrations and with limited quality assurance. The actual injurious agent may be impossible to identify, as is observed in tropical or LMIC regions where traditional remedies are frequently used.[12] The clinical presentation of HDS DILI varies from asymptomatic abnormal liver profiles to mild self-limiting liver injury, to acute liver failure, where transplantation may be warranted. More recent data from LATINDILIN reported 8% of DILI cases due to HDS, with 83% presenting with a hepatocellular injury and 66% with jaundice, and 17% developed acute liver failure.[42] Mortality and risk of acute liver failure was greater with HDS.

Summary

In conclusion, DILI remains a serious and challenging diagnosis in tropical or LMIC countries. The multiple types and phenotypes of DILI vary depending on the drug or toxin and present a diagnostic challenge. Access and availability of the extensive workup needed to assess patients with suspected DILI are limited in many countries. Key to diagnosis is recognition or suspicion of DILI, and key to treatment is stopping the suspected offending drug.

References

1. Chalasani NP, Maddur H, Russo MW, Wong RJ, Reddy KR. ACG Clinical guideline: diagnosis and management of idiosyncratic drug-induced liver injury. *Am J Gastroenterol.* 2021;116(5):878-898.
2. Sonderup MW, Wainwright H, Hall P, Hairwadzi H, Spearman CWN. A clinicopathological cohort study of liver pathology in 301 patients with human immunodeficiency virus/acquired immune deficiency syndrome. *Hepatology.* 2015;61(5):1721-1729.
3. Prahraj D, Anand AC. Tropical liver diseases: an overview. *Clin Liver Dis.* 2021;18(3):138-142.
4. Bessone F, Hernandez N, Lucena MI, et al. The Latin American DILI Registry Experience: a successful ongoing collaborative strategic initiative. *Int J Mol Sci.* 2016;17(3):313.
5. Bessone F, Hernandez N, Mendizabal M, Sanchez A, Paraná R, Arrese M, et al. When the creation of a consortium provides useful answers: experience of The Latin American DILI Network (LATINDILIN). *Clin Liver Dis (Hoboken).* 2019;13(2):51-57.
6. Danan G, Teschke R. RUCAM in drug and herb induced liver injury: the update. *Int J Mol Sci.* 2015; 17(1):14.
7. Davern TJ, Chalasani N, Fontana RJ, et al. Acute hepatitis E infection accounts for some cases of suspected drug-induced liver injury. *Gastroenterology.* 2011;141(5):1665-1672.e1-9.
8. El-Mokhtar MA, Ramadan HKA, Thabet MM, et al. The unmet needs of hepatitis E virus diagnosis in suspected drug-induced liver injury in limited resource setting. *Front Microbiol.* 2021;12:737486.
9. Echevarría JM, González JE, Lewis-Ximenez LL, et al. Hepatitis E virus infection in Latin America: a review. *J Med Virol.* 2013;85(6):1037-1045.
10. Hoofnagle JH, Nelson KE, Purcell RH. Hepatitis E. *N Engl J Med.* 2012;367(13):1237-1244.
11. Lee AU, Lee C. Hepatitis D review: challenges for the resource-poor setting. *Viruses.* 2021;13(10):1912.
12. Hoofnagle JH, Björnsson ES. Drug-induced liver injury: types and phenotypes. *N Eng J Med.* 2019; 381(3):264-273.
13. Reuling IJ, de Jong GM, Yap XZ, et al. Liver injury in uncomplicated malaria is an overlooked phenomenon: an observational study. *EBioMedicine.* 2018;36:131-139.
14. Riebensahm C, Ka D, Sow A, Semmo N, Wandeler G. A closer look at the spectrum of drug-induced liver injury in sub-Saharan Africa. *Expert Rev Clin Pharmacol.* 2019;12(9):875-883.
15. Saukkonen JJ, Cohn DL, Jasmer RM, et al. An official ATS statement: hepatotoxicity of antituberculosis therapy. *Am J Respir Crit Care Med.* 2006;174(8):935-952.
16. Shang P, Xia Y, Liu F, et al. Incidence, clinical features and impact on anti-tuberculosis treatment of anti-tuberculosis drug induced liver injury (ATLI) in China. *PLoS One.* 2011;6(7):e21836.
17. Huang YS, Chern HD, Su WJ, et al. Polymorphism of the N-acetyltransferase 2 gene as a susceptibility risk factor for antituberculosis drug-induced hepatitis. *Hepatology.* 2002;35(4):883-839.
18. Ramappa V, Aithal GP. Hepatotoxicity related to anti-tuberculosis drugs: mechanisms and management. *J Clin Exp Hepatol.* 2013;3(1):37-49.
19. Saukkonen J. Challenges in reintroducing tuberculosis medications after hepatotoxicity. *Clin Infect Dis.* 2010;50(6):840-842.

20. Moosa MS, Maartens G, Gunter H, et al. A randomized controlled trial of intravenous N-acetylcysteine in the management of anti-tuberculosis drug-induced liver injury. *Clin Infect Dis.* 2021;73(9): e3377-e3383.
21. Meintjes G, Sonderup MW. A practical approach to the diagnosis and management of paradoxical tuberculosis immune reconstitution inflammatory syndrome: TB-associated immune reconstitution inflammatory syndrome is seen after the initiation of antiretroviral therapy. *Contin Med Educ.* 2011;29(10):410-415.
22. Dwyer-Lindgren L, Cork MA, Sligar A, et al. Mapping HIV prevalence in sub-Saharan Africa between 2000 and 2017. *Nature.* 2019;570(7760):189-193.
23. Ogedegbe AO, Sulkowski MS. Antiretroviral-associated liver injury. *Clin Liver Dis.* 2003;7(2):475-499.
24. Núñez M. Clinical syndromes and consequences of antiretroviral-related hepatotoxicity. *Hepatology.* 2010;52(3):1143-1155.
25. Dieterich DT, Robinson PA, Love J, Stern JO. Drug-induced liver injury associated with the use of nonnucleoside reverse-transcriptase inhibitors. *Clin Infect Dis.* 2004;38(suppl 2):S80-S89.
26. Wooltorton E. HIV drug nevirapine (Viramune): risk of severe hepatotoxicity. *CMAJ.* 2004;170(7):1091.
27. Manosuthi W, Sukasem C, Lueangniyomkul A, et al. CYP2B6 haplotype and biological factors responsible for hepatotoxicity in HIV-infected patients receiving efavirenz-based antiretroviral therapy. *Int J Antimicrob Agents.* 2014;43(3):292-296.
28. Apostolova N, Gomez-Sucerquia LJ, Gortat A, Blas-Garcia A, Esplugues JV. Autophagy as a rescue mechanism in Efavirenz-induced mitochondrial dysfunction: a lesson from hepatic cells. *Autophagy.* 2011;7(11):1402-1404.
29. Sonderup MW, Maughan D, Gogela N, et al. Identification of a novel and severe pattern of efavirenz drug-induced liver injury in South Africa. *AIDS.* 2016;30(9):1483-1485.
30. Maughan D, Sonderup M, Gogela N, et al. A natural history of efavirenz drug-induced liver injury. *S Afr Med J.* 2021;111(12):1190-1196.
31. Sharma M, Saravolatz LD. Rilpivirine: a new non-nucleoside reverse transcriptase inhibitor. *J Antimicrob Chemother.* 2013;68(2):250-256.
32. Sulkowski MS. Drug-induced liver injury associated with antiretroviral therapy that includes HIV-1 protease inhibitors. *Clin Infect Dis.* 2004;38(suppl 2):S90-S97.
33. Hauser A, Kusejko K, Johnson LF, et al. Impact of scaling up dolutegravir on antiretroviral resistance in South Africa: a modeling study. *PLoS Med.* 2020;17(12):e1003397.
34. Wang B, Abbott L, Childs K, et al. Dolutegravir-induced liver injury leading to sub-acute liver failure requiring transplantation: a case report and review of literature. *Int J STD AIDS.* 2018;29(4):414-417.
35. Chalasani N, Bonkovsky HL, Fontana R, et al. Features and outcomes of 899 patients with drug-induced liver injury: the DILIN prospective study. *Gastroenterology.* 2015;148(7):1340-1352.e7.
36. Lucena MI, Molokhia M, Shen Y, et al. Susceptibility to amoxicillin-clavulanate-induced liver injury is influenced by multiple HLA class I and II alleles. *Gastroenterology.* 2011;141(1):338-347.
37. Cirulli ET, Nicoletti P, Abramson K, et al. A missense variant in PTPN22 is a risk factor for drug-induced liver injury. *Gastroenterology.* 2019;156(6):1707-1716.e2.
38. Rapoport GL, Castano JJJ, Shakhatreh M, Zamir A. S3498 severely abnormal liver enzymes secondary to Bactrim. *Am J Gastroenterol.* 2020;115:S1.
39. Anania FA, Rabin L. Terbinafine hepatotoxicity resulting in chronic biliary ductopenia and portal fibrosis. *Am J Med.* 2002;112(9):741-742.
40. García Rodríguez LA, Duque A, Castellsague J, Pérez-Gutthann S, Stricker BH. A cohort study on the risk of acute liver injury among users of ketoconazole and other antifungal drugs. *Br J Clin Pharmacol.* 1999;48(6):847-852.
41. Navarro VJ, Barnhart H, Bonkovsky HL, et al. Liver injury from herbals and dietary supplements in the U.S. Drug-Induced Liver Injury Network. *Hepatology.* 2014;60(4):1399-1408.
42. Bessone F, García-Cortés M, Medina-Caliz I, et al. Herbal and dietary supplements-induced liver injury in Latin America: experience from the LATINDILI Network. *Clin Gastroenterol Hepatol.* 2022;20(3): e548-e563.

CHAPTER 25

Congestive Hepatopathy

Hailemichael Desalegn Mekonnen

KEY POINTS

- Systemic changes in the circulation and local factors could affect the hepatic venous circulation and lead to congestive hepatopathy or ischemic insult.
- The hepatic artery autoregulates blood flow via the hepatic arterial buffer response (HABR) and maintains a constant hepatic blood circulation. There is no autoregulation from the portal venous system.
- Rheumatic heart disease, constrictive pericarditis, Chagas disease, and endomyocardial fibrosis are important causes of right heart failure leading to congestive hepatopathy in the tropics.
- Clinical manifestations include abdominal and leg swelling with hepato-jugular reflux. Splenomegaly occurs in long-standing cases of cardiac cirrhosis.
- Chest x-ray could help diagnose chronic pericarditis, with characteristic calcifications of the pericardium. Echocardiography is important to diagnose underlying causes of right-side heart failure. Abdominal ultrasound can show signs of hepatic congestion.
- Management of the underlying cardiac condition is the cornerstone of therapy.

Introduction

The liver is affected by changes that occur due to disturbances in the circulatory system, including vascular insult. It receives approximately 25% of the cardiac output and it is the largest solid internal organ in the body.[1] Chronic changes of increased central venous pressure due to heart failure or other cardiac disorders lead to increased blood flow in the hepatic venous circulation, which can induce congestive hepatopathy.[2] Such circulatory changes could also occur due to local changes in the liver, including sinusoidal obstruction syndrome, portal vein thrombosis, Budd-Chiari syndrome, and peliosis hepatis, among others.[3]

Pathogenesis

To understand the pathogenesis of congestive hepatopathy, it is important to discern the hepatic circulation. The liver is a unique organ that receives a dual blood supply: a well-oxygenated arterial blood from the hepatic artery, which comprises 25% of the volume, and the other 75% is deoxygenated blood from the portal vein.[4] The hepatic artery is the dominant artery autoregulating blood flow via the hepatic arterial buffer response (HABR). When there is decreased portal flow, this will activate HABR as compensatory upregulation of hepatic arterial flow and vice versa. This autoregulation preserves a constant level of total hepatic blood flow by maintaining hepatic oxygenation and clearance. This autoregulation by HABR can compensate for up to 60%

decrease in portal blood flow.[5] What about the regulation in the portal venous flow? There is no autoregulation for the portal venous system unlike the arterial blood flow. The portal vein is formed behind the junction of the head and neck of the pancreas, formed by the splenic and mesenteric venous system. So the mesenteric circulation provides a gradient between portal and hepatic venous pressures.[6]

Any cause of right ventricular heart failure can precipitate hepatic congestion and affect the autoregulation system. These include conventional conditions like constrictive pericarditis, tricuspid regurgitation, mitral stenosis (rheumatic heart disease), cardiomyopathy, and cor pulmonale. Tropical causes of cardiac illness include more neglected entities such as Chagas disease and endomyocardial fibrosis (EMF). Moreover, schistosomiasis, caused by *Schistosoma mansoni*, a parasitic disease that is abundant in sub-Saharan Africa, especially in the Nile-basin countries, is an important cause of pulmonary hypertension. Pulmonary arterial hypertension has been reported in 5% to 10% of patients with hepatosplenic schistosomiasis. In patients with advanced hepatosplenic schistosomiasis autopsy studies have identified restrictive pattern of right ventricular dysfunction as well as EMF.[7]

Complications of hepatic congestion occur through the effects of decreasing hepatic blood flow, lowering arterial oxygen saturation, and an increase in hepatic venous pressures, thereby causing hepatic injury. These changes are characteristically seen on histology at zone III of the liver. Zone III has the lowest perfusion due to its distance from the portal triad. It plays a role in hematology with clotting factor and protein synthesis.[8] The increase in hepatic venous pressure transmits to the hepatic veins and sinusoids, thereby decreasing portal venous flow. It also causes a series of changes: sinusoidal congestion, dilation of sinusoidal fenestrae, and exudation of protein and fluid into the space of Disse, then impairment in diffusion of oxygen and nutrients to the hepatocytes. It is important to note that chronic congestion can cause perivenular fibrosis and, ultimately, lead to the development of cirrhosis.[9]

EPIDEMIOLOGY

The true prevalence of congestive hepatopathy is difficult to estimate. However, in resource-limited countries, where uncorrected rheumatic heart disease and constrictive pericardial disease are more frequent, the prevalence is thought to be higher. Fontan-associated liver disease (FALD) can also manifest with hepatopathy, hepatic fibrosis, and eventually cirrhosis. Fontan procedure is performed for patients with tricuspid atresia and as a final-stage palliation for pediatric patients with univentricular physiology heart disease. The procedure is an operation to connect a single working heart ventricle to the systemic vascular system while allowing passive venous return to the pulmonary arteries.[9] As patients after Fontan procedure could reach adolescence, it is important to look for signs of liver disease in such patients. FALD is in the spectrum of congestive hepatopathy, related to chronically elevated central venous pressures, stemming from passive venous congestion and impaired hepatic blood flow.[10]

Clinical Presentation

Initially, patients with congestive hepatopathy are usually asymptomatic.[11] When symptomatic, dull right abdominal pain or jaundice may be the only symptoms. Jaundice is seen in less than 10% of cases. On physical examination, clinical signs of cirrhosis are generally absent (unless the patient developed cirrhosis). Signs of right-side heart failure are important to elicit. In cases of tricuspid regurgitation pulsatile liver may be noticed. It is important to remember that loss of the pulsatile nature of the liver may signal development of cardiac cirrhosis.[12] Asymptomatic elevation of liver enzymes is the most common finding. Specific laboratory abnormalities include mild elevation of serum transaminases (2–3 X ULN), increased indirect bilirubin (total bilirubin usually less than 3 mg/dL), and low albumin (30%–50% of patients). The hypoalbuminemia is not related to liver failure and in most cases it is due to malnutrition or protein losing enteropathy. As evident in an old study of 175 patients, with severe right-side heart failure, liver panels (ALT, AST, ALP, albumin, bilirubin) could be normal in most patients with either acute or chronic disease. The PT, International Normalized Ratio (INR) is abnormal in 75% of patients (due to congestion of zone III where clotting factors are produced) and returns back to normal levels very slowly with improvement of heart failure.[13]

Diagnosis

The diagnosis of congestive hepatopathy requires a proper evaluation of underlying risk factor for right-side heart failure. Patients may not have signs of portal hypertension until late in the disease course, when they develop cirrhosis. At that time, hepatosplenomegaly, upper GI bleeding, and ascites will be seen. Signs of right-side heart failure are important to make the diagnosis, with tender hepatomegaly, hepatojugular efflux, and peripheral edema being characteristic findings. In early stages pulsatile liver may be auscultated and its absence likely suggests progression to cardiac cirrhosis. Patients with congestive hepatopathy will have a normal liver parenchyma and during the early periods, the synthetic function might not be affected (although, as mentioned above, PT or INR might be elevated due to congestion). Overt clinical ascites is rare, but serum-ascites-albumin gradient is usually >1.1 g/dL.

Some causes that should be excluded include diseases associated with cardiomyopathy such as amyloidosis and hemochromatosis. Liver pathology (biopsy) is not always needed to reach the diagnosis. The diagnosis can be confirmed in a patient with an underlying right-side heart disease presenting with signs of portal hypertension and characteristic imaging signs (Figure 25.1).[14]

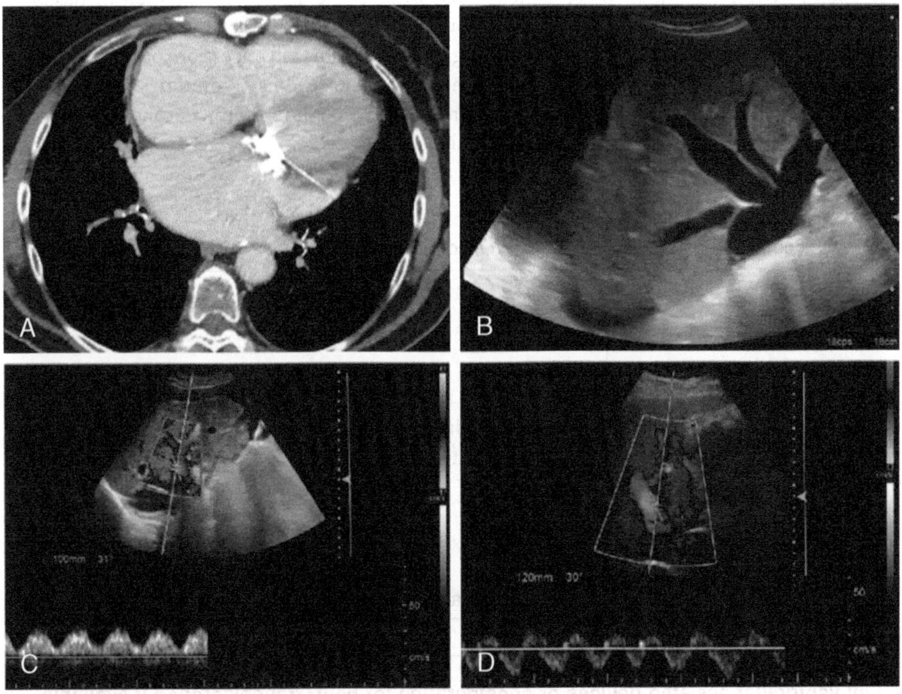

Figure 25.1 Imaging signs of congestive hepatopathy.[14] (A) Cardiomegaly; (B) dilated suprahepatic vein in a patient with congestive hepatopathy; (C) Doppler ultrasound in the dilated suprahepatic veins; (D) hepatopetal flow in the portal vein.

Common ultrasound (US) findings of CH include a dilated inferior vena cava and dilated hepatic veins; the degree of dilatation correlates with the severity of heart failure; absent or diminished respiratory variation can be seen when there is increased venous pressure; and spectral Doppler US analysis can show loss of the normal triphasic hepatic venous waveform due to poor antegrade venous flow.[15]

If a biopsy is obtained, the gross pathologic appearance of the liver is described as "nutmeg liver," characterized by dark centrilobular zones (due to sinusoidal congestion) alternating with pale periportal zones. On histology, zone III predominant sinusoidal dilation, congestion, and hepatocyte atrophy are noted. Cardiac cirrhosis is a histologic diagnosis when the fibrosis becomes extensive with bridging to adjacent lobules and the replacement of normal architecture with regenerative nodules.[8]

Management

Management of congestive hepatopathy should be directed or in consultation with cardiology experts. The most important focus for patients with congestive hepatopathy is management of the underlying cardiac condition, including optimization of cardiac output (Figure 25.2). Diuresis should be provided cautiously and correction of the hemodynamic status could reverse the early changes of congestive hepatopathy. The most dreadful complication could occur due to overzealous use of diuresis, one that could precipitate hepatic ischemia and risk fulminant hepatic failure.[8,16] Patients with FALD should undergo regular surveillance for hepatocellular carcinoma as they are at increased risk.[17]

ACE inhibitors (ACEi) are useful in this setting as they decrease left ventricular filling pressure. Caution should be used with some ACEi in liver dysfunction. Lisinopril and captopril seem safer choice in this regard. In those patients that cannot tolerate ACEi angiotensin receptor blockers (ARVBs) can be used, also with caution, as losartan is also metabolized in the liver.[18] Diuretics should be used in those with clinical signs or symptoms of congestion, particularly loop diuretics, always keeping in mind the recommendation of not overusing diuretics.[19] If arrhythmias are present, antiarrhythmic such as amiodarone can be helpful. If amiodarone is used for a prolonged time, one has to address for potential hepatotoxicity.[20]

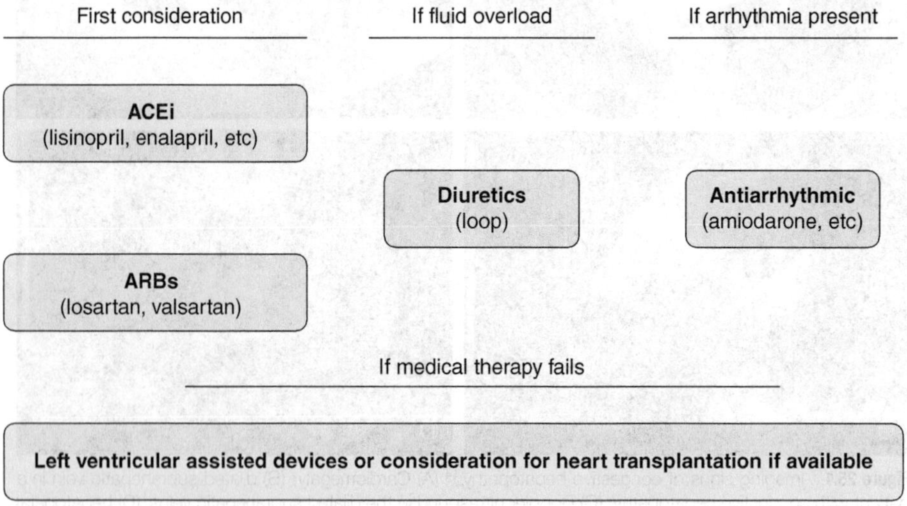

Figure 25.2 Considerations for the management of congestive hepatopathy. (Adapted from Ref. 18.)

In general, the severity of the underlying cardiac disease determines the treatment outcome and successful management of the underlying cardiac condition could potentially reverse the liver fibrosis.[14] In this regard, we recommend early treatment of cardiac disease, that is, long-standing rheumatic heart disease which is a major cause of congestive hepatopathy and cardiac failure in resource-limited countries.

References

1. Ford RM, Book W, Spivey JR. Liver disease related to the heart. *Transplant Rev (Orlando)*. 2015;29(1): 33-37.
2. Weisberg IS, Jacobson IM. Cardiovascular diseases and the liver. *Clin Liver Dis*. 2011;15(1):1-20.
3. DeLeve LD. Vascular liver diseases. *Curr Gastroenterol Rep*. 2003;5(1):63-70.
4. Lautt WW. Hepatic circulation: physiology and pathophysiology. In: Granger N, Granger JP, eds. *Colloquium Series on Integrated Systems Physiology: From Molecule to Function*. (Vol. 1, No. 1). Morgan & Claypool Publishers; 2009:1-174.
5. Lautt WW. Mechanism and role of intrinsic regulation of hepatic arterial blood flow: hepatic arterial buffer response. *Am J Physiol*. 1985;249(5):G549-G556.
6. Carneiro C, Brito J, Bilreiro C, et al. All about portal vein: a pictorial display to anatomy, variants and physiopathology. *Insights Imaging*. 2019;10(1):1-8.
7. Groom ZC, Protopapas AD, Zochios V. Tropical diseases of the myocardium: a review. *Int J Gen Med*. 2017;10:101-111.
8. Hilscher M, Sanchez W. Congestive hepatopathy. *Clin Liver Dis*. 2016;8(3):68.
9. Lemmer A, VanWagner LB, Ganger D. Assessment of advanced liver fibrosis and the risk for hepatic decompensation in patients with congestive hepatopathy. *Hepatology*. 2018;68(4):1633-1641.
10. Emamaullee J, Zaidi AN, Schiano T, et al. Fontan-associated liver disease: screening, management, and transplant considerations. *Circulation*. 2020;142(6):591-604.
11. Morales A, Hirsch M, Schneider D, González D. Congestive hepatopathy: the role of the radiologist in the diagnosis. *Diagn Interv Radiol*. 2020;26(6):541.
12. Sessa A, Allaire M, Lebray P, et al. From congestive hepatopathy to hepatocellular carcinoma, how can we improve patient management? *JHEP Rep*. 2021;3(2):100249.
13. Richman SM, Delman AJ, Grob D. Alterations in indices of liver function in congestive heart failure with particular reference to serum enzymes. *Am J Med*. 1961;30(2):211-225.
14. Zhang Y, Fang XM. Hepatocardiac or cardiohepatic interaction: from traditional Chinese medicine to Western medicine. *Evid Based Complement Alternat Med*. 2021;2021:6655335.
15. Wells ML, Fenstad ER, Poterucha JT, et al. Imaging findings of congestive hepatopathy. *Radiographics*. 2016;36(4):1024-1037.
16. Kisloff B, Schaffer G. Fulminant hepatic failure secondary to congestive heart failure. *Am J Dig Dis*. 1976;21(10):895-900.
17. Rychik J, Atz AM, Celermajer DS, et al. Evaluation and management of the child and adult with Fontan circulation: a scientific statement from the American Heart Association. *Circulation*. 2019;140(6): e234-e284.
18. Sessa A, Allaire M, Lebray P, et al. From congestive hepatopathy to hepatocellular carcinoma, how can we improve patient management? *JHEP Rep*. 2021;3(2):100249.
19. Fredrick MJ, Pound DC, Hall SD, Brater DC. Furosemide absorption in patients with cirrhosis. *Clin Pharmacol Ther*. 1991;49(3):241-247.
20. Lewis JH, Ranard RC, Caruso A, et al. Amiodarone hepatotoxicity: prevalence and clinicopathologic correlations among 104 patients. *Hepatology*. 1989;9(5):679-685.

CHAPTER 26

Acute Liver Failure

Chimaobi M. Anugwom ■ Opeyemi O. Owoseni ■ Thomas M. Leventhal

KEY POINTS

- Determining the cause of acute liver failure (ALF) involves evaluating for common etiologies like toxins and drugs or uncommon ones such as Yellow fever or hepatitis E
- Transfer of patients to a transplant center, when possible, is imperative and is strongly associated with survival
- Optimal intensive care is important and necessary in all patients with ALF
- N-acetyl cysteine (NAC) has been shown to be beneficial in all patients with ALF, including those not due to acetaminophen
- A careful system-based approach with a multidisciplinary team of the hepatologist, critical care specialist, neuro-intensivist, and nephrologist (when available) is vital in the management of ALF

Introduction

Acute liver failure (ALF) is a rare but specific syndrome resulting from acute liver injury, in the absence of prior liver disease, with consequent development of altered mentation and coagulopathy. Its onset is usually rapid and associated with high mortality rates. In resource-rich countries the incidence of ALF is estimated to be about 10 cases per million people per year.[1-3] The incidence in resource-limited settings varies greatly, with some studies suggesting rates as high as 80 cases per million people per year, though there is paucity of data from these regions of the world.[4]

ALF is generally defined by the following:

1. Acute liver injury that develops within 26 weeks from inciting event
2. Coagulopathy, defined as an international normalized ratio (INR) >1.5
3. Hepatic encephalopathy
4. Absence of chronic liver disease (CLD), except Wilson disease, autoimmune hepatitis, and hepatitis B. Acute mortality in most CLD is dramatically lower than ALF, but it is important to recognize that these particular CLDs can have acute episodes of hepatocellular necrosis leading to true ALF.

To assist with determination of etiology, O'Grady categorized ALF slightly differently based on the interval between the onset of jaundice and encephalopathy as: hyperacute (0–7 days), acute (8–28 days), and subacute (>28 days to less than 26 weeks).[5]

Etiology of ALF

MEDICATIONS

- Drug-induced liver injury (especially paracetamol/acetaminophen) constitutes the most common etiology of ALF in the Western world.
- In Africa and Asia excessive (intentional or accidental) consumption of acetaminophen is not as common. Medications such as antitubercular drugs (isoniazid), antibiotics (especially amoxicillin-clavulanate), and the inhaled anesthetic halothane are more likely to be the etiology of ALF.[6,7] A position paper from the Latin America Drug Induced Liver Injury (LATIN-DILI) registry notes amoxicillin-clavulanate as a major cause of liver damage in the region.[8]

TOXINS

- Consumption of local herbs and roots for medical purposes is associated with development of ALF in Africa.
- Some herbal medicines also contain adulterants and contaminants such as cadmium and lead that may potentiate liver injury.
- Exposure to toxic agents such as Amanita or Aflatoxin may result in ALF:
- *Amanita phalloides*, or death cap, is a mushroom that is native to Europe but is now found in the Americas as well as some parts of Africa such as in South Africa and Tanzania, usually among pines and oak trees.[9]
- Aflatoxin is produced by certain molds (*Aspergillus* species) in improperly stored grains and nuts. At high doses it can cause hepatic necrosis and ALF, especially in children. As a potent carcinogen, exposure over time increases the risk for gallbladder cancer and hepatocellular carcinoma.[10]

INFECTIONS

- Most infectious causes of ALF are due to viruses with a predilection for the liver.[11]
- A study from Johns Hopkins University School of Medicine suggested that the leading causes of ALF globally are hepatitis B virus (HBV) and hepatitis A virus (HAV) infection.[12]
- An informal survey of practicing hepatologists in Nigeria showed that HBV is a prominent cause of ALF in Nigeria.
- Hepatitis E virus (HEV) infection is another important cause in the tropics, with most cases being reported from Asia.
- Much less common viral precipitants of ALF include: parvovirus, yellow fever virus, and hemorrhagic fever viruses such as Lassa, Marburg, and Ebola.
- Clinically severe malaria infections have also been reported in a study from Sudan as potential causes of ALF.[6]

OTHER CAUSES

- Though not common in the tropics, autoimmune hepatitis, Budd-Chiari syndrome, Wilson disease, and Reye syndrome are etiologies of ALF that may be considered.

Presentation

Symptoms: Non-specific symptoms include: abdominal pain, abdominal swelling, malaise, nausea, and vomiting. Symptoms specific for liver dysfunction (secondary to coagulopathy and encephalopathy) include yellowness of the skin, tremors, drowsiness, confusion, epistaxis, hematemesis, and melena.

Signs: Jaundice, right upper quadrant tenderness, bruising, disorientation, asterixis.

Laboratory findings: Evidence of liver injury (elevated aspartate aminotransferase, alanine aminotransferase and serum bilirubin), but more importantly, synthetic dysfunction shown by increased prothrombin time (PT)/INR. Other findings include low pH and high levels of ammonia and lactate.

The multiple systemic clinical manifestations of ALF are shown in Figure 26.1.

Diagnosis

Diagnosis of ALF is achieved through the combination of clinical signs (hepatic encephalopathy, jaundice) and laboratory evidence (elevated PT/INR, elevated liver enzymes). Using a combination of a thorough history (with attention to social history, medication exposures, use of herbal/traditional pharmacologic remedies, and family history), physical examination, and careful evaluation with laboratory tests and radiographic studies, the cause of ALF can often be elucidated.

There may be times when the cause of ALF is not readily apparent, though. In these scenarios a liver biopsy may be useful to further delineate etiology. However, it is recommended that liver biopsies be carried out only if the diagnosis will affect clinical management. If the INR is less than 2, and platelet count >50,000, percutaneous liver biopsy or plugged percutaneous liver biopsy can be attempted in stable select patients. In those with more consumptive coagulopathy and platelet count <50,000 and in unstable patients, a transjugular liver biopsy is preferred; however, this modality may not be readily available in resource-limited regions. Furthermore, routine correction of platelets with infusions and INR with fresh frozen plasma prior to liver biopsy is not recommended.[13-15]

Table 26.1 shows the different causes of ALF with corresponding screening/first-tier and confirmatory/second-tier testing.

A plausible flow chart for evaluation of liver injury (as shown in Figure 26.2) can be employed to ensure judicious use of resources as the work-up for ALF is undertaken.

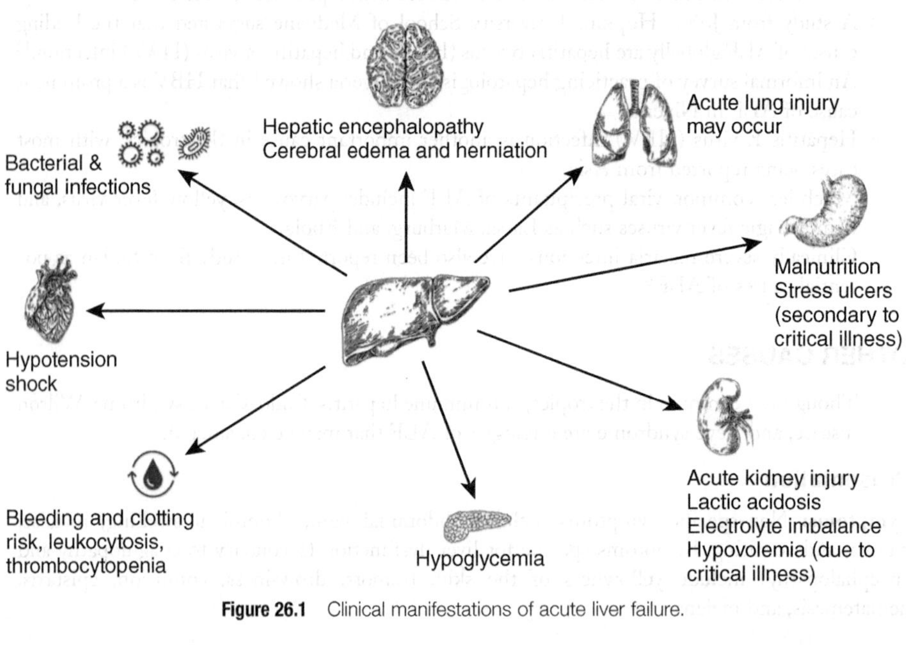

Figure 26.1 Clinical manifestations of acute liver failure.

TABLE 26.1 ■ Screening and Confirmatory Testing for Etiology of Acute Liver Failure

Etiology	Screening/First-Tier Test	Confirmatory/Second-Tier Test
Paracetamol/acetaminophen	History of exposure	Acetaminophen serum level*
Ischemia	Blood pressure trend, abdominal ultrasound with doppler	Rapid improvement of liver enzymes, echocardiogram
Amanita phalloides	History of exposure	—
Hepatitis A	IgM anti-HAV	HAV RNA
Hepatitis E	IgM anti-HEV	HEV RNA
Hepatitis B	IgM anti-HBc, HBsAg	HBV DNA
Drug-induced liver injury	History of exposure, diagnosis of exclusion	Liver biopsy
Autoimmune hepatitis	ANA, ASMA/F-actin, serum IgG	Liver biopsy
Wilson disease	Slit lamp examination of the eyes, ALP/bilirubin ratio <4, hemolysis, ceruloplasmin/urinary copper†	Liver biopsy, quantitative liver copper measurement
HELLP syndrome, acute fatty liver of pregnancy	Abdominal ultrasound	Liver biopsy
Herpes simplex virus	IgM anti-HSV 1/2	Blood HSV DNA
Budd-Chiari syndrome	Liver ultrasound with Doppler	Hepatic venogram

*Acetaminophen level may be normal in some cases.

†Ceruloplasmin and urinary copper may be falsely deranged in ALF. Prior laboratory tests may be helpful.

ALP—Alkaline phosphatase; ANA—antinuclear antibody; ASMA—anti-smooth muscle antibody; HAV—hepatitis A virus; HBV—hepatitis B virus; HEV—hepatitis E virus; HSV—herpes simplex virus

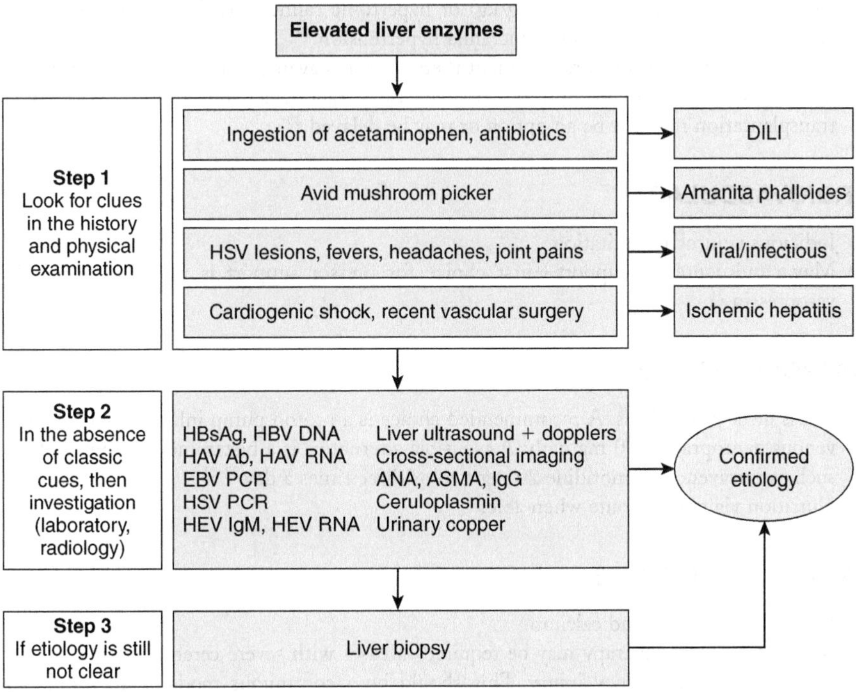

Figure 26.2 Suggested flow chart for evaluation of liver injury.

Management

The mortality associated with ALF is quite high without liver transplantation and varies by etiology of ALF. In the tropics and other resource-limited regions the treatment of ALF may be limited to supportive and expert intensive care.[16,17] Where available, referral for liver transplantation evaluation is the treatment of choice, as transplant is required in cases who continue to worsen clinically or do not respond to supportive measures.

GENERAL

- Transfer to a liver transplant center (if available, and if nearby) is imperative to survival of these patients.
- Adequate intensive care is necessary and all patients with ALF should receive intensive care unit level of care with system-based approach to management.
- N-acetylcysteine (NAC) has been shown to improve the transplant-free survival of patients, even in non-acetaminophen causes of ALF.[18] This is usually administered as a 150 mg/kg dose in 5% dextrose solution as a loading dose, followed by 50 mg/kg given over 4 hours, and then 100 mg/kg over 16 hours. Based on this data, and the low risk of adverse effects associated with NAC, it should be considered in all patients with ALF.

NEUROLOGICAL

- Keep head-of-bed at 30°.
- Maintain the patient's neck in neutral position.
- Allow spontaneous hyperventilation and hypothermia.
- Consider IV mannitol (0.25-0.5 g/kg) or hypertonic saline (goal Na ~145–150) to treat cerebral edema with resultant intracranial hypertension.[19]
- Consider continuous renal replacement therapy (when available, for removal of serum ammonia) and therapeutic hypothermia (to decrease metabolic demand) for severe cases where transplantation may not be an option or may be delayed.[20]

CARDIOVASCULAR

- Judicious volume resuscitation.
- May require pressor support—first choice for pressor support is norepinephrine, then vasopressin.[21]

GASTROINTESTINAL

- Stress ulcer prophylaxis. A recommended choice is a proton pump inhibitor such as intravenous pantoprazole 40 mg daily. A plausible alternative is a histamine-2 receptor blocker such as intravenous famotidine 20 mg two or three times a day.[22-24]
- Nutrition via enteral route when able.

RENAL/ELECTROLYTES

- Replete phosphorus and calcium.
- Renal replacement therapy may be required in cases with severe cerebral edema or in the presence of acute kidney injury. This should be a continuous modality to avoid rapid electrolyte/volume shifting.[25]

ENDOCRINE

- Close blood glucose monitoring.

HEMATOLOGIC

- Clotting and bleeding risk are both increased.
- In ALF, INR is a marker of liver synthetic dysfunction and *not* bleeding risk.
- Bleeding in persons with ALF is often related to thrombocytopenia/impaired platelet function.
- Avoid unnecessary use of blood products to correct INR (or PT).[26]

INFECTIONS

- Routine surveillance with cultures every 2 to 3 days, together with prompt aggressive treatment.
- Consider empiric antibiotics and antifungals, though these do not improve outcomes.[27]

References

1. Simões C, Santos S, Vicente M, Sousa Cardoso F. Epidemiology of acute liver failure from a regional liver transplant center in Portugal. *GE Port J Gastroenterol.* 2018;26(1):33-39.
2. Weiler N, Schlotmann A, Schnitzbauer AA, Zeuzem S, Welker MW. The epidemiology of acute liver failure. *Dtsch Arztebl Int.* 2020;117(4):43-50.
3. Lee WM. Acute liver failure in the United States. *Semin Liver Dis.* 2003;23(3):217-226.
4. Ho CM, Lee CH, Wang JY, Lee PH, Lai HS, Hu RH. Nationwide longitudinal analysis of acute liver failure in Taiwan. *Medicine (Baltimore).* 2014;93(4):e35.
5. O'Grady JG, Schalm SW, Williams R. Acute liver failure: redefining the syndromes. *Lancet.* 1993; 342(8866):273-275.
6. Mudawi HM, Yousif BA. Fulminant hepatic failure in an African setting: etiology, clinical course, and predictors of mortality. *Dig Dis Sci.* 2007;52(11):3266-3269.
7. Devarbhavi H, Aithal G, Treeprasertsuk S, et al. Drug-induced liver injury: Asia Pacific Association of Study of Liver consensus guidelines. *Hepatol Int.* 2021;15(2):258-282.
8. Bessone F, Hernandez N, Tagle M, et al. Drug-induced liver injury: a management position paper from the Latin American Association for Study of the liver. *Ann Hepatol.* 2021;24:100321.
9. Garcia J, Costa VM, Carvalho A, et al. Amanita phalloides poisoning: mechanisms of toxicity and treatment. *Food Chem Toxicol.* 2015;86:41-55.
10. Williams JH, Phillips TD, Jolly PE, Stiles JK, Jolly CM, Aggarwal D. Human aflatoxicosis in developing countries: a review of toxicology, exposure, potential health consequences, and interventions. *Am J Clin Nutr.* 2004;80(5):1106-1122.
11. Deepak NA, Patel ND. Differential diagnosis of acute liver failure in India. *Ann Hepatol.* 2006;5(3): 150-156.
12. McDowell Torres D, Stevens RD, Gurakar A. Acute liver failure: a management challenge for the practicing gastroenterologist. *Gastroenterol Hepatol (N Y).* 2010;6(7):444-450.
13. Neuberger J, Patel J, Caldwell H, et al. Guidelines on the use of liver biopsy in clinical practice from the British Society of Gastroenterology, the Royal College of Radiologists and the Royal College of Pathology. *Gut.* 2020;69(8):1382-1403.
14. Orthup PG, Garcia-Pagan JC, Garcia-Tsao G, et al. Vascular liver disorders, portal vein thrombosis, and procedural bleeding in patients with liver disease: 2020 practice guidance by the American Association for the Study of Liver Diseases. *Hepatology.* 2021;73(1):366-413.
15. Kamphuisen PW, Wiersma TG, Mulder CJ, de Vries RA. Plugged-percutaneous liver biopsy in patients with impaired coagulation and ascites. *Pathophysiol Haemost Thromb.* 2002;32(4):190-193.
16. Alam S, Azam G, Mustafa G, et al. Natural course of fulminant hepatic failure: the scenario in Bangladesh and the differences from the west. *Saudi J Gastroenterol.* 2009;15(4):229-233.

17. Cainelli F, Nardo B, Viderman D, Dzudzor B, Tachi K, Vento S. Treatment of acute liver failure in resource-constrained settings without transplantation facilities can be improved. *Front Med (Lausanne).* 2016;3:31.
18. Lee WM, Hynan LS, Rossaro L, et al. Intravenous N-acetylcysteine improves transplant-free survival in early stage non-acetaminophen acute liver failure. *Gastroenterology.* 2009;137(3):856-864.e1.
19. Canalese J, Gimson AE, Davis C, Mellon PJ, Davis M, Williams R. Controlled trial of dexamethasone and mannitol for the cerebral oedema of fulminant hepatic failure. *Gut.* 1982;23(7):625-629.
20. Cardoso FS, Gottfried M, Tujios S, Olson JC, Karvellas CJ. Continuous renal replacement therapy is associated with reduced serum ammonia levels and mortality in acute liver failure. *Hepatology.* 2018; 67(2):711-720.
21. Eefsen M, Dethloff T, Frederiksen HJ, Hauerberg J, Hansen BA, Larsen FS. Comparison of terlipressin and noradrenalin on cerebral perfusion, intracranial pressure and cerebral extracellular concentrations of lactate and pyruvate in patients with acute liver failure in need of inotropic support. *J Hepatol.* 2007; 47(3):381-386.
22. Barkun AN, Bardou M, Pham CQ, Martel M. Proton pump inhibitors vs. histamine 2 receptor antagonists for stress-related mucosal bleeding prophylaxis in critically ill patients: a meta-analysis. *Am J Gastroenterol.* 2012;107(4):507-521.
23. Ye Z, Reintam Blaser A, Lytvyn L, et al. Gastrointestinal bleeding prophylaxis for critically ill patients: a clinical practice guideline. *BMJ.* 2020;368:l6722.
24. Stravitz RT, Kramer AH, Davern T, et al. Intensive care of patients with acute liver failure: recommendations of the U.S. Acute Liver Failure Study Group. *Crit Care Med.* 2007;35(11):2498-2508.
25. Leventhal TM, Liu KD. What a nephrologist needs to know about acute liver failure. *Adv Chronic Kidney Dis.* 2015;22(5):376-381.
26. Stravitz RT, Lisman T, Luketic VA, et al. Minimal effects of acute liver injury/acute liver failure on hemostasis as assessed by thromboelastography. *J Hepatol.* 2012;56(1):129-136.
27. Olson J, Lee WM. AASLD position paper: the management of acute liver failure. *Hepatology.* 2005; 41(5):1179-1197.

CHAPTER 27

Liver Transplantation in Tropical Settings

Elizabeth S. Aby ■ Wendy C. Spearman ■ John R. Lake

KEY POINTS

- An improved awareness of tropical infectious diseases among practitioners who care for liver transplant recipients is imperative given globalization.
- A careful history is essential to recognize which donors and transplant recipients should be screened for tropical infectious diseases.
- Prevention strategies, such as pre-transplant vaccination for vaccine-preventable infections, are needed to help mitigate post-transplant infectious complications.
- Depending on the setting, diseases like Chagas, strongyloidiasis, malaria, or schistosomiasis should be considered.

Introduction

Globalization, along with expansion of transplant programs across the world, has led to the enhanced scrutiny of tropical infectious diseases among liver transplant donors and recipients (Tables 27.1 and 27.2). Given the changes in the transplant landscape, the impact of tropical diseases on post-transplant patients needs to be carefully considered. Moreover, etiology of liver disease varies across different geographical settings, and interaction between infections (e.g., hepatitis B and schistosomiasis) adds further complexity to transplantation in tropical settings. This chapter will review the management of Chagas disease, malaria, leishmaniasis, strongyloidiasis, and schistosomiasis pre- and post-liver transplantation.

Chagas Disease

Chagas disease is caused by a protozoan parasite, *Trypanosoma cruzi*, transmitted by the infected feces of triatomine insects through penetration of the parasite into a bite wound, skin lesions, or intact mucous membranes.[1] Chagas disease is endemic in 21 Latin American countries.[2] Transmission can occur via organ transplantation, including liver transplantation.[3-5]

SCREENING

As part of the pre-transplant screening process, recipients, living donors, and deceased donors should be tested for Chagas seropositivity if they are from endemic countries, as well as those at increased epidemiological risk (such as those who were born in an endemic area).[6,7]

TABLE 27.1 ■ Tropical Parasitic Infections in Solid Organ Transplant Recipients

Helminths	*Cyclospora*
Echinococcus	*Cystoisospora belli*
Filariasis	*Entamoeba histolytica*
Strongyloides	*Giardia*
Schistosoma	*Leishmania*
Protozoa	***Microsporidia***
Babesia	*Plasmodium*
Blastocystis hominis	*Toxoplasma gondii*
Clonorchis sinensis	*Trypanosoma cruzi*
Cryptosporidium	

TABLE 27.2 ■ Tropical Non-Parasitic Infections (Viral, Bacterial, and Fungal) in Solid Organ Transplant Recipients

Bacteria	Hantavirus
Brucellosis	Hepatitis A
Leprosy	Hepatitis B
Leptospirosis	Hepatitis C
Mycobacterium	Hepatitis D
Fungi	Hepatitis E
Blastomycosis	Human immunodeficiency virus
Coccidioidomycosis	Human T-lymphotropic virus type-1/2
Histoplasmosis	Measles
Paracoccidioidomycosis	Rabies virus
Viruses	West Nile viruses
Dengue	Yellow fever

DIAGNOSIS AND TREATMENT

Reactivation or transmission can occur without clinical symptoms.[6] Asymptomatic parasitemia may progress to symptomatic disease with several different presentations, from a nonspecific febrile syndrome to Chagas meningoencephalitis, or tumor-like brain lesions (Chagomas).[6]

Given that reactivation and transmission can occur without symptoms, a strict monitoring protocol is necessary to detect subclinical reactivation and treat it preemptively. For instance, the Chagas Disease Argentine Collaborative Transplant Consortium recommends that all transplant recipients who are infected with *T. cruzi* should be monitored for reactivation every 1 to 2 weeks for the first 6 months and then monthly thereafter with Strout test and polymerase chain reaction (PCR).[8]

Parasitemia (without clinical manifestations) can be detected with positive PCR and/or Strout tests. In immunocompromised patients, serology is not useful for monitoring for reactivation.[8] Treatment with benznidazole yields excellent outcomes for those with subclinical parasitemia or non-severe clinically apparent disease.[1] Benznidazole is the first-line treatment over nitroimidazole, given a better side effect profile.[9] During reactivation episodes, maintenance immunosuppression, for example, use of mycophenolate mofetil, should be minimized; however, given the excellent response to treatment, the graft should not be put at risk for rejection.[8]

PREVENTION

Given that *de novo* Chagas disease can occur post-transplant if living in or traveling to endemic regions, individuals should be aware of risk factors for acquisition, such as prolonged stays, rural areas, and staying in thatched huts.[10]

Malaria

Malaria is a mosquito-borne illness caused by *Plasmodium* parasites, mainly *Plasmodium falciparum* and *Plasmodium vivax*, transmitted by *Anopheles* mosquitoes.[11] Malaria can also be transmitted through blood transfusions, needlestick injury, and following solid organ transplantation, although this is rare.[12,13]

SCREENING

For donors from endemic regions and those who have recently traveled to endemic areas, the best screening strategy is one that can detect low-level parasitemia. Detection of *Plasmodium* via PCR should be considered given it is more sensitive and specific than microscopy[14]; however, this strategy is limited given the associated expense, and it requires expertise and specialized equipment.[15] The gold standard for diagnosing malaria remains microscopic observation of thick or thin blood smears.[16] Rapid diagnostic tests can also be considered when microscopic evaluation is unavailable.

DIAGNOSIS AND TREATMENT

Post-transplant patients are at risk for reactivation of latent *P. vivax* or *Plasmodium ovale* due to loss of natural immunity in the setting of immunosuppression or recrudescence of asymptomatic infection.[14]

Malaria symptoms are often nonspecific and can include fever, chills, malaise, myalgias, and headache. Severe disease, on the other hand, can present with altered consciousness, anemia, thrombocytopenia, renal failure, hypotension, respiratory distress, and disseminated intravascular coagulation. Disease severity is related to a multitude of factors, including immunosuppression status, *Plasmodium* species, onset of antimalarial therapy, and parasitemia.[14,17] A high index of suspicion should be maintained for individuals presenting with pyrexia of unknown origin if previous malaria infection or recent exposure to a malaria-endemic region.

When a *Plasmodium* infection is diagnosed, antimalarial treatment should be instituted based on the *Plasmodium* species and the drug resistance patterns in the geographical region. Based on the current Centers for Disease Control and Prevention guidance, for those with uncomplicated malaria, there are several treatment options. Chloroquine or hydroxychloroquine are recommended for *Plasmodium malariae.* If *P. ovale* or *P. vivax* is acquired in an area without chloroquine resistance, chloroquine or hydroxychloroquine are recommended, and, if not glucose-6-phosphate-dehydrogenase deficient, adding primaquine or tafenoquine is recommended. Chloroquine or hydroxychloroquine are also recommended for *Plasmodium knowlesi.* For those with uncomplicated *P. vivax* that is acquired in an area with chloroquine resistance, several regimens are recommended—artemether-lumefantrine or atovaquone-proguanil or quinine in addition to one of the following: tetracycline or doxycycline or clindamycin; or, if no other options, mefloquine. For those with *P. falciparum* in an area with no chloroquine resistance, chloroquine or hydroxychloroquine are recommend. If *P. falciparum* is acquired in an area with chloroquine resistance, one of the following options can be used: artemether-lumefantrine or atovaquone-proguanil or quinine (in addition to tetracycline or doxycycline or clindamycin), or, if no other options, mefloquine; artemether-lumefantrine is the preferred treatment. For those with severe malaria or inability to tolerate oral medications, intravenous artesunate is recommended (further information on treatment is available in a different chapter in the book).

For post-transplant patients, holding mycophenolate mofetil temporarily could be considered.

PREVENTION

Following transplantation, it is important to engage in appropriate prevention strategies when traveling to malaria-endemic areas, including mosquito exposure prevention measures and chemoprophylaxis depending on the malaria risk. Before traveling to endemic areas, post-transplant patients should discuss appropriate measures with their transplant physician, especially given the known interactions between antimalarial medications and transplant medications, such as calcineurin inhibitors, mTOR inhibitors, and trimethoprim-sulfamethoxazole.[15] Consultation with a travel clinic, specifically skilled in assessing the need for infectious disease prophylaxis, might be of benefit.

Leishmaniasis

Leishmaniasis is a parasitic disease caused by an intracellular parasite via the bite of a sand fly, *Phlebotomus* and *Lutzomyia*.[18] Leishmaniasis is endemic to Asia, Africa, the Americas, and the Mediterranean region.[16]

SCREENING

Routine serologic screening of organ donors from endemic countries is not currently advised. If a donor is known to have leishmaniasis, it is advised that the recipient be carefully monitored in the post-transplant period.

DIAGNOSIS AND TREATMENT

Post-transplant patients can acquire leishmaniasis through primary infection, post-transplant, reactivation of latent infection, receipt of an infected organ, or blood transfusion.[16,19] Infected patients can present in one of three ways—visceral, cutaneous, or mucocutaneous disease—which is impacted by the infecting organism and the host immune response. Impaired host cellular immunity impacts the development of infection and the severity of disease.[20]

Cutaneous leishmaniasis, the most common manifestation, is generally characterized by solitary papules, often at the site of inoculation. The mucocutaneous form, on the other hand, typically develops after resolution of the primary cutaneous lesion and most commonly involves the mucous membranes of the nose and mouth.[21] Visceral leishmaniasis often presents with fever, hepatosplenomegaly, and pancytopenia.[22]

The diagnosis of visceral leishmaniasis requires histopathology or culture, often from the bone marrow. The sensitivity of bone marrow biopsy has been reported to be 98% in organ transplant patients.[23] The protozoan can also be found in scrapings of cutaneous or mucosal ulcerations.

The treatment of leishmaniasis is determined by host and parasite factors. For those with visceral leishmaniasis, the use of liposomal amphotericin B is associated with an efficacy of greater than 90%.[24] Alternative therapies include antimonials, paromomycin or miltefosine. When selecting therapies, it is important to be aware of the potential interaction, such as the potential for additive nephrotoxicity when tacrolimus is used along with amphotericin B; however, liposomal preparations should be associated with less toxicity.[25]

PREVENTION

Precautions should be taken to avoid sand fly bites in endemic areas given that there are no vaccines or drugs available to prevent infection.

Strongyloidiasis

Strongyloides is an intestinal nematode that is endemic worldwide but more prevalent in tropical or subtropical areas, such as sub-Saharan Africa, Latin America, and Southeast Asia.[26] In liver transplant recipients strongyloidiasis can be related to donor-derived transmission or as reactivation of latent disease.[10]

SCREENING

For those living in endemic areas, transplant candidates, deceased donors, and living donors should be screened for *Strongyloides* with enzyme-linked immunosorbent assay testing for *Strongyloides* immunoglobulin G (given it is more sensitive than stool exams).[7,10] Transmission of *Strongyloides* via transplantation has been described and associated with morbidity and mortality.[27,28] The mortality rate in hyperinfection syndrome and disseminated infection in transplanted patients has been estimated to be 50% and 70%, respectively.[29]

DIAGNOSIS AND TREATMENT

While infection with *Strongyloides* is often asymptomatic or minimally symptomatic in immunocompetent individuals, it can present with more significant symptoms in those who are immunosuppressed. *Strongyloides stercoralis* can result in hyperinfection syndrome following solid organ transplantation, such as liver transplantation.[27,28] Those with *Strongyloides* hyperinfection syndrome and disseminated disease can present in a similar fashion to classic strongyloidiasis, with symptoms such as nausea, emesis, diarrhea, cough, fever, and shortness of breath, but they can also present with more significant manifestations, such as a shock, respiratory distress, disseminated intravascular coagulation, meningitis, and renal failure.[30] Susceptibility to hyperinfection syndrome is related to immunosuppression, especially with high-dose corticosteroids.[27,31]

Post-transplant patients infected with *Strongyloides* should be treated with ivermectin. For those with hyperinfection or disseminated disease, treatment is recommended until visible organisms are cleared followed by an additional 1 to 2 weeks of ivermectin.[10] When using ivermectin, it is important to consider potential interactions with immunosuppressive agents. For instance, ivermectin is a cytochrome P450 inducer and thus can alter calcineurin inhibitor drug levels.[32]

PREVENTION

A short course of ivermectin or thiabendazole should be considered for seropositive patients pre-transplant.[7,10] If screening is not feasible pre-transplantation, a short course of empiric ivermectin can be considered post-transplant followed by close monitoring. Liver transplant recipients in endemic regions should be advised to wear footwear and avoid walking barefoot.

Schistosomiasis

Schistosomiasis is caused by parasitic flatworms (blood flukes) in the genus *Schistosoma* endemic to the Middle East, South America, Southeast Asia, and, particularly, sub-Saharan Africa.[33]

The specific clinical disease varies by species of *Schistosoma*. In liver transplant recipients schistosomiasis can be related to a reactivation of previous infection or a *de novo* infection.[34,35]

SCREENING

Screening of living organ donors and potential recipients should be considered for individuals who have lived in and/or traveled to endemic countries and have been exposed to fresh water at risk for schistosomiasis. Screening of at-risk donors should be done by serologic testing, stool examination, or histologic examination of the explant.[10] However, schistosomiasis is not often diagnosed pre-transplant given that individuals are often asymptomatic. If a live donor is found to have schistosomiasis, a single dose of praziquantel is recommended prior to transplantation.[10] Alternative therapies include oxamniquine and the antimalarial, artemether.

DIAGNOSIS AND TREATMENT

Acute schistosomiasis often is asymptomatic; therefore many infected individuals are unaware of their infection. However, intestinal schistosomiasis can present with abdominal discomfort, anorexia, and diarrhea, and schistosomiasis can impact the urinary system and present with symptoms such as dysuria and hematuria.[16] Schistosomiasis can be diagnosed based on serology (either serum or blood), tissue biopsy, stool examination, or urine testing. However, false negatives can occur with stool and urine testing.[16] While serologic testing has increased sensitivity, it is also associated with false negatives and does not differentiate between current and prior infections.[10,16]

The risk of reactivation is thought to be related to immunosuppressive therapy post-liver transplant.[34,35] Adult schistosomes do not replicate within the host; therefore transmission by organ transplantation would only be non-replicating adult worms.

For those diagnosed with schistosomiasis post liver transplant, praziquantel is the first-line therapy and is associated with good outcomes.[34,35] When using praziquantel while a patient is on cyclosporine, it is critical to be aware that cyclosporine may decrease the metabolism of praziquantel, leading to higher praziquantel drug levels and increased risk for toxicity. Previous *in vitro* and animal studies have demonstrated that cyclosporine may have anti-schistosomal properties, especially with *Schistosoma mansoni*.[36]

PREVENTION

Liver transplant recipients should be advised to avoid contact with fresh water in endemic regions, which includes swimming, bathing, and wading.

Challenges

While the use of liver transplantation for the treatment of end-stage liver disease has gained acceptance in countries across the globe and the rates of transplantation have increased, challenges remain.[37]

A challenge that faces all countries, not only those in tropical settings, are multifactorial barriers to transplant access, which include but are not limited to initial recognition of end-stage liver disease, referral to specialized centers for liver transplant evaluation, and the economic cost of liver transplantation. Streamlining referral patterns for liver transplantation will have a key role in optimizing peri-transplant outcomes. Potential strategies to improve referral patterns include orientation programs for providers who care for patients with liver disease and increased exposure to transplantation during medical training.[37]

Furthermore, some countries face issues with low rates of organ donation, which limits the ability to serve the population of patients who might benefit from liver transplantation.[38] Strategies such as government-funded advertising campaigns may help individuals better understand the process and benefits of organ donation. For instance, in Brazil, the main strategy for increasing organ donation has been raising public awareness through national educational campaigns, which included media coverage of the campaigns and high-profile successful surgeries.[39]

Many tropical countries also face economic challenges for therapies post liver transplantation. Immunosuppression and other medical therapies, such as hepatitis B immunoglobulin (HBIG) in the post-transplant setting for hepatitis B virus (HBV) prophylaxis, can be costly. Some centers have developed strategies to navigate concerns regarding HBIG cost, such as stratifying patients based on risk. Low-risk patients, those with undetectable HBV DNA at the time of liver transplantation either in the absence of antiviral therapy or while receiving entecavir or tenofovir, do not receive HBIG.[40,41] High-risk patients receive intravenous HBIG during the first year and then HBIG is stopped.[40,41] Other centers have evaluated replacing the use of HBIG with HBV vaccines or potent antiviral therapy alone.[42]

Finally, in order to improve outcomes, countries need to understand transplant outcomes; therefore a centralized system to report transplant outcomes is recommended to track outcomes and identify areas for improvement.

An exhaustive review of the peri-transplant challenges faced in tropical settings is beyond the scope of this chapter. The field of liver transplantation is constantly evolving, and thus collaboration and idea sharing among centers across the globe is critical to improving access to transplantation as well as post-transplant outcomes.

Conclusion

With the ease of air travel, increased emigration from endemic areas, and expansion of solid organ transplantation to much of the world, a heightened awareness of tropical infectious diseases among liver transplant donors and recipients is imperative.

In this chapter we have discussed Chagas disease, malaria, leishmaniasis, strongyloidiasis, and schistosomiasis, but it is important to be aware that other diseases, unusual in the West, may afflict liver transplant recipients, for example, Zika. Knowledge of donor risks for transmission and unusual clinical presentations should serve well to assure good clinical outcomes for those unfortunate recipients who might acquire such infections.

References

1. Bern C. Chagas' disease. *NEJM.* 2015;373(5):456-466. doi:10.1056/NEJMRA1410150.
2. Macado C, Levi J. Transplant-associated and blood transfusion-associated tropical and parasitic infections. *Infect Dis Clin North Am.* 2012;26(2):225-241. doi:10.1016/j.idc.2012.02.008.
3. McCormack L, Quiñónez E, Goldaracena N, et al. Liver transplantation using Chagas-infected donors in uninfected recipients: a single-center experience without prophylactic therapy. *Am J Transplant.* 2012;12(10):2832-2837.
4. Huprikar S, Bosserman E, Patel G, et al. Donor-derived *Trypanosoma cruzi* infection in solid organ recipients in the United States, 2001-2011. *Am J Transplant.* 2013;13(9):2418-2425.
5. Barcan L, Luna C, Clara L, et al. Transmission of *T. cruzi* infection via liver transplantation to a nonreactive recipient for Chagas' disease. *Liver Transpl.* 2005;11:1112-1116.
6. Radisic MV, Repetto SA. American trypanosomiasis (Chagas disease) in solid organ transplantation. *Transpl Infect Dis.* 2020;22(6):1-12. doi:10.1111/tid.13429.
7. Malinis M, Boucher H, AST Infectious Diseases Community of Practice. Screening of donor and candidate prior to solid organ transplantation: guidelines from the American Society of Transplantation Infectious Diseases Community of Practice. *Clin Transplant.* 2019;33(9):e13548. doi:10.1111/ctr.13548.

8. Consortium CDACT, Casadei D. Chagas' disease and solid organ transplantation. *Transplant Proc.* 2010;42(9):3354-3359. doi:10.1016/j.transproceed.2010.09.019.
9. Bern C, Montgomery S, Herwaldt B, et al. Evaluation and treatment of chagas disease in the United States: a systematic review. *JAMA.* 2007;298:2171-2181.
10. Clemente W, Pierrotti L, Abdala E, et al. Recommendations for management of endemic diseases and travel medicine in solid-organ transplant recipients and donors: Latin America. *Transplantation.* 2019;103(1):e38.
11. Phillips M, Burrows J, Manyando C, et al. Malaria. *Nat Rev Dis Prim.* 2017;3:17050.
12. Rosso F, Agudelo Rojas O, Suarez Gil C, et al. Transmission of malaria from donors to solid organ transplant recipients: a case report and literature review. *Transpl Infect Dis.* 2021;23:e13660. doi:10.1111/tid.13660.
13. Mantilla-Flórez Y, Barragán B, Tuta-Quintero E, Pérez-Díaz C. *Plasmodium vivax* infection due to percutaneous exposure in non-endemic area. *Infect Dis Heal.* 2020;25(1):60-62.
14. Pierrotti L, Levi M, Di Santi S, et al. Malaria disease recommendations for solid organ transplant recipients and donors. *Transplantation.* 2018;102(2S suppl 2):S16-S26. doi:10.1097/TP.0000000000002017.
15. Buchan C, Kotton C. Travel medicine, transplant tourism, and the solid organ transplant recipient: guidelines from the American Society of Transplantation Infectious Diseases Community of Practice. *Clin Transpl.* 2019;33(9):1-16.
16. Schwartz BS, Mawhorter SD. Parasitic infections in solid organ transplantation. *Am J Transplant.* 2013;13(suppl 4):280-303. doi:10.1111/ajt.12120.
17. Rodriguez M, Tome S, Vizcaino L, et al. Malaria infection through multiorgan donation: an update from Spain. *Liver Transpl.* 2007;13(9):1302-1304. doi:10.1002/lt.21219.
18. Torres-Guerrero E, Quintanilla-Cedillo M, Ruiz-Esmenjaud J, Arenas R. Leishmaniasis: a review. *F1000Res.* 2017;6:750. doi:10.12688/f1000research.11120.1.
19. Dhaliwal A, Chauhan A, Aggarwal D, et al. Donor acquired visceral leishmaniasis following liver transplantation. *Frontline Gastroenterol.* 2021;12:690-694. doi:10.1136/flgastro-2020-101659.
20. Pearson R, De Sousa A, Jeronimo S. *Leishmania* species: visceral (kala azar), cutaneous, and mucosal leishmaniasis. In: Bennett JE, Dolin R, Blaser MJ, eds. *Principles and Practice of Infectious Diseases.* Philadelphia, PA: Elsevier; 2020:2831-2845.
21. Reithinger R, Dujardin J, Louzir H, et al. Cutaneous leishmaniasis. *Lancet Infect Dis.* 2007;7(9): 581-596. doi:10.1016/S1473-3099(07)70209-8.
22. Veroux M, Corona D, Giuffrida G, et al. Visceral leishmaniasis in the early post-transplant period after kidney transplantation: clinical features and therapeutic management. *Transpl Infect Dis.* 2010;12: 387-391.
23. Antinori S, Cascio A, Parravicini C, et al. Leishmaniasis among organ transplant recipients. *Lancet Infect Dis.* 2008;8:191-199.
24. Burza S, Croft S, Boelaert M, et al. Leishmaniasis. *Lancet.* 2018;392:951-970.
25. Paterson D, Singh N. Interactions between tacrolimus and antimicrobial agents. *Clin Infect Dis.* 1997;25(6):1430-1440.
26. Berk S, Verghese A, Alvarez S, et al. Clinical and epidemiologic features of strongyloidiasis. A prospective study in rural Tennessee. *Arch Intern Med.* 1987;147:1257-1261.
27. Vilela E, Clemente W, Mira R, et al. *Strongyloides stercoralis* hyperinfection syndrome after liver transplantation: case report and literature review. *Transpl Infect Dis.* 2009;11:132-136.
28. Ofosu A, Higgins J, Frye J, et al. Strongyloides superinfection after liver transplantation. *Dig Dis Sci.* 2021;66(7):2178-2182. doi:10.1007/s10620-020-06696-3.
29. Patel G, Arvelakis A, Sauter B, et al. Strongyloides hyperinfection syndrome after intestinal transplantation. *Transpl Infect Dis.* 2008;10:137-141.
30. Kassalik M, Mönkemüller K. *Strongyloides stercoralis* hyperinfection syndrome and disseminated disease. *Gastroenterol Hepatol (N Y).* 2011;7(11):766-768.
31. Morgan J, Schaffner W, Stone W. Opportunistic strongyloidiasis in renal transplant recipients. *Transplantation.* 1986;42(5):518-524.
32. González Canga A, Sahagún Prieto A, Diez Liébana M, et al. The pharmacokinetics and interactions of ivermectin in humans: a mini-review. *AAPS J.* 2008;10(2):42-46.
33. McManus D, Dunne D, Sacko M, et al. Schistosomiasis. *Nat Rev Dis Prim.* 2018;4:13. doi:10.1038/s41572-018-0013-8.

34. Hoare M, Gelson W, Davies S, et al. Hepatic and intestinal schistosomiasis after orthotopic liver transplant. *Liver Transpl.* 2005;11(12):1603-1607.
35. Ahmed K, Safdar K, Kemmer N, et al. Intestinal schistosomiasis following orthotopic liver transplantation: a case report. *Transpl Proc.* 2007;39:3502-3504.
36. Kotton C, Lattes R, AST Infectious Diseases Community of Practice. Parasitic infections in solid organ transplant recipients. *Am J Transplant.* 2009;9(suppl 4):S234-S251.
37. Narasimhan G, Kota V, Rela M. Liver transplantation in India. *Liver Transpl.* 2016;22(7):1019-1024.
38. McCaughan G, Munn S. Liver transplantation in Australia and New Zealand. *Liver Transpl.* 2016;22(6):830-838.
39. Bittencourt P, Farias A, Couto C. Liver transplantation in Brazil. *Liver Transpl.* 2016;22(9):1254-1258.
40. Degertekin B, Han S, Keeffe E, et al. Impact of virologic breakthrough and HBIG regimen on hepatitis B recurrence after liver transplantation. *Am J Transplant.* 2010;10(8):1823.
41. Nath D, Kalis A, Nelson S, Payne W, Lake J, Humar A. Hepatitis B prophylaxis post-liver transplant without maintenance hepatitis B immunoglobulin therapy. *Clin Transpl.* 2006;20(2):206.
42. Gane E, Patterson S, Strasser S, McCaughan G, Angus P. Combination of lamivudine and adefovir without hepatitis B immune globulin is safe and effective prophylaxis against hepatitis B virus recurrence in hepatitis B surface antigen-positive liver transplant candidates. *Liver Transpl.* 2013;19(3):268-274.

SECTION V

Rare Tropical Liver Diseases

CHAPTER 28

Melioidosis and the Liver

Bart J. Currie

KEY POINTS

- Melioidosis is caused by *Burkholderia pseudomallei* and occurs in specific endemic locations, mostly tropical
- Melioidosis has diverse presentations, with pneumonia being the most common
- Liver abscesses can occur and all cases of melioidosis should have abdominal imaging
- Drainage of liver abscesses may be required, and prolonged antibiotic therapy is necessary to prevent relapsed disease

Introduction

Melioidosis is an infection with the environmental bacterium *Burkholderia pseudomallei*, which is variably present in soil and ground water in many tropical and some subtropical locations.[1] As laboratory diagnostic capabilities improve, endemic disease is being increasingly recognized beyond the highly endemic regions of Southeast Asia and northern Australia.[2] In addition, melioidosis is an uncommon but important cause of fever in travelers visiting from or returning from endemic countries. Over the last decade, a small number of cases of melioidosis in the United States have been linked to importation of commercial products contaminated with *Burkholderia pseudomallei* and in 2022 *B. pseudomallei* was for the first time found in the environment of the southern USA and linked to two endemic cases of melioidosis. Melioidosis causes disease in both humans and animals, with a wide diversity of severity and organ involvement. Single or multiple liver abscesses may be present concomitant with pneumonia or other clinical presentations.[3]

EPIDEMIOLOGY

Figure 28.1 shows the currently recognized global distribution of melioidosis. The majority of those infected with *B. pseudomallei* remain asymptomatic, with only positive serology indicating prior infection. The clinical presentation, severity, and outcome of melioidosis are determined by several factors. Most important are the host risk factors specific for melioidosis, with diabetes being the dominant risk factor and present in around half of all cases.[4] Other risk factors include hazardous alcohol use, chronic renal disease, chronic lung disease, and immunosuppression, especially use of high-dose and/or prolonged corticosteroids. Around 20% of cases of melioidosis have no identified risk factor, and in these cases mortality approaches zero with early diagnosis, appropriate antibiotics, and access to state-of-the-art intensive care management. This underlies the concept of *B. pseudomallei* as an opportunistic pathogen, but the reality is that in many countries endemic for melioidosis diagnosis and treatment remain challenging, and the overall mortality can be over 50%.[5]

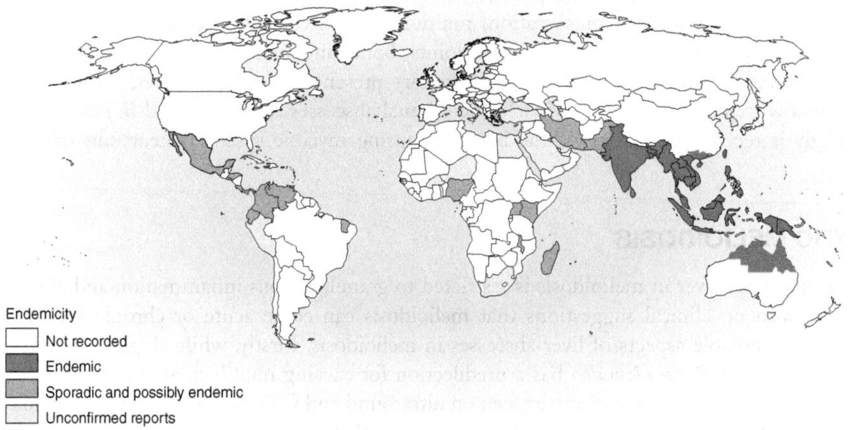

Figure 28.1 Known global distribution of melioidosis. (From Bennet JE, Dolin R, Blaser MJ. Mandell, Douglas, and Bennett's Principles and Practice of Infectious Diseases, 9th edition, Volume 1. © 2020, Elsevier.)

In addition to the bacterial inoculum size, the mode of infection is also important. Most cases follow percutaneous inoculation such as penetrating injuries or cuts and sores exposed to soil, but highest mortality is seen with inhalational melioidosis, which can follow severe weather events such as typhoons, cyclones, and hurricanes, with aerosolization of *B. pseudomallei.* Ingestion of *B. pseudomallei* occurs in animals and in humans in endemic locations where water supplies are from ground water that is not chlorinated, such as bores and water wells.[6]

Almost 90% of all cases are acute presentations, with an incubation period of 1 to 21 days (median 4 days).[4] Around 10% present with chronic melioidosis, which is defined as symptoms being present for 2 months or longer. Activation from latency, analogous to tuberculosis, is much less common than previously thought and represents under 5% of all cases, with the longest documented time between infection and disease onset being 29 years.[7]

PRESENTATION

The clinical spectrum of melioidosis, a "the great mimicker," is very broad. Over half of all cases are bacteremic and up to a quarter need intensive care management for severe sepsis. Community-acquired pneumonia is the presentation for 50% of cases, ranging from a chronic illness mimicking tuberculosis clinically and on CXR, to severe pneumonia with progressive septic shock, which accounts for 75% of intensive care cases.[3,4] In children, and those with no risk factors, the most common presentation is a single nonhealing skin ulcer or abscess, which clinically cannot be differentiated from staphylococcal or streptococcal pyoderma. Blood cultures in these cases are almost always negative, fever and systemic symptoms are often absent, and inflammatory markers such as increased white cell count and C-reactive protein may be normal. Such cutaneous melioidosis accounts for 13% of melioidosis cases in Australia.

Other presentations include genitourinary melioidosis, with prostate abscesses especially common, parotid abscesses, septic arthritis, osteomyelitis, lymphadenopathy sometimes with discharging abscesses, and neurological melioidosis with either brain abscesses or encephalomyelitis.

Bacteremic sepsis without an underlying focus is also seen, especially in immunocompromised patients, and can mimic febrile neutropenia.

Regardless of the primary presentation, multiorgan involvement is common and usually reflects bacteremic spread to internal organs, joints, bone, and muscle. Secondary pneumonia occurs in around 20% of those with another primary presentation. Spleen, liver, prostate, and kidney abscess are commonly seen. Muscle and adrenal abscesses also occur, and *B. pseudomallei* increasingly is recognized as one of the bacteria causing mycotic (pseudo)aneurysms of large arteries.

HEPATIC MELIOIDOSIS

Involvement of the liver in melioidosis is restricted to granulomatous inflammation and abscess formation, with no clinical suggestions that melioidosis can cause acute or chronic hepatitis. There are two notable aspects of liver abscesses in melioidosis. Firstly, while single or multiple abscesses can occur, *B. pseudomallei* has a predilection for causing multiloculated liver abscesses with multiple internal thin septations, as seen on ultrasound and CT scan, described as the "honeycomb" sign (Figure 28.2).[8-10] While it has been noted that other bacteria can also cause these appearances, such an image finding in someone from a melioidosis-endemic location should prompt further microbiological sampling to confirm a diagnosis.

Secondly, the occurrence of liver abscesses in melioidosis is far greater in Asian countries such as Thailand, Cambodia, and India than in northern Australia, where liver abscesses were present in only 3% of melioidosis cases.[4,9,10] It is hypothesized that the high rate of liver abscesses seen in Asia reflects, in part, exposure to unchlorinated water supplies, with subsequently a higher rate of infection attributed to ingestion of *B. pseudomallei*.[5,6] This implies that the liver abscesses seen in Southeast Asia, including the "honeycomb" abscesses, can result from a primary gastrointestinal melioidosis focus with portal tract bacterial spread to the liver in addition to bacteremic spread.[5]

Diagnosis

Clinical suspicion and a history of travel from an endemic region necessitate investigation for melioidosis, which requires culture of *B. pseudomallei* to confirm a diagnosis of melioidosis. Clinical samples should include blood and urine cultures and samples from the clinical focus such as sputum and aspirated pus sent to the microbiology laboratory for microscopy and culture.[1,3] The laboratory should be informed to look specifically for melioidosis as selective media such as Ashdown's agar or liquid broth may be required for samples such as sputum, swabs, pus, and urine. In bacteremic cases *B. pseudomallei* does grow readily in standard blood culture systems.

Identification of cultured organisms also requires careful laboratory assessment as automated systems and newer technologies including MALDI-TOF MS can give incorrect speciation. While PCR is being increasingly used to confirm the identification of *B. pseudomallei* from cultured bacteria, direct PCR from clinical samples has low sensitivity. A lateral flow immunoassay targeting capsular polysaccharide antigen shows promise for the rapid diagnosis of melioidosis directly from clinical samples and is also useful for confirming culture isolate identity.[11] It has been successfully used directly on pus aspirated from a liver abscess (Figure 28.3).

Serology cannot differentiate melioidosis from prior infection and seropositivity rates can exceed 50% in endemic regions. However, positive serology in someone not normally residing in an endemic region is an indicator for further targeted cultures to establish if the diagnosis is melioidosis.

Where available, all cases of melioidosis, irrespective of primary presentation, should have abdominal imaging to look for internal abscesses. This can be CT scan of abdomen and pelvis, or abdominal ultrasound in children and women of childbearing age.

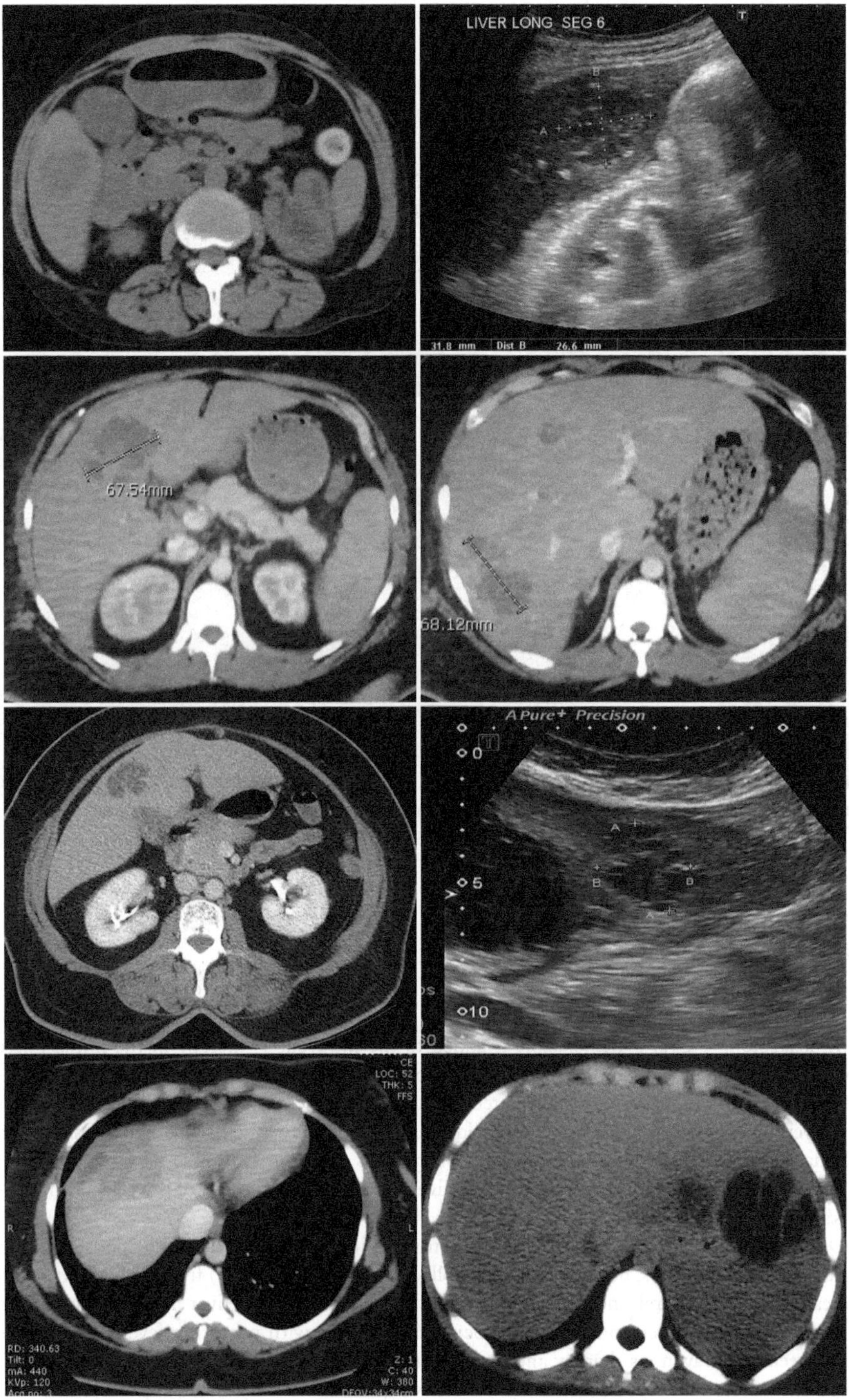

Figure 28.2 The radiological diversity of melioidosis liver abscesses.

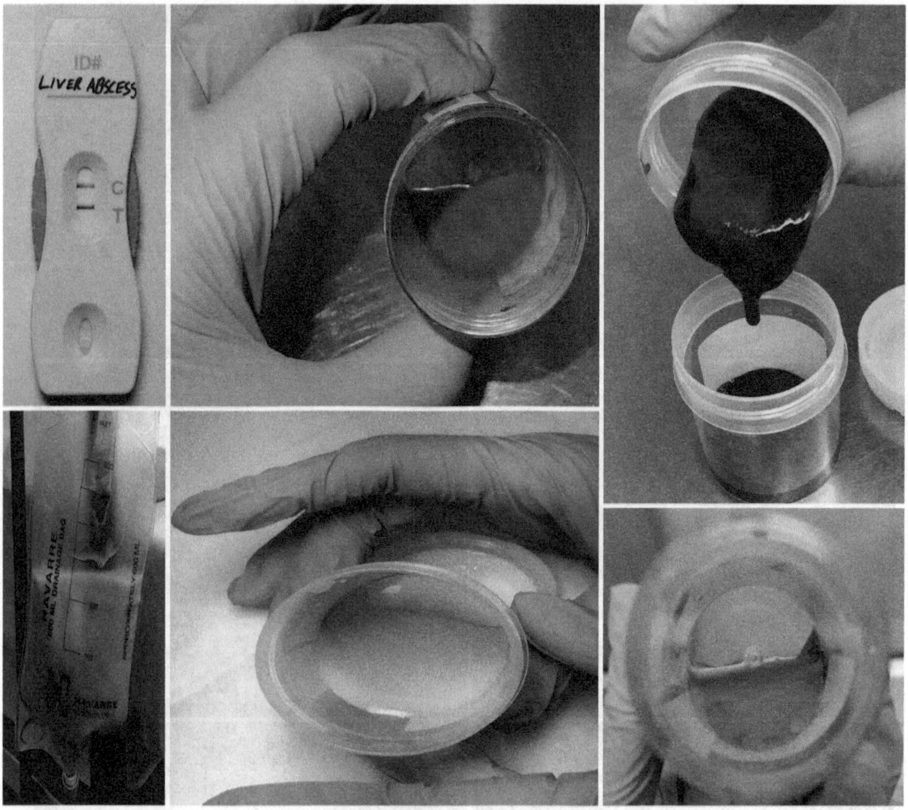

Figure 28.3 The diversity of pus appearance and volume in melioidosis liver abscesses. The pus is non-odorous and is positive on the recently developed melioidosis antigen-capture lateral flow immunoassay.

Management

Antibiotic treatment of melioidosis consists of an initial intensive phase of intravenous ceftazidime or meropenem, followed by an eradication phase of oral trimethoprim/sulfamethoxazole (cotrimoxazole).[1,12] Oral cotrimoxazole is added to the intravenous therapy in the initial phase when there are internal abscesses such as liver abscess and in various other scenarios. If cotrimoxazole is contraindicated or not tolerated because of adverse drug reactions, then alternatives are doxycycline and amoxicillin/clavulanic acid. The duration of the intensive phase is a minimum of 10 days, with duration determined by the clinical focus and severity of melioidosis and extending to 4 weeks or longer. For melioidosis with liver abscesses, a minimum of 4 weeks of intravenous therapy is recommended.

Drainage of internal abscesses for source control is important and should be considered for single large liver abscesses, but other internal collections (baring prostate) frequently resolve with medical therapy and rarely need to be drained. With multiloculated liver abscesses, aspiration drainage of pus for source control may be beneficial in those with persisting fever despite more than a week of intravenous therapy and placement of a drainage catheter is useful in some cases to optimize clearance of pus (Figure 28.3). Following abscess drainage, the "clock" is reset for a further 4 weeks of intravenous therapy.

Following the intravenous therapy, eradication therapy with cotrimoxazole for a duration of usually 3 months is necessary, with 6 months recommended for neurological melioidosis and melioidosis osteomyelitis and potentially lifelong therapy for melioidosis aneurysms requiring vascular grafting.

References

1. Wiersinga WJ, Virk HS, Torres AG, et al. Melioidosis. *Nat Rev Dis Primers.* 2018;4:17107. doi:10.1038/nrdp.2017.107.
2. Chewapreecha C, Holden MTG, Vehkala M, et al. Global and regional dissemination and evolution of *Burkholderia pseudomallei. Nat Microbiol.* 2017;2:16263. doi:10.1038/nmicrobiol.2016.263.
3. Wiersinga WJ, Currie BJ, Peacock SJ. Melioidosis. *N Engl J Med.* 2012;367:1030-1039.
4. Currie BJ, Mayo M, Ward LM, et al. The Darwin Prospective Melioidosis Study: a 30-year prospective, observational investigation. *Lancet Infect Dis.* 2021;21:1737-1746. doi:10.1016/S1473-3099(21)00022-0.
5. Currie BJ. Melioidosis: evolving concepts in epidemiology, pathogenesis and treatment. *Semin Respir Crit Care Med.* 2015;36:111-25.
6. Limmathurotsakul D, Kanoksil M, Wuthiekanun V, et al. Activities of daily living associated with acquisition of melioidosis in northeast Thailand: a matched case-control study. *PLoS Negl Trop Dis.* 2013;7:e2072.
7. Chodimella U, Hoppes WL, Whalen S, et al. Septicemia and suppuration in a Vietnam veteran. *Hosp Pract.* 1997;32:219-221.
8. Apisarnthanarak A, Apisarnthanarak P, Mundy LM. Computed tomography characteristics of *Burkholderia pseudomallei* liver abscess. *Clin Infect Dis.* 2006;42:989-993.
9. Khiangte HL, Vimala LR, Eapen A, et al. A retrospective case-control study to evaluate the diagnostic accuracy of honeycomb sign in melioid liver abscess. *Am J Trop Med Hyg.* 2018;99:852-857.
10. Vatcharapreechasakul T, Suputtamongkol Y, Dance DA, Chaowagul W, White NJ. *Pseudomonas pseudomallei* liver abscesses: a clinical, laboratory, and ultrasonographic study. *Clin Infect Dis.* 1992;14:412-417.
11. Houghton RL, Reed DE, Hubbard MA, et al. Development of a prototype lateral flow immunoassay (LFI) for the rapid diagnosis of melioidosis. *PLoS Negl Trop Dis.* 2014;8(3):e2727. doi:10.1371/journal.pntd.0002727.
12. Sullivan RP, Marshall CS, Anstey NM, et al. 2020 Review and revision of the 2015 Darwin melioidosis treatment guideline; paradigm drift not shift. *PloS Negl Trop Dis.* 2020;14(9):e0008659. doi:10.1371/journal.pntd.0008659.

CHAPTER 29

Histoplasmosis

Kathleen A. Linder ■ Carol A. Kauffman

KEY POINTS

- Histoplasmosis is caused by the dimorphic fungus *Histoplasma capsulatum*, which is highly endemic in certain regions of North and Latin America
- Liver involvement is seen primarily in patients who have disseminated infection, which occurs most often in immunocompromised individuals, especially those with HIV and CD4 <150 cells/μL
- Isolated granulomatous hepatitis due to histoplasmosis is rare
- Detection of *H. capsulatum* cell wall antigens in urine or serum is a rapid and sensitive method for probable diagnosis. Confirmed diagnosis is proven when the organism is grown in culture or the characteristic yeast form is seen on histopathological examination of involved tissues
- The treatment for severe disseminated histoplasmosis is intravenous liposomal amphotericin B; for mild to moderate infection, the treatment is oral itraconazole.

Introduction

Histoplasmosis is caused by the environmental fungus *Histoplasma capsulatum*.

H. capsulatum is a dimorphic fungus; it occurs as a mold in the environment but becomes a yeast in tissues at 37°C. The infecting form is the mold, which produces conidia that are inhaled into the alveoli.

The vast majority of persons infected with *H. capsulatum* have no symptoms and do not seek medical attention. However, exposure to a large inoculum of conidia can lead to severe pulmonary infection. Additionally, when the person exposed to *H. capsulatum* is immunocompromised, the immune system cannot halt the infection, and even a small inoculum can lead to severe infection with widespread dissemination.

Liver disease related to histoplasmosis is seen primarily in patients who have disseminated infection. Rarely, cases of isolated granulomatous hepatitis have been described.

Epidemiology

H. capsulatum occurs as a mold in the soil; growth is enhanced in soil with a high nitrogen content, which explains the propensity of finding the organism in areas that contain bird and bat excrement. The highest risk of developing infection with *H. capsulatum* occurs with activities associated with disturbing the soil, such as spelunking in caves in which large numbers of bats have roosted, performing demolition of old buildings, and landscaping.[1] In these situations outbreaks are frequently described. However, the organism is common enough in highly endemic areas that most cases are sporadic and not associated with activities such as those noted above.

The major endemic areas of *H. capsulatum* are in the Americas, although the organism has been isolated and cases described sporadically in China, India, Thailand, southern Europe, and Africa.[2] The Ohio and Mississippi River Valleys have high endemicity; less often, cases are reported in the mid-Atlantic coastal states, rural New York, and elsewhere. In Central America and northern areas of South America increasing rates of infection with HIV have led to an increase in cases of disseminated histoplasmosis, with high mortality rates that may even surpass those ascribed to tuberculosis in some countries.[3,4]

PRESENTATION

Most patients who are infected with histoplasmosis have few signs and symptoms of infection. Most infections with *H. capsulatum* are self-limited pulmonary infections that rarely come to the attention of physicians and, if seen, are usually misdiagnosed as viral or bacterial pneumonia. Often fungal pneumonia is not considered, and the patient recovers quickly. More severe pulmonary infection occurs in immunosuppressed persons and those who have been exposed to a large inoculum of organisms.

Disseminated histoplasmosis is almost always seen in persons who are immunocompromised, especially those with HIV and CD4 cells $<150/\mu L$.[5] It is this form of infection in which liver involvement can be seen. Patients with disseminated histoplasmosis present with fever, fatigue, anorexia, and weight loss. Skin lesions that are ulcerated or papular and painful oral ulcerations can occur. Examination demonstrates hepatosplenomegaly and, in some patients, diffuse lymphadenopathy.[6] Patients can present with overwhelming infection accompanied by shock, respiratory distress, hepatic failure, and coagulopathy. Adrenal insufficiency, a life-threatening complication of disseminated histoplasmosis, should be considered in patients who have orthostatic hypotension, hyperkalemia, hyponatremia, and eosinophilia.

Liver involvement has been found at autopsy in as many as 90% of patients with disseminated histoplasmosis.[7,8] However, specific symptoms and signs of liver involvement, other than hepatomegaly, are uncommon. In most patients ALT and AST are mildly elevated (occasionally with AST higher than ALT). Alkaline phosphatase is more predictably elevated, and bilirubin is usually only mildly abnormal. Liver biopsy shows granulomas, often necrotizing, and/or aggregates of lymphocytes and macrophages; the organism can be visualized within these areas using methenamine silver stains[9] (Figure 29.1). Uncommonly, patients with disseminated histoplasmosis can present primarily with symptoms and signs of liver disease that may include jaundice and manifestations of portal hypertension.[10-12] Most, but not all, of these patients are immunocompromised. Isolated granulomatous hepatitis presenting as fever of unknown origin also has been attributed to histoplasmosis in a few cases.[13-15]

Diagnosis

The most important first step in diagnosis is to know the typical clinical findings that suggest the possibility of histoplasmosis and then to assess the results of routinely obtained laboratory tests that could point toward possible histoplasmosis. Findings seen frequently in disseminated histoplasmosis include pancytopenia, elevated alkaline phosphatase, and elevated erythrocyte sedimentation rate, C-reactive protein, and ferritin.

A proven diagnosis of histoplasmosis is established by isolating the organism in culture or by visualizing it on histopathological examination of infected tissues.[16] Culture may take as long as 4 to 6 weeks; the organism grows in the mold form at room temperature. Blood cultures, especially if performed by the lysis centrifugation technique, can yield *H. capsulatum* in patients who have disseminated disease.[17] Histopathology reveals granulomatous inflammation, and the organism is seen as ovoid budding 2 to 4 μm yeasts.

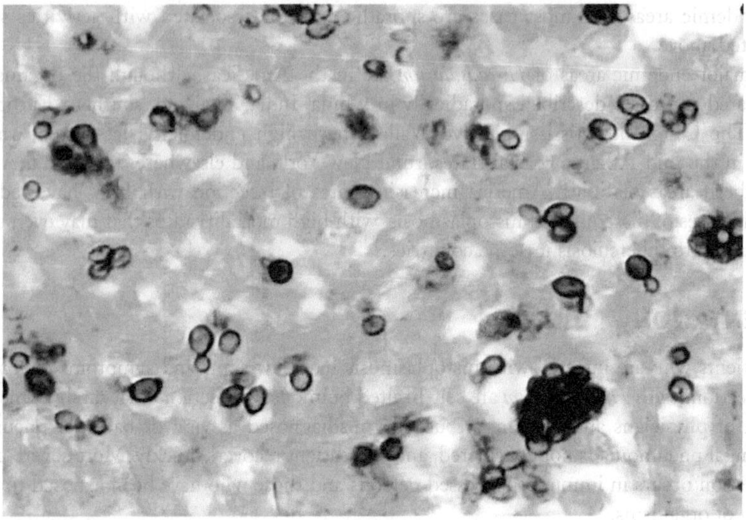

Figure 29.1 Biopsy sample from liver of a patient who was taking immunosuppressive drugs to prevent rejection of a kidney transplant and who developed disseminated histoplasmosis showing many budding yeasts, 2 to 4 μm in diameter, stained with methenamine silver stain.

Probable histoplasmosis can be diagnosed by detection of *Histoplasma* cell wall antigens in urine or serum.[16] The enzyme immunoassay (EIA) from MiraVista Laboratories (Indianapolis, IN, USA) shows a sensitivity as high as 90% in patients with disseminated histoplasmosis, most of whom had HIV.[17] An EIA from IMMY (Norman, OK, USA) is more readily available in Latin America and has comparable sensitivity to the MiraVista EIA in persons with disseminated infection.[18]

Detection of antibodies against *H. capsulatum* can be helpful for diagnosis, but immunocompromised patients are often unable to produce antibodies.

Management

Guidelines for the management of histoplasmosis have been published by the Infectious Diseases Society of America.[19] All patients with disseminated histoplasmosis, including most patients with liver involvement, should be treated with an antifungal agent. Infrequently, patients have only mild to moderate infection, and they can be treated with oral itraconazole. Patients who are severely ill and/or immunocompromised patients should be treated initially with a lipid formulation of intravenous amphotericin B (3–5mg/kg/day); if not available, amphotericin B deoxycholate (0.7–1.0 mg/kg/day) can be substituted but is more toxic.

Following improvement, generally after about 2 weeks, step-down treatment can be given with oral itraconazole, 200 mg three times daily for 3 days, then 200 mg twice daily for 12 months. Alternative oral agents for step-down therapy include posaconazole and voriconazole, but experience is limited to small uncontrolled series and individual case reports. All patients treated with an azole agent should have serum drug levels measured to ensure absorption and to avoid toxicity.

References

1. Benedict K, Mody RK. Epidemiology of histoplasmosis outbreaks, United States, 1938–2013. *Emerg Infect Dis.* 2016;22:370-378.
2. Scully MC, Baddley JW. Epidemiology of histoplasmosis. *Curr Fungal Infect Rep.* 2018;12:51-58.

3. Nacher M, Adenis A, McDonald S, et al. Disseminated histoplasmosis in HIV-infected patients in South America: a neglected killer continues on its rampage. *PLoS Negl Trop Dis.* 2013;7:e2319.
4. Adenis AA, Valdes A, Cropet C, et al. Burden of HIV-associated histoplasmosis as compared to tuberculosis in Latin America: a modelling study. *Lancet Infect Dis.* 2018;18:1150-1159.
5. Nacher M, Valdes A, Adenis A, et al. Disseminated histoplasmosis in HIV-infected patients: a description of 34 years of clinical and therapeutic practice. *J Fungi (Basel).* 2020;6(3):164.
6. Assi MA, Sandid MS, Baddour LM, et al. Systemic histoplasmosis: a 15-year retrospective institutional review of 111 patients. *Medicine (Baltimore).* 2007;86:162-169.
7. Goodwin RA, Shapiro JL, Thurman GH, et al. Disseminated histoplasmosis: clinical and pathologic correlations. *Medicine (Baltimore).* 1980;59:1-33.
8. Sayeed M, Benzamin M, Nahar L, et al. Hepatic histoplasmosis: an update. *J Clin Transpl Hepatol.* 2022;10:726-729. doi:10.14218/JCTH.2020.00080.
9. Lamps LW, Molina CP, West AB, et al. The pathologic spectrum of gastrointestinal and hepatic histoplasmosis. *Am J Clin Pathol.* 2000;113:64-72.
10. Nahar L, Benzamin MD, Sarkar N, et al. An 8-year Bangladeshi girl with disseminated histoplasmosis, presented as chronic liver disease with portal hypertension: a rare case report. *BMC Pediatr.* 2020;20: 284-287.
11. Rihana NA, Kandula M, Velez A, et al. Histoplasmosis presenting as granulomatous hepatitis: case report and review of the literature. *Case Rep Med.* 2014;2014:879535 doi:10.1155/2014/879535.
12. Washburn L, Galvan NT, Dhingra S, et al. Histoplasmosis hepatitis after orthotopic liver transplantation. *J Surg Case Rep.* 2017;2017(12):rjx232.
13. Zoutman DE, Ralph ED, Frei JV. Granulomatous hepatitis and fever of unknown origin: an 11-year experience of 23 cases with three years' follow-up. *J Clin Gastroenterol.* 1991;13:69-75.
14. Sartin JS, Walker RC. Granulomatous hepatitis: a retrospective review of 88 cases at the Mayo Clinic. *Mayo Clin Proc.* 1991;66:914-918.
15. Kibria R, Bari K, Ali SA, et al. "Ohio river valley fever" presenting as isolated granulomatous hepatitis: a case report. *South Med J.* 2009;102:656-658.
16. Donnelly JP, Chen SC, Kauffman CA, et al. Revision and update of the consensus definitions of invasive fungal disease from the European Organization for Research and Treatment of Cancer and the Mycoses Study Group Education and Research Consortium. *Clin Infect Dis.* 2020;71:1367-1376.
17. Azar MM, Hage CA. Laboratory diagnostics for histoplasmosis. *J Clin Microbiol.* 2017;55:1612-1620.
18. Martínez-Gamboa A, Niembro-Ortega MD, Torres-González P, et al. Diagnostic accuracy of antigen detection in urine and molecular assays testing in different clinical samples for the diagnosis of progressive disseminated histoplasmosis in patients living with HIV/AIDS: a prospective multicenter study in Mexico. *PLoS Negl Trop Dis.* 2021;15(3):e0009215.
19. Wheat LJ, Freifeld AG, Kleiman MB, et al. Clinical practice guidelines for the management of patients with histoplasmosis: 2007 update by the Infectious Diseases Society of America. *Clin Infect Dis.* 2007; 45:807-817.

CHAPTER 30

Brucellosis and the Liver

Eduardo Gotuzzo ■ Mariana Martel

KEY POINTS

- The most common infection is produced by *Brucella melitensis*, whose reservoir is mainly sheep and goats
- Most affected areas are the Mediterranean, Latin America, and regions of Asia
- Presenting symptoms include fever, joint pain, and hepatosplenomegaly. These symptoms can sometimes repeat sporadically in what is known as "undulant fever"
- When *Brucella* affects the liver, increase in alkaline phosphatase is the most common expression, and granulomas are frequently found in histology
- Treatment includes tetracyclines in addition to a second antibiotic

Introduction and Epidemiology

Brucellosis is a zoonosis (bacterial) with great impact on the economy and the public health of the regions of the world where it is present. Its incidence is largely unknown because it is not a notifiable disease. However, there is an action plan underway for the inclusion of neglected infectious diseases into national notification lists that could help revert this problem.[1,2]

The worldwide known ecological environments where this infection can be found are the Mediterranean region (e.g., Spain, Portugal, Italy, Türkiye, Greece, etc.) and some Latin American countries, specifically Mexico and Peru.[3,4] Nonetheless, in recent years brucellosis has been frequently reported in African countries and in some parts of Asia, including some regions of China.[5,6]

This zoonosis has three important strains: *Brucella melitensis*,[7] whose reservoir is goats and sheep; *Brucella abortus*, with cattle being the most important reservoir; and *Brucella suis*, with pigs being the major reservoir. There are other animals that can also be reservoirs for these species, but from an epidemiological point of view, they are less important. There are two strains that can rarely cause human infection: *Brucella canis*, with dogs being the reservoir, and *Brucella ceti*, found in dolphins and whales.

Brucellosis has a severe form caused by *B. melitensis*,[7] described initially by David Bruce on the Island of Malta,[8] that can become chronic and has higher mortality. *B. abortus* produces a milder form, less severe, and almost never chronic. Finally, *B. suis* produces an abscess-like lesion that causes a different reaction in the organism and whose incidence has been diminishing due to the vaccination of pigs.

Clinical Presentation

B. melitensis is the strain with the greatest impact in the world and produces three different clinical forms, two of which are very well recognized. The first form is the acute form that induces fever,

TABLE 30.1 ■ **Clinical Differences Among Different Forms of Brucellosis**

	Acute Brucellosis	Undulant Fever	Chronic Brucellosis
Age	Young adults, children	Young adults, children	Adults >40 years old
Fever	+++	++	Rare
Arthritis	Peripheric	Sacroiliitis > Peripheric	Spondylitis
Splenomegaly	>70%	±40%	Uncommon
Hepatomegaly	>70%	50%	20%–30%
Depression	No	Occasional	Frequent
Uveitis	No	Uncommon	Occasional (5%)

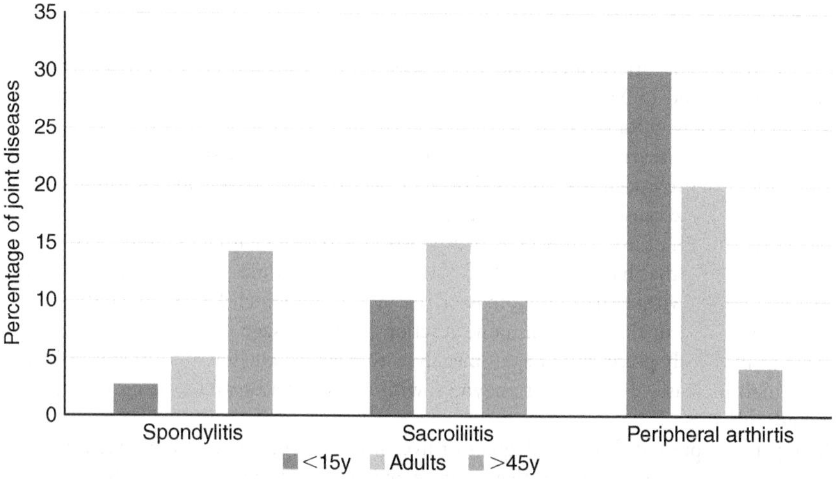

Figure 30.1 The difference between three clinical forms of *Brucella melitensis* in joint affection according to age.

malaise, intense sweating (mainly at night), rapid weight loss, and the presence of hepatosplenomegaly.[9] These patients also complain of joint syndromes (arthralgia and/or arthritis) according to age.[10]

The second form is called "undulant fever," which was described by Sir D. Bruce as the nowadays typical history of self-limiting fever in undulating periods that lasts for 1 or 2 weeks, associated with arthralgia, malaise, the presence of discrete hepatomegaly, and intermittent joint pain. These febrile periods disappear after approximately 1 year.

Lastly, there is the third form, which is the chronic form and is the least mentioned in the literature. It is recognized in endemic areas and resembles "a chronic fatigue syndrome." The patients do not have fever, but a sensation of fever and malaise in waves, that is associated with unusual exhaustion, joint involvement, such as arthralgia, and states of depression.

The differences between these three clinical presentations are summarized in Table 30.1 and the difference in joint affection is summarized in Figure 30.1, showing the information gathered throughout many years of investigation by the Alexander von Humboldt Institute of Tropical Medicine.

Diagnosis

The isolation of *Brucella* from blood samples can enable its early detection. The biphasic method, also called the *Ruiz Castañeda* method, allows this as well. Being an intracellular bacterium, the growth of *Brucella* in this medium is noticeable after 3 to 6 days, but from time to time positive results take longer (up to 10 days) and laboratories must be made aware of this. Likewise, bone marrow culture has been very useful in detecting *Brucella* in patients who are taking antibiotics or have chronic forms of the disease. Bone marrow culture is a faster, more efficient, and more useful method to isolate the bacteria.

Serology is very useful in the acute and undulating phase; the tube agglutination test (TAT) offers a sensitivity of 85% (title 1/160) and Rose Bengal has both a high sensitivity and specificity. PCR can also offer results with high sensitivity and specificity, but confirmation studies are necessary.[9,11]

In the chronic form it is recommended to measure IgM levels and perform bone marrow culture, with these being the most useful methods during this presentation.

Brucellosis of the Liver

Brucellosis can cause a variety of chronic liver diseases. There is a form of cirrhosis that has been reported on the Island of Malta, in infected people before there was any antibiotic treatment.[7] This condition is now quite rare.

A much rarer and severe form was extensively described in a classic article on autopsies in Peruvian patients with brucellosis who died of acute liver failure.[12] Severe liver atrophy was found and determined as the cause of death in this cohort.

The classic pattern of liver damage in Brucellosis is associated with a granulomatous reaction on the hepatic tissue that has been widely described. Ultrastructural studies have not shown the presence of *Brucella* within the granulomas or the liver itself, which led to conclude that these structural changes occur due to an immune reaction to the passage of the bacteria through the liver. This form usually presents as hepatomegaly with elevated alkaline phosphatase (ALP) but without a high increase of other liver enzymes, with transaminases values being normal or discreetly high.[13,14]

These patients present different degrees of liver involvement related to an extensive hepatic granulomatosis, which causes progressive jaundice, mainly in the acute phases of the disease, with fever, hepatosplenomegaly, and bacteremia. In our extensive experience, we have found only one patient (a pregnant woman) with fatal acute liver failure secondary to Brusellosis.[7,15]

Because liver damage is one of the main manifestations of brucellosis, it has been recorded in many studies through the passage of time. Table 30.2 summarizes signs, symptoms, and complications of liver involvement due to this infection.

Hepatomegaly is frequent in *Brucella* infection, present in approximately 50% to 70% of cases.[9] Most cases involve increase in alkaline phosphatase. The increase of transaminases that reflect liver damage is also reported, ranging from 27% to 62% for aspartate aminotransferase (AST) and 29% to 62% for alanine aminotransferase (ALT). This is slightly different from the authors' experience, according to which minimal to no increase in AST or ALT is seen.

Ozturk-Engin et al. found scleral icterus as a complication in 23% of their cases.[13] Meanwhile, only one case of liver abscess was reported by Colmenero et al.[20] If liver abscesses are found, *B. suis* should be suspected.

Historically, the formation of hepatic granulomas due to brucellosis was associated with the infection of *B. abortus.* However, different studies performed on patients infected with *B. melitensis* showed that this species was also capable of causing granuloma formation within the liver, as well as diffuse hepatitis with inflammatory infiltration of parenchymal tissue and minimal necrosis. Table 30.3 summarizes important studies that present histological evidence of liver damage, allowing the identification of hepatic granulomas. It can be observed that the main finding is the presence of multiple granulomas and diffuse hepatitis due to *B. melitensis,* which agrees with previously reported information.

TABLE 30.2 ■ **Brucellosis Studies That Report Liver Damage**

Author	Year	Total Number of Participants (*n*)	Signs and Symptoms (*n*)	Complications (*n*)
Gür et al.[16]	2003	283	Hepatomegaly = 78 Increased AST = 124 Increased ALT = 109	Jaundice = 35 Hepatitis = 3
Ma et al.[17]	2021	442	Hepatomegaly = 72 Increased AST = 200 Increased ALT = 143	
Zheng et al.[18]	2018	12842	Hepatomegaly = 2055	Hepatitis = 5779
Hassouneh et al.[19]	2019	28	Hepato-/splenomegaly = 10 Increased AST = 17 Increased ALT = 14	
Colmenero et al.[20]	1996	530	Hepatomegaly = 202 Increased AST = 247 Increased ALT = 261	Hepatitis = 12 Liver abscess = 1
Agin et al.[21]	2020	284	Hepatomegaly = 64 Increased AST = 77 Increased ALT = 83	
Young et al.[22]	2014	20	Increased AST = 10 Increased ALT = 9	
Ozturk-Engin et al.[13]	2014	325	Hepatomegaly = 203	Jaundice = 44 Scleral icterus = 75
Sahinturk et al.[23]	2018	195	Increased AST = 70 Increased ALT = 70	
Jia et al.[14]	2017	590	Hepatomegaly = 176 Increased AST = 179 Increased ALT = 179	Jaundice = 3

ALT, alanine aminotransferase; *AST*, aspartate aminotransferase.

Treatment

Tetracyclines are the drugs of choice for the treatment of brucellosis. For many years, in many studies it has been monotonously demonstrated that there is no resistance by *Brucella* strains to this antibiotic. Tetracyclines should always be used in combination with other antibiotics. Until a few years ago, the guidelines recommended an oral treatment of tetracyclines for 6 weeks, in addition to rifampicin. This combination has the clear drawback that the treated patients present with high degree of relapses. This greater amount of failures is based on the fact that rifampicin reduces the half-life time and concentration of tetracyclines. In the consensus published after the meeting of international experts at Ioannina, Greece, and in a meta-analysis,[31-33] it is shown that the best treatment is to prescribe aminoglycosides (especially parenteral gentamicin) for 1 to 2 weeks, in combination with a tetracycline for 6 weeks. Doxycycline is the most favored tetracycline because it is required only twice a day and has easy gastrointestinal absorption. In the case of severe forms, such as endocarditis, the option of administering a third drug has been considered. The third drug could be cotrimoxazole or rifampin.

In children under 7 years of age and in pregnant women, where the use of tetracyclines should not be included, the combination of oral cotrimoxazole plus rifampin for 6 weeks has been recommended.

TABLE 30.3 ■ **Brucellosis Studies With Histological Evidence of Liver Damage**

Author	Year	Etiologic Diagnosis	Presence of Granulomas	Other Findings
Young et al.[22]	2014	*B. melitensis*	• 2/20 patients with macro-granulomas and non-caseating granulomas • 2/20 with microgranulomas • 16/20 without granulomas	Hepatitis with mild lymphocytic infiltrates causing portal and lobular inflammation.
Akritidis et al.[24]	2007	*B. melitensis*	• 14/14 patients with parenchymal granulomas • 6/14 with granulomas in the portal space	3 patients presented single granulomas: 2 parenchymal and 1 within portal space. Inflammatory infiltration was present in 9/14 patients and mild and localized necrosis was found in the parenchymal tissue of 5/14 patients.
Colmenero et al.[20]	1997	*B. melitensis*	5/8 patients with granulomatous hepatitis	1 patient presented a multilocular liver abscess with calcification within and necrotizing granulomatous inflammation.
Ledro et al.[25]	1983	*B. melitensis*	12/20 patients with granulomas (acute and acute-chronic)	2 patients with chronic brucellosis had normal liver biopsies.
Cervantes et al.[26]	1982	*B. melitensis*	28/40 patients with either multiple or single granulomas	35/40 patients with non-specific reactive hepatitis.
Young et al.[27]	1979	*B. melitensis*	5/5 without granulomas	Diffuse hepatitis with acute and chronic inflammatory cells and necrotic hepatocytes.
		B. abortus	2/2 with non-caseating granulomas	
Recavarren and Gotuzzo[15]	1975	*B. melitensis*	10/10 with granulomatous hepatitis detected by electron microscopy	The parenchymal granulomas found were formed by lymphoid cells and histiocytes and in some cases giant cells. Brucella was not isolated from any tissue sample.
Hunt et al.[28]	1967	*B. abortus*	5/9 patients with active inflammation and granulomas	1 case of cirrhosis due to *B. abortus.* The finding of sinusoidal infiltration with lymphocytes, plasma cells, and polymorphs was common.
Joske et al.[29]	1955	*B. abortus*	5/10 liver biopsies presented granulomas	
Barret et al.[30]	1953	*B. abortus*	10/12 patients with chronic brucellosis presented multiple granulomas	

Tigecycline and meropenem have been shown to have *in vitro* activity, but medical experience with these antibiotics is minimal. Quinolones have shown activity *in vitro* as well, although authors' personal experience with them has been unfavorable.

Finally, control of brucellosis can be achieved, like other zoonoses, by vaccinating the main reservoir (cattle, sheep, pig). In countries where massive vaccination has been carried out for cattle or pigs, brucellosis has disappeared (Argentina, Uruguay, Spain). In Peru, when goat vaccination programs are carried out, the immediate impact they have on human brucellosis prevalence is greatly noticed.

References

1. Pan American Health Organization, World Health Organization: Regional Office for the Amricas. *Plan of Action for the Elimination of Neglected Infectious Diseases and Post-elimination Actions 2016-2022* [Internet]. Iris.paho.org. 2022 [cited 23 July 2022]. Available at: https://iris.paho.org/handle/10665.2/33976.
2. Laine C, Scott H, Arenas-Gamboa A. Human Brucellosis: Widespread information deficiency hinders and understanding of global disease frequency. *PLoS Negl Trop Dis.* 2022;16(5):e0010404. doi:10.1371/journal.pntd.0010404.
3. Pappas G, Akritidis N, Bosilkovsky M, Epameinondas T. Brucellosis. *N Eng J Med.* 2005:352(22):2325-2336. doi:10.1056/NEJMra050570.
4. Franco MP, Mulder M, Gilman R, Smits HL. Human brucellosis. *Lancet Infect Dis.* 2007;7(12):775-786. doi:10.1016/S1473-3099(07)70286-4.
5. Jiang H, O'Callaghan D, Ding J. Brucellosis in China: History progress and challenge. *Infec Dis Poverty.* 2020;9(1):1-4. doi:10.1186/s40249-020-00673-8.
6. Lai S, Zhou H, Xiong, W, et al. Changing epidemiology of human brucellosis, China, 1955-2014. *Emerg Infect Dis.* 2017;23(2):184-194. doi:10.3201/eid2302.151710.
7. Spink WW, Hoffbauer FW, Walker WW, Green RA. Histopathology of the liver in human brucellosis. *J Lab Clin Med.* 1949;34(1):40-58.
8. Bruce D. *Note on the Discovery of a Microorganism in Malta Fever.* London: John Brigg; 1887.
9. Gotuzzo E. Brucellosis. In: Guerrant R, Walker D, Weller P, eds. *Tropical Infectious Diseases: Principles, Pathogens, & Practice.* 2nd ed. Reimp, Philadelphia: Elsevier Churchill Livingstone; 2006:463-470.
10. Gotuzzo E, Alarcón G, Bocanegra T, et al. Articular involvement in human brucellosis: A retrospective analysis of 304 cases. *Semin Arthritis Rheum.* 1982;12(2):245-255. doi:10.1016/0049-0172(82)90064-6.
11. Yagupsky P, Morata P, Colmenero JD. Laboratory diagnosis of human brucellosis. *Clin Microbiol Rev.* 2019;33(1):e00073-19. doi:10.1128/CMR.00073-19.
12. Arias-Stella J. Brucelosis: Contribución al conocimiento patológico. *Anal Fac Med.* 1951;34(3):429-517. doi:10.15381/anales.v34i3.9532.
13. Ozturk-Engin D, Erdem H, Gencer S, et al. Liver involvement in patients with brucellosis: Results of the Marmara study. *Eur J Clin Microbiol Infect Dis.* 2014;33(7):1253-1262. doi:10.1007/s10096-014-2064-4.
14. Jia B, Zhang F, Lu Y, et al. The clinical features of 590 patients with brucellosis in Xinjiang, China with the emphasis on the treatment of complications. *PLoS Negl Trop Dis.* 2017;11(5):e0005577. doi:10.1371/journal.pntd.0005577.
15. Recavarren S, Gotuzzo E. Patogénesis de las hepatitis granulomatosas por Brucella. Estudios ultra estructurales. *Acta Med Per.* 1975;IV:39-50.
16. Gür A, Geyik MF, Dikici B, et al. Complications of brucellosis in different age groups: a study of 283 cases in southeastern Anatolia of Turkey. *Yonsei Med J.* 2003;44(1):33-44. doi:10.3349/ymj.2003.44.1.33.
17. Ma L, Ma J, Chen X, Dong L. A 10-year retrospective comparative analysis of the clinical features of brucellosis in children and adults. *J Infect Dev Ctries.* 2021;15(8):1147-1154. doi:10.3855/jidc.13962.

18. Zheng R, Xie S, Lu X, et al. A Systematic Review and Meta-Analysis of Epidemiology and Clinical Manifestations of Human Brucellosis in China. *Biomed Res Int.* 2018;2018:5712920. doi:10.1155/2018/5712920.
19. Hassouneh L, Quadri S, Pichilingue-Reto P, et al. An Outbreak of Brucellosis: An Adult and Pediatric Case Series. *Open Forum Infect Dis.* 2019;6(10):ofz384. doi:10.1093/ofid/ofz384.
20. Colmenero JD, Reguera JM, Martos F, et al. Complications associated with *Brucella melitensis infection*: a study of 530 cases. *Medicine (Baltimore).* 1996;75(4):195-211. doi:10.1097/00005792-199607000-00003.
21. Agin M, Kayar Y. Demographic, Laboratory, and Clinical Comparison of Pediatric Brucella Cases With and Without Liver Involvement. *Cureus.* 2020;12(10):e10862. doi:10.7759/cureus.10862.
22. Young EJ, Hasanjani Roushan MR, Shafae S, et al. Liver histology of acute brucellosis caused by *Brucella melitensis. Hum Pathol.* 2014;45(10):2023-2028. doi:10.1016/j.humpath.2014.07.007.
23. Sahinturk H, Baran B, Sisman G, Altun R. Liver involvement is associated with blood culture positivity and high agglutination titre in patients with brucellosis in Turkey. *J Med Microbiol.* 2018;67(8):1078-1082. doi:10.1099/jmm.0.000791.
24. Akritidis N, Tzivras M, Delladetsima I, et al. The liver in brucellosis. *Clin Gastroenterol Hepatol.* 2007;5(9):1109-1112. doi:10.1016/j.cgh.2006.08.010.
25. Ledro D, Llamas R, Herrerias JM, et al. The presence of granulomas due to *Brucella melitensis* in hepatitis. *J Infect Dis.* 1983;147(3):606-607. doi:10.1093/infdis/147.3.606a.
26. Cervantes F, Bruguera M, Carbonell J, et al. Liver disease in brucellosis: a clinical and pathological study of 40 cases. *Postgrad Med J.* 1982;58(680):346-350. doi:10.1136/pgmj.58.680.346.
27. Young EJ. *Brucella melitensis* hepatitis: the absence of granulomas. *Ann Intern Med.* 1979;91(3):414-415. doi:10.7326/0003-4819-91-3-414.
28. Hunt CA, Bothwell PW. Histological findings in human brucellosis. *J Clin Pathol.* 1967;20(3):267-272. doi:10.1136/jcp.20.3.267.
29. Joske RA, Finckh E, Hepatic changes in human brucellosis. *Medical Journal of Australia.* 1955;1(8):266-269. doi:10.5694/j.1326-5377.1955.tb88648.x.
30. Barrett GM, Rickards AG. Chronic brucellosis. *Q J Med.* 1953;22(1):23-42. doi:10.1093/oxfordjournals.qjmed.a066665.
31. Ariza J, Bosilkovski M, Cascio A, et al. International Society of Chemotherapy; Institute of Continuing Medical Education of Ioannina. Perspectives for the treatment of brucelosis in the 21st century: the loannina recommendations. *PLoS Med.* 2007;4(12):e317. doi:10.1371/journal.pmed.0040317.
32. Solis Garcia del Pozo J, Solera J. System Review and Meta-Analysis of Randomized Clinical Trials in the Treatment of Human Brucellosis. *PLoS ONE.* 2012;7(2):e32090. doi:10.1371/journal.pone.0032090.
33. Yousefi-Nooraie R, Mortaz-Hejri S, Mehrani M, Sadeghipour P. Antibiotics for treating human brucellosis. *Cochrane Database Syst Rev.* 2012;10(10):CD007179. doi:10.1002/14651858.CD007179.pub2.

CHAPTER 31

Leptospirosis and the Liver

Pravin Amin ■ Vinay Amin

KEY POINTS

- Leptospirosis is a zoonotic infection caused by spirochaete that is ubiquitously seen across the globe in both low-income and high-income countries.
- Hepatic involvement in leptospirosis is not unusual and can fluctuate from an asymptomatic increase in transaminases to more severe icteric hepatitis and, rarely, acute liver failure.
- Liver involvement may be in isolation in milder cases, or as a part of a more severe hepatorenal presentation, or a more sinister multiple organ failure from severe sepsis.
- Diagnosis is based on a high index of clinical suspicion followed by molecular and serological tests, and it can be confirmed by culture of the organism from clinical specimen in appropriate media.
- Histopathologic changes are most marked in the liver, kidneys, lungs, and heart, although in general the structure of the liver is not notably disrupted.
- Leptospirosis is highly susceptible to appropriate therapy with beta-lactam antibiotics or tetracyclines.

Introduction

Leptospirosis is a well-known zoonotic infection caused by pathogenic spirochetes of the genus *Leptospira*. *Leptospira* are bacteria transmitted either indirectly or directly from animals to human beings and rarely between humans. There are around 21 species that are pathogenic to humans. A severe appearance of leptospirosis was first portrayed by Adolf Weil in Germany during an epidemic in 1886, and it is hence referred to also as Weil disease.[1] In humans the range of disease triggered by leptospirosis is exceptionally vast and may vary from subclinical infection to precipitating severe multiorgan dysfunction with high mortality. Leptospirosis has been reported across the globe but is mostly seen in the tropics and subtropical regions where there is considerable rainfall.[2,3]

Epidemiology

Leptospirosis is distributed worldwide and is seen in both high-income and low-income countries. It is estimated that the annual prevalence in tropical climatic zones is above 10 cases per 100,000 population and notably less (0.1–1 per 100,000) in temperate climatic zones.[4] The actual number of infections is probably higher in the tropics and subtropical regions, as the diagnosis may be missed because of the variable presentation. Most of the human cases reported in Asia are from India, Sri Lanka, Thailand, and Indonesia and are seen mainly during the rainy season.

In the Americas it is seen particularly during flooding due to heavy rains in several Latin American countries including Brazil, Nicaragua, Guyana, and others. There are about 58,000 annual deaths from leptospirosis globally.[5]

Etiopathogenesis

Leptospira are spiral-shaped spirochaetes that have high mobility with a unique feature of hooked ends on both sides, which helps distinguish them from other spirochaetes. The high corkscrew motility is due to the presence of the periplasmic endo-flagellum, which separates it from other spirochetes and is responsible for its pathogenesis.[6] *Leptospira* may appear as both Gram-positive and Gram-negative bacteria having lipopolysaccharides, hemolysins, outer membrane proteins, and other surface proteins, increasing its adhesive capabilities and hence its pathogenicity.[7] *Leptospira* are categorized into three groups: (1) Pathogenic leptospires (*L. interrogans, L. weilii, L. noguchii, L. kirschneri, L. borgpetersenii, L. santarosai, L. kmetyi, L. alexanderi, and L. alstonii*); (2) intermediate pathogenic leptospires (*L. wolffii, L. fainei, and L. licerasiae*); and (3) saprophytic leptospires: (*L. biflexa, L. vanthielli, L. yanagawae, L. wolbachii, and L. kmetyi*).[8] The serovar is the basic systematic unit, distinct on the center of antigenic connections and variances. The pathogenic strains are presumed to be serovars of *L. interrogans*, whereas non-pathogenic are delegated as *L. biflexa*, and there are about 250 pathogenic serovars. In urban areas rodents are the universal carriers and leptospires are usually carried in the renal tubules of these mice, which are commonly asymptomatic.[9] These leptospires, when shed in water bodies, especially during floods, may survive in moist soil and water for weeks and months, more so in an alkaline environment. People who are exposed to these infected waters are highly likely to get infected, and the disease can be a risk for sewage workers, farmers, veterinary workers, and gardeners.[8,10] *Leptospira* invades the human body through mucous membranes or grazes and cuts in the skin. The organisms then bind to the extracellular matrix and subsequently invade the host's defense system, producing toxic proteins leading to disruption of the vascular integrity and damaging the cell membrane. These events precede the development of vasculitis involving inflammatory infiltration with neutrophils, monocytes, and histiocytes.[3] Histopathologic changes are markedly evident in the liver, kidneys, lungs, heart, and brain; however, other organs may also be affected by severe infections. In the liver there may be considerable intrahepatic cholestasis with hypertrophy of the Kupffer cells, cell infiltration in portal areas, and sometimes extensive necrosis of hepatocytes leading to hepatic failure.[11,12] The kidneys show evidence of interstitial nephritis, with the microbes being demonstrated in the renal tubules. When the myocardium is affected, there is demonstrable interstitial myocarditis and pulmonary congestion with hemorrhage in the lungs. The lungs may also demonstrate evidence of acute lung injury and hyaline membrane formation. The brain may show perivascular cuffing and the muscles may show focal necrosis, which may explain the extreme myalgia.[3] Spirochetes supposedly release a toxin that can damage muscle directly, and the organisms invade myocytes, causing inflammation and damage.[13]

Clinical Presentation

Clinical symptoms of leptospirosis range from a mild viral fever to a more severe hepatorenal failure or multiple organ failure. The incubation period is generally 2 to 10 days varying from 2 to 30 days. The initial leptospiremia may persist for up to 7 days. The symptoms are usually nonspecific, with fever with or without chills, malaise, cough, chest discomfort, vomiting, abdominal cramps, breathlessness, and frontal headache.[14] The characteristic features of Weil syndrome include jaundice, acute renal failure, cutaneous and pulmonary hemorrhage, and myocarditis with cardiac arrhythmias.[15] One may encounter lymphadenopathy, severe myalgia, arthralgia, evidence of atypical meningitis in about 25% of the cases, and, rarely, skin rashes. In cases of severe leptospirosis ocular signs include conjunctival inflammation and uveitis.[13] Uveitis may last for weeks and months. Leptospirosis demonstrates a biphasic clinical presentation (Figure 31.1), with an acute phase of sepsis, ensued by the immune phase where antibodies are produced against the organism, with *Leptospira* penetrating the tissues, leading to organ dysfunction usually seen after 2 weeks.[13,16] Most of the infections in leptospirosis may be subclinical or of milder intensity. Such patients probably do not look for medical assistance, and these cases may be anicteric. About 10% of cases are icteric leptospirosis and usually represent a more severe form of the disease that could rapidly worsen.[17] About 5% and 15% of cases may be severely ill patients, of which a 5% to 40 % mortality may be seen.[8] The serum bilirubin levels could reach very high levels, and this may take weeks to normalize, and there can be a mild rise of the alkaline phosphatase levels as well. The transaminase levels are usually moderately elevated in multiples of hundreds of IU/L, whereas serum bilirubin may increase up to 30 to 40 mg/dL.[13] The high levels of bilirubin are a result of septic cholestasis. An aspartate transaminase (AST) to alanine transaminase (ALT) ratio (AAR) of >3 may indicate a grave prognosis.[18] Serum amylase levels can rise significantly in a select group of individuals. In a retrospective study from northern India assessing patients with cirrhosis and leptospirosis, it was found that liver involvement and neurological symptoms were more frequent in those with cirrhosis (91.6% vs 61.5% and 54.7% vs 24.8%, respectively).[19]

Diagnostic Studies

Both leukopenia and leukocytosis may be seen along with thrombocytopenia as well as pancytopenia and disseminated intravascular coagulation in severe cases. Liver function tests display an elevation of bilirubin, alkaline phosphatase, and aminotransferases to varying levels.[20] Routine urine examination shows hematuria, pyuria, proteinuria granular, and hyaline casts. In patients with meningoencephalitis leptospires may be isolated from cerebrospinal fluid (CSF), demonstrating elevated opening pressure during a lumbar puncture. CSF examination initially shows elevation of both polymorphs and lymphocytes but subsequently preponderance of lymphocytes. CSF protein may be normal or could be elevated, and CSF glucose levels could even be normal. In icteric patients CSF may appear xanthochromic. Elevated serum amylase and creatinine phosphokinase levels could be seen in a few cases. Renal dysfunction with elevated blood urea and serum creatinine with metabolic acidosis is not uncommon in severe leptospirosis.[21]

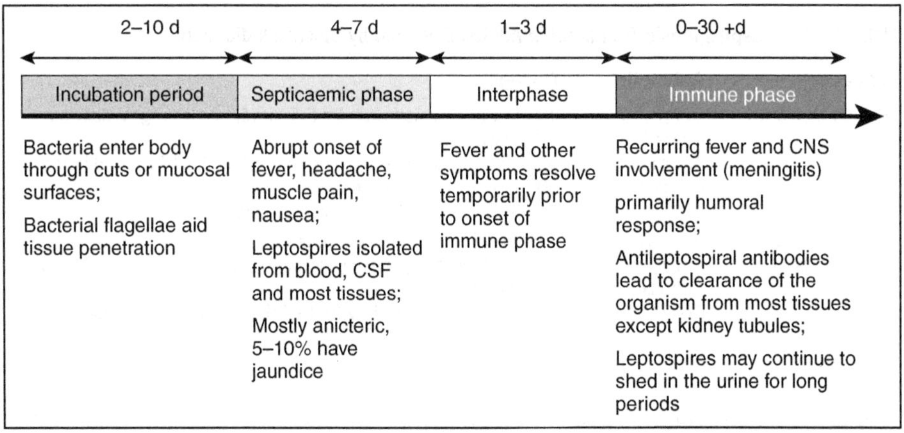
2–10 d
4–7 d
1–3 d
0–30 +d
Incubation period
Septicaemic phase
Interphase
Immune phase
Bacteria enter body through cuts or mucosal surfaces;
Bacterial flagellae aid tissue penetration
Abrupt onset of fever, headache, muscle pain, nausea;
Leptospires isolated from blood, CSF and most tissues;
Mostly anicteric, 5–10% have jaundice
Fever and other symptoms resolve temporarily prior to onset of immune phase
Recurring fever and CNS involvement (meningitis)
primarily humoral response;
Antileptospiral antibodies lead to clearance of the organism from most tissues except kidney tubules;
Leptospires may continue to shed in the urine for long periods

Figure 31.1 Leptospirosis demonstrates a biphasic clinical presentation. (From World Health Organization. Leptospirosis: *Fact Sheet*. WHO; 2009. https://apps.who.int/iris/handle/10665/205437)

The currently available serological tests that assess antibodies against *Leptospira* include the standard microscopic agglutination test (MAT), indirect hemagglutination, and enzyme-linked immunosorbent assay (ELISA) kits to detect IgG and IgM antibodies.[22] The MAT is referred to as a gold-standard assay, which provides both antibody titer and serovar, though of late, its role in diagnosis has been questioned.

Polymerase chain reaction (PCR) and loop-mediated isothermal amplification have also been used as molecular techniques for detecting leptospires because of their high specificity and sensitivity.[23] The limitation of these techniques is the need for cutting-edge and expensive laboratory equipment with highly trained technicians to operate them.

Management

Cases of severe leptospirosis need to be managed in an intensive care unit (ICU) with suitable early antimicrobial agents and appropriate, efficient organ support.[16] The early implementation of effective therapy clearly reduces both morbidity and mortality. The supportive care in the ICU encompasses ventilatory support, hemodynamic support, renal replacement therapy, care of a semicomatose patient, nutritional support, and component therapy to correct hematologic anomalies.[16]

The benchmark for the treatment of leptospirosis involves administering appropriate antibiotics (Table 31.1). These organisms respond well to antibiotics and there have been no reports suggesting the development of resistance to the current array of agents available for therapy. For severe diseases, penicillin, third-generation cephalosporins such as ceftriaxone or cefotaxime, and doxycycline are agents of choice. After initiation of antimicrobial therapy the rapid clearance of spirochetes can lead to an acute inflammatory response in the form of rigors, fever, and hypotension called Jarisch-Herxheimer reaction. Corticosteroids have been used in severe leptospirosis, more so when there is pulmonary involvement; however, there is insufficient data to recommend their regular use.[24-27] In some small studies plasmapheresis has been used as a modality of adjuvant therapy in severe leptospirosis but cannot be advocated as routine therapy due to lack of high-quality data.[28] In cases with fulminant hepatic failure liver transplant has been carried out with mixed results.[29]

TABLE 31.1 ■ **Leptospirosis Treatment in Adults: Selection by Disease Indication**

Indication	Antibiotic	Dosage
Mild leptospirosis	Doxycycline	100 mg orally twice daily for 5–7 days, or 100 mg IV daily for 7 days
	Ampicillin Amoxicillin	500–750 mg orally every 6 hours, or 0.5–1 g IV every 6 hours
	Azithromycin	500 mg orally every 6 hours 1 g orally, then 500 mg daily for 2 days
Moderate to severe leptospirosis	Penicillin G	1.5 million units IV every 6 hours
	Ampicillin	500–750 mg orally every 6 hours, or 0.5–1 g IV every 6 hours
	Ceftriaxone	1–2 g IV daily for 7 days
	Doxycycline	100 mg orally, twice daily for 5–7 days or 100 mg IV daily for 7 days
Prophylaxis	Doxycycline	200 mg orally per week

From Jimenez JIS, Marroquin JLH, Richards GA, Amin P. Leptospirosis: report from the Task Force on Tropical Diseases by the World Federation of Societies of Intensive and Critical Care Medicine. J Crit Care. 2018;43: 361–5. Elsevier.

References

1. Vinetz JM. Leptospirosis. *Curr Opin Infect Dis.* 2001;14(5):527-538.
2. Sanders EJ, Rigau-Perez JG, Smits HL, et al. Increase of leptospirosis in dengue-negative patients after a hurricane in Puerto Rico in 1996 [correction of 1966]. *Am J Trop Med Hyg.* 1999;61(3):399-404.
3. Levett PN. Leptospirosis. *Clin Microbiol Rev.* 2001;14(2):296-326.
4. World Health Organization. *Leptospirosis: Fact Sheet.* WHO; 2009. Available at: https://apps.who.int/iris/handle/10665/205437.
5. Costa F, Hagan JE, Calcagno J, et al. Global morbidity and mortality of leptospirosis: a systematic review. *PloS Negl Trop Dis.* 2015;9(9):e0003898.
6. Slamti L, de Pedro MA, Guichet E, Picardeau M. Deciphering morphological determinants of the helix-shaped *Leptospira. J Bacteriol.* 2011;193(22):6266-6275.
7. Haake DA. Spirochaetal lipoproteins and pathogenesis. *Microbiology (Reading).* 2000;146(Pt 7):1491-1504.
8. Karpagam KB, Ganesh B. Leptospirosis: a neglected tropical zoonotic infection of public health importance-an updated review. *Eur J Clin Microbiol Infect Dis.* 2020;39(5):835-846.
9. WHO. *Leptospirosis: Fact Sheet.* 2018. Available at: https://apps.who.int/iris/handle/10665/205437.
10. Costa F, Ribeiro GS, Felzemburgh RD, et al. Influence of household rat infestation on *Leptospira* transmission in the urban slum environment. *PLoS Negl Trop Dis.* 2014;8(12):e3338.
11. Shintaku M, Itoh H, Tsutsumi Y. Weil's disease (leptospirosis) manifesting as fulminant hepatic failure: report of an autopsy case. *Pathol Res Pract.* 2014;210(12):1134-1137.
12. De Brito T, Machado MM, Montans SD, Hoshino S, Freymuller E. Liver biopsy in human leptospirosis: a light and electron microscopy study. *Virchows Arch Pathol Anat Physiol Klin Med.* 1967;342(1):61-69.
13. Bharti AR, Nally JE, Ricaldi JN, et al. Leptospirosis: a zoonotic disease of global importance. *Lancet Infect Dis.* 2003;3(12):757-771.
14. Lin PC, Chi CY, Ho MW, Chen CM, Ho CM, Wang JH. Demographic and clinical features of leptospirosis: three-year experience in central Taiwan. *J Microbiol Immunol Infect.* 2008;41(2):145-150.
15. Vinetz JM, Glass GE, Flexner CE, Mueller P, Kaslow DC. Sporadic urban leptospirosis. *Ann Intern Med.* 1996;125(10):794-798.
16. Jimenez JIS, Marroquin JLH, Richards GA, Amin P. Leptospirosis: report from the task force on tropical diseases by the World Federation of Societies of Intensive and Critical Care Medicine. *J Crit Care.* 2018;43:361-365.
17. Heath Jr CW, Alexander AD, Galton MM. Leptospirosis in the United States. Analysis of 483 cases in man, 1949, 1961. *N Engl J Med.* 1965;273(17):915-922 concl.
18. Chang ML, Yang CW, Chen JC, et al. Disproportional exaggerated aspartate transaminase is a useful prognostic parameter in late leptospirosis. *World J Gastroenterol.* 2005;11(35):5553-5556.
19. Goyal O KD, Goyal P, Chhina RS. Hepatic dysfunction and predictors of mortality in Leptospirosis: a re-emerging tropical disease in northern India. *Trop Gastroenterol.* 2016;37(4):248-257.
20. Edwards GA, Domm BM. Human leptospirosis. *Medicine (Baltimore).* 1960;39:117-156.
21. Farr RW. Leptospirosis. *Clin Infect Dis.* 1995;21(1):1-8.
22. Jacob SM, Geethalakshmi S, Karthikeyan S, et al. A 3-year retrospective analysis on the prevalence of antileptospiral antibodies among children in Chennai City, India. *J Med Microbiol.* 2018;67(12):1706-1710.
23. Gravekamp C, Van de Kemp H, Franzen M, et al. Detection of seven species of pathogenic leptospires by PCR using two sets of primers. *J Gen Microbiol.* 1993;139(8):1691-1700.
24. Kularatne SA, Budagoda BD, de Alwis VK, et al. High efficacy of bolus methylprednisolone in severe leptospirosis: a descriptive study in Sri Lanka. *Postgrad Med J.* 2011;87(1023):13-17.
25. Thunga G, John J, Sam KG, et al. Role of high-dose corticosteroid for the treatment of leptospirosis-induced pulmonary hemorrhage. *J Clin Pharmacol.* 2012;52(1):114-116.
26. Azevedo AF, Miranda-Filho Dde B, Henriques-Filho GT, Leite A, Ximenes RA. Randomized controlled trial of pulse methyl prednisolone × placebo in treatment of pulmonary involvement associated with severe leptospirosis. [ISRCTN74625030]. *BMC Infect Dis.* 2011;11:186.
27. Rodrigo C, Lakshitha de Silva N, Goonaratne R, et al. High dose corticosteroids in severe leptospirosis: a systematic review. *Trans R Soc Trop Med Hyg.* 2014;108(12):743-750.
28. Trivedi SV, Vasava AH, Bhatia LC, Patel TC, Patel NK, Patel NT. Plasma exchange with immunosuppression in pulmonary alveolar haemorrhage due to leptospirosis. *Indian J Med Res.* 2010;131:429-433.
29. Lebreton T, Aubrun F, Mabrut JY, Heyer L, Perrin C. Liver transplantation for acute liver failure attributed to leptospirosis: a report of two cases. *Case Rep Crit Care.* 2019;2019:5189542.

CHAPTER 32

The Liver in Q Fever

Pirathaban Sivabalan ■ Mohammed Alizzi ■ Robert Norton

KEY POINTS

- Q fever is a zoonotic infection caused by *Coxiella burnetii*
- Two types of clinical entities exist: acute Q fever and chronic Q fever (alternatively known as persistent focalized infection)
- Isolated hepatitis can occur in acute Q fever
- Most cases of hepatitis in chronic Q fever are associated with endocarditis
- Diagnosis can be made via serology and molecular assays of Q fever
- Most common pathological finding in acute Q fever hepatitis is the presence of "doughnut granuloma," which is not pathognomonic for this condition
- In chronic Q fever liver biopsy generally displays a nonspecific reactive hepatitis with lymphocytic infiltration with foci of spotty necrosis
- Infection due to Q fever can trigger autoimmune antibodies, which may potentiate autoimmune liver diseases
- Treatment is with doxycycline for acute Q fever, and prolonged synergistic therapy with doxycycline and hydroxychloroquine for chronic Q fever

Background

Q fever is a zoonotic infection with a worldwide distribution, excluding New Zealand.[1] The causal agent is the intracellular Gram-negative bacterium *Coxiella burnetii*.[2] It is traditionally an occupational hazard more frequently seen in farmers, veterinarians, and abattoir workers, with cattle, sheep, and goats being the most common reservoirs.[1,3,4] However, it is now appreciated that the organism is identifiable in a wide variety of vertebrates such as domestic and feral dogs, cats, birds, macropods, possums, and invertebrates (predominantly ticks).[5,6] The predominant transmission route of the organism to humans is via inhalation of aerosols or dust contaminated by secretions from infected animals, including birth products, urine, and feces.[4] In Australia, Q fever is the most commonly reported zoonosis and is a notifiable disease in all states and territories.[4,7]

Historical Overview

Q or "query" fever was first recognized as a human disease in Australia in the mid-1930s.[1,3,8,9] The term "query" was used at the time, as the causative agent was unknown. It was first described by Edward Holbrook Derrick in 1935.[10] He reported nine patients, out of whom one developed jaundice. Derrick had difficulty in isolating an etiological agent and initially hypothesized the causative pathogen to be a virus, before Macfarlane Burnet postulated its potential rickettsial origin.[1] Subsequent work demonstrated that the liver of guinea pigs infected with the serum of patients with the disease showed large quantities of the presumptive infecting agent.[10] It was not until 1937 that the true pathogen of Q fever was discovered when Burnet and Mavis Freeman isolated the bacterium from one of Derrick's patients,[11] initially being identified as a species of *Rickettsia*. A connection was made in 1938 when Cox and Davis isolated the infectious agent from ticks in Montana, United States.[1,11] Initially named *Rickettsia burnetii*, this was soon changed in 1938 after a proposition to create a new genus, *Coxiella*. The renaming of the etiological agent to *C. burnetii* honors both Cox and Burnet for their pioneering research leading to this discovery.[1] Nowadays, *C. burnetii* is no longer regarded as closely related to *Rickettsiae* and is rather considered a proteobacterium given its similarities to *Legionella* and *Francisella*.[12]

Acute Q Fever and Its Impact on the Liver

Acutely, Q fever may present as a flu-like illness, pneumonia, hepatitis, or prolonged fever. Cases can either be mild or asymptomatic. Occasionally, it may present as meningoencephalitis, as myocarditis, or with a rash.[1] Isolated hepatitis is a common presentation of acute Q fever. This is the commonest presentation in countries where the disease is endemic, such as Australia,[13] Spain, France, Israel, Portugal, and Taiwan.[14-18]

There is a marked geographical difference in the association of hepatitis with acute Q fever. Hepatitis was the main clinical presentation in reports from France and Southern Spain. Pneumonia, however, predominates in the Spanish Basque region.[19] Possible reasons for this discrepancy include varying routes of infection (aerosol versus ingestion), host-pathogen differences, and variations in the infecting dose.

One of the largest Q fever outbreaks occurred in the Netherlands between 2007 and 2009.[19] Wielders et al. examined this outbreak and found moderately elevated liver chemistry tests (ALT or bilirubin) in hospitalized acute Q fever patients but no cases of significant hepatitis. This Dutch study defined hepatitis due to acute Q fever as a twofold increase in the reference value for alanine aminotransferase (ALT; 45 U/L for males, 35 U/L for females) in combination with a twofold increase in bilirubin (34 mmol/L). In this study of 183 patients, only 2 (1.1%) presented with jaundice, but 25% had elevation of bilirubin levels.

The presence of headache has been proposed in early reports for differentiating acute hepatitis due to Q fever from viral hepatitis.[20] This, however, is nonspecific and has been reported in only 33.9% of proven Q fever cases in the Dutch study.[19] Other accompanying findings are anorexia, vomiting, diarrhea, and painful hepatomegaly.[14-17] Jaundice, as previously mentioned, is rare, but it has been reported in severe hepatitis, especially in Taiwan, where hyperbilirubinemia was found in more than one-third of cases.[18] In that study patients with jaundice presented a significant delay in reduction of fever after initiation of antibiotic therapy compared to patients without jaundice. The French National Reference Centre for Q Fever reported on a cohort of 1806 patients with acute Q fever. Hepatitis was reported as the most frequent clinical form of acute Q fever (46.3%), although a definition of hepatitis was not provided.[21] The prognosis of acute hepatitis with *C. burnetii* infection is good. Fatal cases due to hepatic insufficiency are very rare.[22-26]

Diagnosis of Acute and Chronic Q Fever

Diagnosis of acute Q fever is via the isolation of *C. burnetii* and/or detection of *C. burnetii* by nucleic acid amplification test (NAAT) and/or seroconversion or fourfold or greater increase in *C. burnetii* antibody titer to phase II antigen via complement fixation or indirect immunofluorescence IgG antibody assay in paired sera. However, the diagnosis of chronic Q fever is challenging. It is acknowledged that the term "chronic" Q fever is not universally accepted. An alternative term used is "persistent focalised infection".[21] Usually, the diagnosis of chronic Q fever relies on serology and/or the detection of DNA in blood or tissue via polymerase chain reaction (PCR). PCR techniques for detecting *C. burnetii* have been shown to have low sensitivity, particularly as illness progresses, with no detection after day 17.[27,28] Thus serology is a pivotal tool for diagnosis. During acute infection, antibodies to phase II antigens are detected first, followed by phase I antibodies. Persisting high levels of antibodies to phase I antigens are thought to be triggered by continuous antigenic stimulation and are considered indicative of chronic Q fever. Chronic Q fever can occur several months or years after acute infection. If an acute Q fever case progresses to chronic disease, phase I IgG titer will continue to rise and might exceed the phase II titer. It is possible for a patient with previously diagnosed acute Q fever who no longer has clinical symptoms to have increased phase I IgG titers for several months that subsequently decrease or stabilize without ever progressing to chronic disease. A cutoff for phase I IgG ≥1:800 or 1:1,024 (depending on the cut-off values used by the individual laboratory and national consensus guidelines) using an immunofluorescence assay (IFA) has been internationally accepted in the serological diagnosis of chronic Q fever.[27,29] However, this value of a phase 1 antibody titer is variable and frequently not reproducible between laboratories.

After primary infection, approximately 1% to 5% can progress to chronic Q fever. Common manifestations of this include endocarditis and infection of vascular aneurysms and prostheses. Arthritis, osteomyelitis, and hepatitis are rare manifestations of chronic Q fever, and at times a primary focus may not be identifiable.[5,30-33] Cases of chronic Q fever with hepatic involvement are commonly also associated with endocarditis, but isolated cases of hepatitis have been described.[1] Rarely Q fever has been reported to cause hepatic fibrosis and cirrhosis.[34,35] One of the largest studies of chronic Q fever, the Dutch National Chronic Q Fever Study Database, did not report any cases of chronic hepatitis associated with chronic Q fever.[36]

Diagnosis of liver involvement in chronic Q fever is usually via a combination of investigations. Other than serology and molecular assays, evaluation of liver enzymes and synthetic function would be an initial step.[37] Liver biopsy can be performed, which can show a variety of features that will be later discussed in this chapter. Positron emission tomography-computed tomography (PET-CT) can also be used in assessing infiltration of infection into the liver.[38]

Pathophysiology of Q Fever Hepatitis

The liver could act as a reservoir for Q fever. The three main manifestations of Q fever hepatitis are: (1) an initial infectious hepatitis-like picture, (2) hepatitis as an incidental finding in a patient with acute Q fever, and (3) fevers of unknown origin with characteristic granulomas on liver biopsy.[35] As seen in Figure 32.1, the most common pathological finding in the liver in acute Q fever is doughnut granuloma. This is demonstrated by a central fat vacuole, a fibrin ring, activated macrophages, and lymphocytes.[39] However, atypical pathological aspects have been reported including epithelioid granulomas with eosinophilic infiltration, extensive extravasated fibrin without ring granulomas, and acute cholangitis without granulomas.[39] Other, less specific hepatic lesions such as portal triaditis, Kupffer cell hyperplasia, and moderate fatty change have been described.[40] Kupffer cells are considered to be the target cells for *C. burnetii* infection in liver tissue. This may initiate local inflammation and the formation of granulomas.[40] Doughnut granulomas are not specific for Q fever and can be seen in various diseases such as tuberculosis, cytomegaloviral hepatitis, Epstein-Barr virus hepatitis, and others.[39]

C. burnetii is not generally detected in the liver, although isolation or visualization by direct antigen immunofluorescence has occasionally been successful. The predominant histological pattern of the liver in chronic Q fever corresponds to a nonspecific reactive hepatitis with

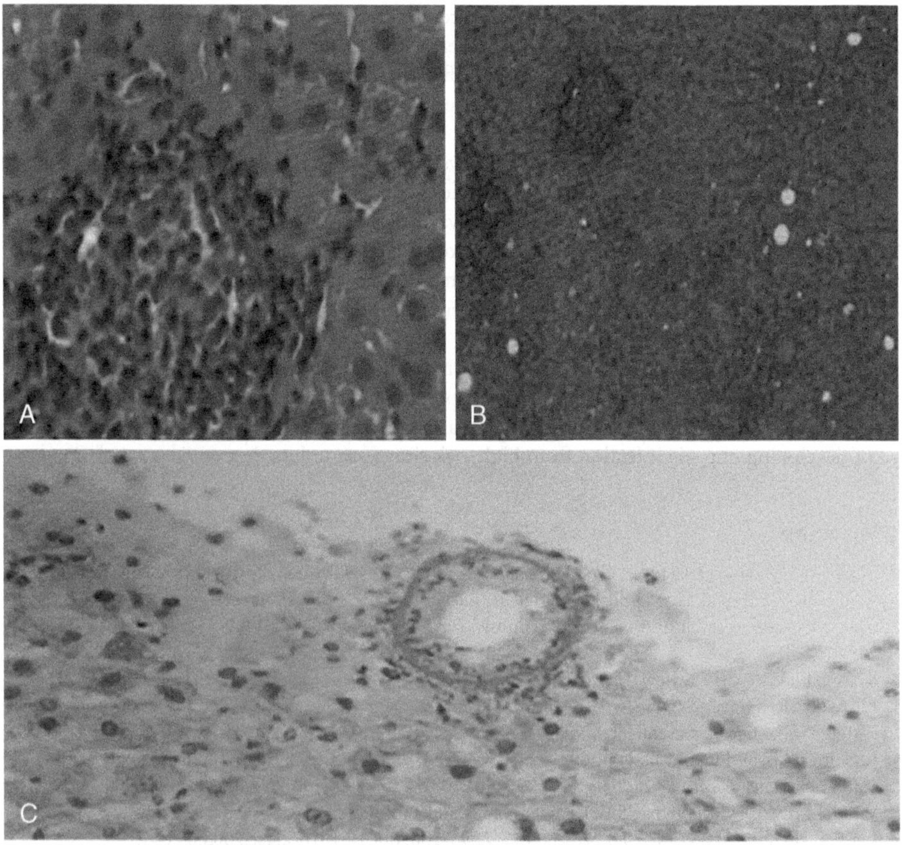

Figure 32.1 Liver biopsy of patient with Q fever hepatitis. A: Top left, granuloma; B: top right, granuloma with central lipid vacuoles; C: bottom-fibrin ring.

lymphocytic infiltration with foci of spotty necrosis. Granulomas have rarely been reported in chronically infected patients, and the typical doughnut granulomas have never been reported in chronic Q fever.[40]

Autoimmune hepatitis needs to be considered in Q fever–infected patients with transaminitis and with a prolonged fever and who do not respond to appropriate antibiotic therapy. These patients may exhibit anti-smooth muscle antibodies and are rapidly cured by short-term corticosteroid therapy.[28] Q fever is known to affect the body's own immune response and frequently patients with hepatitis exhibit autoantibodies, including those to smooth muscle, anticardiolipin, antiphospholipid, circulating anticoagulant, and antinuclear antibodies.[40]

Treatment and Prevention

Acute Q fever usually resolves spontaneously within 2 to 6 weeks. The value of treating nonpregnant adults who have spontaneously recovered has been debated. First-line therapy is a 14-day course of doxycycline. In pregnancy doxycycline is contraindicated, so trimethoprim plus sulfamethoxazole is recommended instead. Although it has been associated with congenital abnormalities when used during pregnancy, the benefit of treatment outweighs potential harms, and concomitant use of folic acid reduces the risk.[41]

Treatment of chronic Q fever usually requires prolonged synergistic combination therapy of doxycycline with hydroxychloroquine.[41] Other agents that can be potentially used include trimethoprim-sulfamethoxazole, rifampin, and ofloxacin. Duration of therapy is generally 18 to 24 months, depending on site of infection and serologic response,[1] with surgery being required in some cases to reduce microbial burden.

Several vaccines have been developed and have generally been administered to individuals at high risk of acquiring Q fever. The types of vaccines include whole-cell vaccine for Q fever, which has been developed in Australia, and an acellular vaccine that is available in the United States.[42,43] Prior to vaccination, individuals should have serology and a skin test to determine if there is a history of previous exposure. One study showed that the vaccine provided more than 93% protective efficacy, and the incidence of Q fever in vaccinated individuals was 5.4 per 100,000 person-years of follow-up.[44]

Other preventative measures involve minimizing exposure. Such measures include educating the public on sources of infection, appropriate disposal of birth products, consumption of pasteurized milk products, quarantine of imported animals, and exclusion of individuals who are at high risk of developing chronic infection from high-risk situations unless they are immune.[8]

References

1. Maurin M, Raoult D. Q fever. *Clin Microbiol Rev.* 1999;12(4):518-553. doi:10.1128/CMR.12.4.518.
2. Porter SR, Czaplicki G, Mainil J, Guattéo R, Saegerman C. Q fever: current state of knowledge and perspectives of research of a neglected zoonosis. *Int J Microbiol.* 2011;2011:248418. doi:10.1155/2011/248418.
3. Marrie TJ. Q fever: a review. *Can Vet J.* 1990;31(8):555-563.
4. Eastwood K, Graves S, Massey P, Bosward K, van den Berg D, Hutchinson P. Q fever: a rural disease with potential urban consequences. *Aust J Gen Pract.* 2018;47(3):112-116. doi:10.31128/afp-08-17-4299.
5. Raoult D, Tissot-Dupont H, Foucault C, et al. Q fever 1985-1998. Clinical and epidemiologic features of 1,383 infections. *Medicine (Baltimore).* 2000;79(2):109-123. doi:10.1097/00005792-200003000-00005.
6. Woldehiwet Z. Q fever (coxiellosis): epidemiology and pathogenesis [published correction appears in Res Vet Sci. 2004;77(3):269]. *Res Vet Sci.* 2004;77(2):93-100. doi:10.1016/j.rvsc.2003.09.001.
7. Australian Government. *Australian National Notifiable Diseases Case Definitions—Q Fever.* Canberra: Department of Health; Updated March 12, 2004. Available at: www.health.gov.au/internet/main/publishing.nsf/content/cda-surveil-nndss-casedefs-cd_qfev.htm. Accessed June 1, 2021.
8. Centers for Disease Control and Prevention. *Q Fever.* Updated June 27, 2019. Available at: https://www.cdc.gov/qfever/stats/index.html. Accessed June 1, 2021.
9. Eldin C, Mélenotte C, Mediannikov O, et al. From Q fever to *Coxiella burnetii* infection: a paradigm change. *Clin Microbiol Rev.* 2017;30(1):115-190. doi:10.1128/CMR.00045-16.
10. Derrick EH. "Q fever" A new fever entity. Clinical features, diagnosis and laboratory investigation. *Med J Aust.* 1937;2(8):281-299. Available at: https://doi.org/10.5694/j.1326-5377.1937.tb43743.x.
11. Burnet F, Freeman M. Experimental studies on the virus of "Q" fever. *Med J Aust.* 1937;2(8):299-305. doi:10.5694/j.1326-5377.1937.tb43744.x.
12. Honarmand H. Q fever: an old but still a poorly understood disease. *InterdiscipPerspect Infect Dis.* 2012;2012:1-8. doi:10.1155/2012/131932.
13. Gale M, Ketheesan N, Govan B, Kennedy L, Norton R. Q fever cases at a North Queensland centre during 1994–2006. *Intern Med J.* 2007;37(9):644-646. doi:10.1111/j.1445-5994.2007.01441.x.
14. Edouard S, Mahamat A, Demar M, Abboud P, Djossou F, Raoult D. Comparison between emerging Q fever in French Guiana and endemic Q fever in Marseille, France. *Am J Trop Med Hyg.* 2014;90:915-919. doi:10.4269/ajtmh.13-0164.
15. Ergas D, Keysari A, Edelstein V, Sthoeger Z. Acute Q fever in Israel: clinical and laboratory study of 100 hospitalized patients. *Isr Med Assoc J.* 2006;8(5):337-341. Available at: https://pubmed.ncbi.nlm.nih.gov/16805234/. Accessed July 14, 2021.
16. Palmela C, Badura R, Valadas E. Acute Q fever in Portugal: epidemiological and clinical features of 32 hospitalized patients. *Germs.* 2012;2:43-59. doi:10.11599/germs.2012.1013.

17. Espejo E, Gil-Diaz A, Oteo JA, et al. Clinical presentation of acute Q fever in Spain: seasonal and geographical differences. *Int J Infect Dis.* 2014;26:162-164. doi:10.1016/j.ijid.2014.06.016.
18. Chang K, Yan JJ, Lee HC, Liu KH, Lee NY, Ko WC. Acute hepatitis with or without jaundice: a predominant presentation of acute Q fever in southern Taiwan. *J Microbiol Immunol Infect.* 2004;37:103-108.
19. Wielders CC, Wuister AM, de Visser VL, et al. Characteristics of hospitalized acute Q fever patients during a large epidemic, The Netherlands. *PLoS One.* 2014;9(3):e91764. doi:10.1371/journal.pone.0091764.
20. Alkan WJ, Evenchik Z, Eshchar J. Q fever and infectious hepatitis. *Am J Med.* 1965;38:54-61. doi:10.1016/0002-9343(65)90159-2.
21. Melenotte C, Protopopescu C, Million M, et al. Clinical features and complications of *Coxiella burnetii* infections from the French National Reference Center for Q Fever. *JAMA Netw Open.* 2018;1(4):e181580. doi:10.1001/jamanetworkopen.2018.1580.
22. Dugdale C, Chow B, Yakirevich E, Kojic E, Knoll B. Prolonged pyrexia and hepatitis: Q fever. *Am J Med.* 2014;127:928-930. doi:10.1016/j.amjmed.2014.06.003.
23. Oh M, Baek S, Lee SO, Yu E, Ryu JS. A case of acute Q fever hepatitis diagnosed by F-18 FDG PET/CT. *Nucl Med Mol Imaging.* 2012;46:125-128. doi:10.1007/s13139-012-0130-3.
24. Berkovitch M, Aladjem M, Beer S, Cohar K. A fatal case of Q fever hepatitis in a child. *Helv Paediatr Acta.* 1985;40:87-91.
25. Isaksson HJ, Hrafnkelsson J, Hilmarsdottir I. Acute Q fever: a cause of fatal hepatitis in an Icelandic traveller. *Scand J Infect Dis.* 2001;33:314-315. doi:10.1080/003655401300077441.
26. Lin PH, Lo YC, Chiang FT, et al. Acute Q fever presenting as fever of unknown origin with rapidly progressive hepatic failure in a patient with alcoholism. *J Formos Med Assoc.* 2008;107:896-901. doi:10.1016/S0929-6646(08)60207-7.
27. Fenollar F, Fournier PE, Raoult D. Molecular detection of Coxiella burnetii in the sera of patients with Q fever endocarditis or vascular infection. *J Clin Microbiol.* 2004;42(11):4919-4924. doi:10.1128/JCM.42.11.4919-4924.2004.
28. Schneeberger P, Hermans M, van Hannen E, Schellekens J, Leenders A, Wever P. Real-time PCR with serum samples is indispensable for early diagnosis of acute Q fever. *Clin Vaccine Immunol.* 2010;17(2):286-290. doi:10.1128/cvi.00454-09.
29. Raoult D, Marrie T, Mege J. Natural history and pathophysiology of Q fever. *Lancet Infect Dis.* 2005;5(4):219-226.
30. Botelho-Nevers E, Fournier PE, Richet H, et al. *Coxiella burnetii* infection of aortic aneurysms or vascular grafts: report of 30 new cases and evaluation of outcome. *Eur J Clin Microbiol Infect Dis.* 2007;26(9):635-640. doi:10.1007/s10096-007-0357-6.
31. Million M, Thuny F, Richet H, Raoult D. Long-term outcome of Q fever endocarditis: a 26-year personal survey. *Lancet Infect Dis.* 2010;10(8):527-535. doi:10.1016/S1473-3099(10)70135-3.
32. Brouqui P, Dupont HT, Drancourt M, et al. Chronic Q fever. Ninety-two cases from France, including 27 cases without endocarditis. *Arch Intern Med.* 1993;153(5):642-648. doi:10.1001/archinte.153.5.642.
33. Frankel D, Richet H, Renvoisé A, Raoult D. Q fever in France, 1985-2009. *Emerg Infect Dis.* 2011;17(3):350-356. doi:10.3201/eid1703.100882.
34. Raoult D, Marrie TJ. Q fever. *Clin Infect Dis.* 1995;20(3):489.
35. Marrie TJ, Raoult D. Q fever: a review and issues for the next century. *Int J Antimicrob Agents.* 1997;8(3):145-161. doi:10.1016/s0924-8579(96)00369-x.
36. Kampschreur LM, Delsing CE, Groenwold RH, et al. Chronic Q fever in the Netherlands 5 years after the start of the Q fever epidemic: results from the Dutch chronic Q fever database. *J Clin Microbiol.* 2014;52(5):1637-1643. doi:10.1128/JCM.03221-13.
37. Dupuis G, Péter O, Lüthy R, Nicolet J, Peacock M, Burgdorfer W. Serological diagnosis of Q fever endocarditis. *Eur Heart J.* 1986;7(12):1062-1066. doi:10.1093/oxfordjournals.eurheartj.a062016.
38. Golden MJ, Fair JR. Q Fever masquerading as prostate cancer metastases. *Clin Nucl Med.* 2012;37(5):511-513. doi:10.1097/RLU.0b013e31823ea70a.
39. Lee M, Jang JJ, Kim YS, et al. Clinicopathologic features of Q fever patients with acute hepatitis. *Korean J Pathol.* 2012;46(1):10.
40. Levy P, Raoult D, Razongles JJ. Q-fever and autoimmunity. *Eur J Epidemiol.* 1989;5(4):447-453. doi:10.1007/BF00140139.
41. Tgldcdp.tg.org.au. *Therapeutic Guidelines.* 2019. Available at: https://tgldcdp.tg.org.au/viewTopic?topicfile=q-fever#toc_d1e47. Accessed December 21, 2021.

42. Ackland JR, Worswick DA, Marmion BP. Vaccine prophylaxis of Q fever: a follow-up study of the efficacy of Q-Vax (CSL) 1985–1990. *Med J Aust.* 1994;160:704.
43. Waag DM, England MJ, Tammariello RF, et al. Comparative efficacy and immunogenicity of Q fever chloroform:methanol residue (CMR) and phase I cellular (Q-Vax) vaccines in cynomolgus monkeys challenged by aerosol. *Vaccine.* 2002;20(19–20):2623-2634. doi:10.1016/s0264-410x(02)00176-7.
44. Woldeyohannes S, Perkins N, Baker P, Gilks C, Knibbs L, Reid S. Q fever vaccine efficacy and occupational exposure risk in Queensland, Australia: a retrospective cohort study. *Vaccine.* 2020;38(42): 6578-6584. doi:10.1016/j.vaccine.2020.08.006.

CHAPTER 33

Hepatic Manifestations of the Dengue Infection

Kittiyod Poovorawan

KEY POINTS

- Dengue is a common mosquito-borne viral infection
- Liver involvement and abnormal liver function tests are common with various degrees of hepatocellular injury from mild to acute liver failure
- The most common hepatic manifestation of dengue is hepatomegaly
- Acute liver failure is a severe complication and is associated with high mortality
- N-acetylcysteine is potentially beneficial for the treatment of dengue-related severe liver injury

Introduction

Dengue is a common mosquito-borne viral infection affecting people in tropical areas. Dengue is caused by a virus of the Flaviviridae family and there are four dengue virus serotypes, namely dengue viruses 1 to 4 (DENV-1 to DENV-4). The global incidence of dengue has increased in recent decades. The estimation of apparent dengue infection is approximately 96 million cases annually worldwide.[1] About half of the world's population is now at risk with risk of infection existing in 129 countries; most of the actual burden is in Asia.[2] Patients with dengue may develop dysfunction of multiple organs including that of heart, muscle, kidney, liver, and brain.[3] Liver involvement is common among dengue viral infections.

Clinical Presentation

The majority of dengue-infected cases are asymptomatic, and among symptomatic cases, the clinical spectrum can be mild to severe, including undifferentiated fever, dengue fever, dengue hemorrhagic fever, and life-threatening dengue shock syndrome. The most common symptom of dengue is fever with myalgia, arthralgia, headache, especially retro-orbital type pain, nausea, and vomiting. Symptoms of typical dengue fever usually last 5 to 7 days.

The most common hepatic manifestation of dengue is hepatomegaly, which is sometimes painful, especially in children and young adults. Hepatomegaly can be observed in approximately 10% to 20% of dengue cases; however, this finding has been observed more often in severe liver injury and liver failure cases.[4] Ultrasonography might reveal hepatomegaly, some amount of ascites, and edematous gallbladder (Figure 33.1). Jaundice is not a common presentation of dengue, and it is likely to be found only in severe cases late in the course of the illness. Abnormal liver

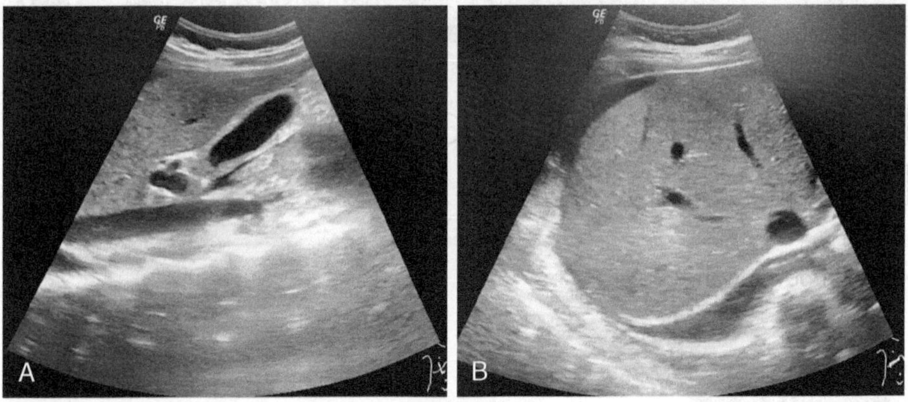

Figure 33.1 Liver ultrasonography of dengue hemorrhagic fever patient revealed edematous gallbladder (A), hepatomegaly and amount of ascites (B). (Case record from Bangkok Hospital for Tropical Diseases, Faculty of Tropical Medicine, Mahidol University.)

function tests are a common laboratory finding in the majority of cases. Mild elevation of alanine aminotransferase up to two to five times the upper limit of normal with a relatively normal level of serum alkaline phosphatase is observed in most cases. However, approximately 10% to 20% of hospitalized dengue cases can show more than 10 times the elevation of alanine aminotransferase.[5,6] Like most systemic tropical infections, aspartate aminotransferase is usually at a higher level than alanine aminotransferase, approximately two times/ratio in dengue.[4,6] In comparison to other mosquito-borne viral infections, for example chikungunya, hepatocellular injury is more common and prominent in dengue infection.

Dengue and COVID-19

In the context of the COVID-19 pandemic, dengue viruses and the virus that causes COVID-19 (SARS-CoV-2) can cause similar symptoms in the early stages of infection. The common dengue symptoms fever, headache, and muscle pain. Nausea, vomiting, and diarrhea are occasionally present in both infections. However, respiratory symptoms are relatively rare in dengue infection and providers should be cautious, especially in dengue and COVID-19 co-endemic areas.

Pathophysiology of Liver Injury in Dengue

The mechanism of liver injury caused by dengue is categorized into three main paths: First, direct viral effects, as hepatocytes and Kupffer cells are prime targets for dengue viral infection and replication; second, dysregulated host immune response against the virus involving secondary liver damage; and third, liver injury related to hemodynamic instability.[7]

Liver pathology of severe dengue infection demonstrates diffuse hemorrhage and an edematous liver. The most common cell affected by the dengue virus are hepatocytes, Kupffer, and endothelial cells.[8] Microscopic findings include microsteatosis, macrosteatosis, and nuclear degeneration, which are more prominent around the portal spaces. Focal areas of necrosis with nuclear vacuolar degeneration, swollen mitochondria, presence of mononuclear infiltrate, and increased macrophage cells are frequent findings.

Apart from viral injury related to the infection, various predisposing factors might also impact the presentation and severity of liver involvement in dengue infection including chronic liver diseases and alcohol consumption.[9]

Acute Liver Failure in Dengue Infection

Acute Liver failure secondary to dengue infection is a rare but serious complication.[10] This complication usually occurs during the second week of illness.[11] The incidence of acute liver failure is reported to be 0.3% to 4.4% among symptomatic dengue patients (Table 33.1).

A retrospective cohort study among 1926 serologically confirmed dengue patients hospitalized at the Hospital for Tropical Diseases, Bangkok, Thailand, found that the incidence of dengue-associated acute liver failure was 0.31%. Dengue-associated acute liver failure was more common among young adults.[4] Increased levels of alanine aminotransferase and aspartate aminotransferase were also more prominent among young adults than older ones.[12] The median duration from onset of fever to development of acute liver failure was 7.5 days. There are no specific risk factors for severe liver injury from dengue infection, but patients with the severe stage of dengue had a higher risk of developing severe hepatitis and acute liver failure.[4] Therefore patients with warning signs of severe dengue including severe stomach pain, persistent vomiting, bleeding, difficult or rapid breathing, fatigue, and irritability should be closely observed. Among those dengue patients with severe hepatitis assessment of Model for End-Stage Liver Disease (MELD) score is recommended to predict development of acute liver failure.[5]

Diagnosis

Dengue is a systemic viral infection whose clinical presentation can be unspecific. Laboratory diagnosis methods should be performed to confirm dengue virus infection. The confirmation test can be detection of the virus, viral nucleic acid, antigens, or antibodies. Viral antigens (dengue nonstructural protein 1, NS1 antigen) and antibodies are used as the standard of care

TABLE 33.1 ■ **Incidence and Clinical Outcome of Acute Liver Failure Secondary to Dengue Infection**[4,11,13,14]

Study, Author, Year	Country	Study Period	Study Population	Age of Population	Incidence Rate (%)	Mortality Rate (%)
Prospective observational study, Itha et al., 2005	India (dengue outbreak at that time)	September 2003–December 2003	*N* = 45 serologically confirmed dengue patients	>18 years male and female	4.44	100
The prospective observational study, Trung et al., 2010	Vietnam	2006–2008	*N* = 644 serologically confirmed dengue patients	>14 years male and female	0.77	20
Retrospective study, Devarbhavi et al., 2020	India	2014–2017	*N* = 10,108 serologically confirmed dengue patients	>10 years male and female	0.35	58.3
Retrospective cohort study, Kye Mon, et al., 2016	Thailand	2011–2015	*N* = 1,926 serologically confirmed dengue patients	≥15 years male and female	0.31	66.7

N = number.

tests. After the onset of illness, the NS1 antigen by immunoassay can be detected in serum for 4 to 5 days. After 4 days of illness, IgM antibody testing can be used as the serologic diagnosis of dengue infection. However, cross-reactivity with other flaviviruses should be of concern.

Management

Currently, there is no specific antiviral medicine to treat dengue. Most cases will recover with supportive care. In dengue hemorrhagic fever patients intravenous fluids need to be used and adjusted to maintain adequate intravascular circulation. Liver injury related to dengue usually resolves spontaneously after clinical recovery within a few weeks. N-acetylcysteine, which is beneficial for the treatment of various acute liver injuries, especially paracetamol overdose toxicity, has a potential role in the treatment of dengue-induced acute liver failure. Some clinical case reports suggest clinical and biochemical improvements by using N-acetylcysteine among dengue-related severe liver injuries.[13,14] However, randomized clinical trials are required to confirm the efficacy.

Conclusion

Liver involvement and abnormal liver function test in dengue are common. There is a wide range of hepatocellular injury, from mild hepatitis to acute liver failure. Acute liver failure is rare in patients with dengue, but it is associated with a high mortality rate. Acute liver failure secondary to dengue is associated with severe dengue and occurs more often in young adults than in older patients. N-acetylcysteine is potentially beneficial for the treatment of dengue-related severe liver injury.

References

1. Bhatt S, Gething PW, Brady OJ, et al. The global distribution and burden of dengue. *Nature.* 2013; 496(7446):504-507. doi:10.1038/nature12060.
2. Brady OJ, Gething PW, Bhatt S, et al. Refining the global spatial limits of dengue virus transmission by evidence-based consensus. *PLoS Negl Trop Dis.* 2012;6(8):e1760. doi:10.1371/journal.pntd.0001760.
3. Umakanth M, Suganthan N. Unusual manifestations of dengue fever: A review on expanded dengue syndrome. *Cureus.* 2020;12(9):e10678. doi:10.7759/cureus.10678.
4. Kye Mon K, Nontprasert A, Kittitrakul C, Tangkijvanich P, Leowattana W, Poovorawan K. Incidence and clinical outcome of acute liver failure caused by dengue in a hospital for tropical diseases, Thailand. *Am J Trop Med Hyg.* 2016;95(6):1338-1344. doi:10.4269/ajtmh.16-0374.
5. Teerasarntipan T, Chaiteerakij R, Komolmit P, Tangkijvanich P, Treeprasertsuk S. Acute liver failure and death predictors in patients with dengue-induced severe hepatitis. *World J Gastroenterol.* 2020;26(33): 4983-4995. doi:10.3748/wjg.v26.i33.4983.
6. Fernando S, Wijewickrama A, Gomes L, et al. Patterns and causes of liver involvement in acute dengue infection. *BMC Infect Dis.* 2016;16:319. doi:10.1186/s12879-016-1656-2.
7. Mrzljak A, Tabain I, Premac H, et al. The role of emerging and neglected viruses in the etiology of hepatitis. *Curr Infect Dis Rep.* 2019;21(12):51. doi:10.1007/s11908-019-0709-2.
8. Povoa TF, Alves AM, Oliveira CA, Nuovo GJ, Chagas VL, Paes MV. The pathology of severe dengue in multiple organs of human fatal cases: Histopathology, ultrastructure and virus replication. *PLoS One.* 2014;9(4):e83386. doi:10.1371/journal.pone.0083386.
9. Debes JD, Ashhab A. Acute liver failure and dengue: Alcohol matters. *Am J Trop Med Hyg.* 2017;96(3): 760. doi:10.4269/ajtmh.16-0985a.
10. Gasperino J, Yunen J, Guh A, Tanaka KE, Kvetan V, Doyle H. Fulminant liver failure secondary to haemorrhagic dengue in an international traveller. *Liver Int.* 2007;27(8):1148-1151. doi:10.1111/j.1478-3231.2007.01543.x.

11. Trung DT, Thao le TT, Hien TT, et al. Liver involvement associated with dengue infection in adults in Vietnam. *Am J Trop Med Hyg.* 2010;83(4):774-780. doi:10.4269/ajtmh.2010.10-0090.
12. Chhong LN, Poovorawan K, Hanboonkunupakarn B, et al. Prevalence and clinical manifestations of dengue in older patients in Bangkok Hospital for Tropical Diseases, Thailand. *Trans R Soc Trop Med Hyg.* 2020;114(9):674-681. doi:10.1093/trstmh/traa043.
13. Itha S, Kashyap R, Krishnani N, Saraswat VA, Choudhuri G, Aggarwal R Profile of liver involvement in dengue virus infection. *Natl Med J India.* 2005;18:127.
14. Devarbhavi H, Ganga D, Menon M, Kothari K, Singh R Dengue hepatitis with acute liver failure: Clinical, biochemical, histopathological characteristics and predictors of outcome. *J Gastroenterol Hepatol.* 2020;35:1223-1228.
15. Tafere GG, Wondafrash DZ, Demoz FB. Repurposing of N-acetylcysteine for the treatment of dengue virus-induced acute liver failure. *Hepat Med.* 2020;12:173-178. doi:10.2147/HMER.S263840.
16. Dissanayake D, Gunaratne W, Kumarihamy K, Kularatne SAM, Kumarasiri PVR. Use of intravenous N-acetylcysteine in acute severe hepatitis due to severe dengue infection: A case series. *BMC Infect Dis.* 2021;21(1):978. doi:10.1186/s12879-021-06681-9.

CHAPTER 34

Leishmaniasis in Tropical Diseases

Wanessa T. Clemente ■ Francisco Penna Guilherme Cancela

KEY POINTS

- Visceral leishmaniasis (VL) is a widely distributed endemic disease, but there are limited studies on patients with liver diseases or severe hepatic dysfunction.
- Recurrence of disease is not unusual, especially in the immunocompromised.
- The most common clinical manifestation of VL is fever, often associated with visceromegaly and cytopenia. The liver is frequently involved, although is unlikely for VL to present with severe liver impairment.
- Definitive diagnosis requires demonstration of the parasite by microscopy, histopathology, or culture (needle aspiration or biopsy, usually bone marrow or spleen).
- Liposomal amphotericin is highly effective and is the preferred treatment in severe cases and immunocompromised persons.

Global Epidemiology

Leishmaniasis is caused by infection with *Leishmania* parasites widely distributed in tropical, subtropical, and temperate countries, with 0.2–0.4 million new visceral leishmaniasis (VL) cases and 0.7–1.2 million new cutaneous leishmaniasis (CL) cases per year worldwide. The leishmaniases are a group of diseases caused by protozoan parasites from more than 20 *Leishmania* species. The visceral presentation is a life-threatening infection. Specifically, more than 90% of VL cases globally occur in six countries: Bangladesh, Brazil, Ethiopia, India, South Sudan, and Sudan. In Europe, the Mediterranean area is considered endemic for *Leishmania infantum*, and cases have been reported in Spain, France, Italy, and Portugal.[1,2]

Typically, leishmania, a protozoa parasite, is transmitted by the bite of an infected female sandfly. However, the protozoan can also be transmitted via intravenous drug use, blood transfusion, organ transplantation, congenital infection, and laboratory accidents, although these modes of transmission are relatively rarely reported. The most important *Leishmania* species related to VL are *Leishmania donovani* and *Leishmania infantum* (syn. *L. chagasi* in Latin America), but species that cause CL (e.g., *Leishmania tropical*) can eventually visceralize, particularly in the immunocompromised host.[3] *L. donovani* and *L. infantum* belong to the *L. donovani* complex, and while closely related, they present some epidemiological differences. *L. donovani* shows an anthroponotic transmission mode (from human to human), while L. *infantum*, on the other hand, is zoonotic. Likewise, *L. donovani* is found only in the Old World (mainly India and East Africa) and *L. infantum* in the Mediterranean region and Latin America (Figure 34.1). In non-endemic regions leishmaniasis cases may reflect travel and immigration patterns.[1,2]

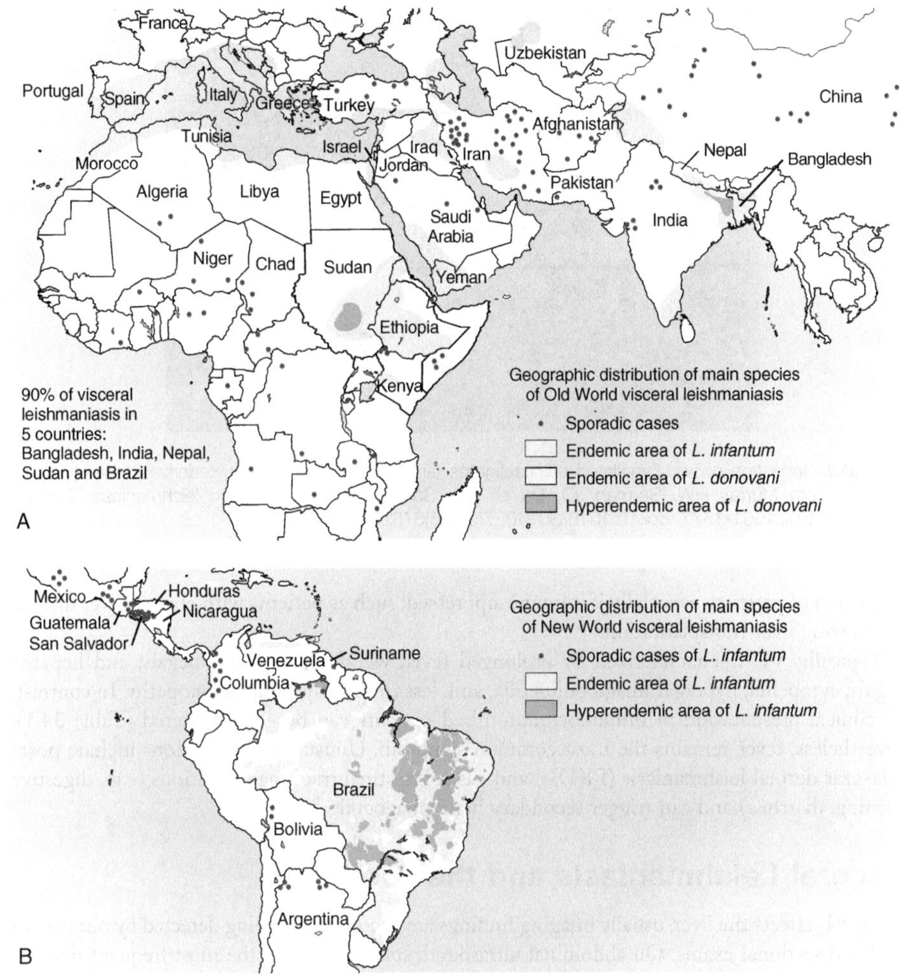

Figure 34.1 Visceral leishmaniasis in the Old World and New World.[2]

Clinical Features and Imaging

There is a high prevalence of asymptomatic human carriers of *L. infantum* in endemic areas, which suggests that this disease presents a latent behavior. Whereas most immunocompetent individuals will not develop clinical disease after this parasitic infection, medication-related or acquired development of immunosuppression can result in variable disease presentation. In this context it can be seen in HIV and non-HIV-related immunosuppressive conditions, such as transplantation, rheumatology, oncology, and hematology. Thus it is recommended that patients living in or returning from areas endemic for leishmaniasis consider this diagnosis.[1–4]

Leishmania amastigotes invade and replicate within host macrophages, and subsequently, the parasites can disseminate and infect cells of the reticuloendothelial system in various tissues, including the liver (Figure 34.2). However, the infection becomes symptomatic in only a small

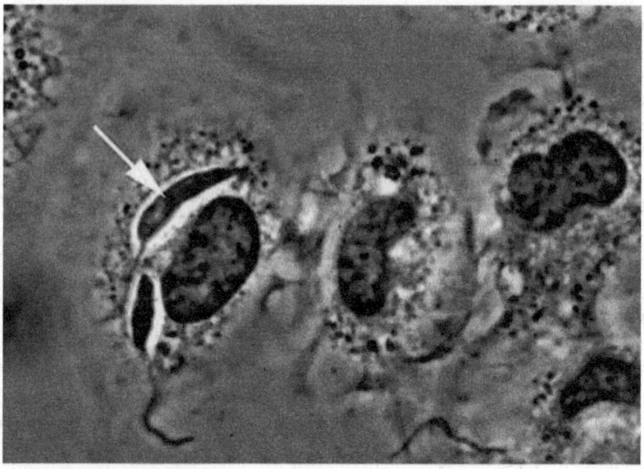

Figure 34.2 Ingestion of two flagellated promastigotes (arrow) by human monocytederived macrophages. (Adapted from Murray HW, Berman JD, Davies CR, Saravia NG. Advances in leishmaniasis. *Lancet*. 2005;366(9496):1561-1577. doi:10.1016/S0140-6736(05)67629-5)

proportion of patients, especially if immunosuppressed, such as patients with chronic liver disease or following liver transplantation[4]

Typically, VL is characterized by prolonged fever, weight loss, splenomegaly, and hepatomegaly, cytopenia, hypergammaglobulinemia, and, less frequently, lymphadenopathy. In contrast, the clinical presentation in immunocompromised patients can be greatly altered (Table 34.1). Nevertheless, fever remains the most common symptom. Unusual manifestations include post-Kala-azar dermal leishmaniasis (PKDL) and gastrointestinal tract manifestations (e.g., digestive bleeding, diarrhea) and can trigger secondary hemophagocytic.[3]

Visceral Leishmaniasis and the liver

When VL affects the liver, usually imaging findings are encountered, being detected by ultrasound (US) and sectional exams. On abdominal ultrasound, splenomegaly is the most frequent finding, found in 36% to 100% of cases, associated or not with hepatomegaly. Other alterations described in the liver are hyperechoic, homogeneous, and granular aspects, as well as the presence of multiple hypoechoic and even nodular areas in the parenchyma. Findings of portal hypertension may also be present.[23] On the other hand, in cross-sectional imaging exams common findings are enlarged liver and spleen, with hypodense nodular lesions in late phases on CT with contrast or heterogeneous parenchyma on T2 with hypointense nodular lesions on MRI.[24] The degree of elevation in liver enzymes is relative to the severity of the disease. However, AST and ALT levels are usually <3ULN with a higher AST to ALT ratio. A recent study from Ethiopia reported mean ALT of 67 IU/L and ALT of 48 IU//L with minimal elevaiton of bilirrubin in VL.[25]

Laboratory Diagnosis

The diagnostic strategy should be based on a combination of methods to increase performance, including (when available) microscopy, culture, molecular, and serologic testing. Usually, the diagnostic confirmation is based on the demonstration of *Leishmania* parasites via microscopic examination or culture of sample tissues. The sensitivity varies depending on the material. In high-income countries, or whenever it is available, molecular-based tests should be used, as they

TABLE 34.1 ■ **Clinical Manifestation of Visceral Leishmaniasis in Liver Disease Patients**

Number of Cases	Clinical Scenario	Country	Clinical Manifestation and Laboratory Findings	Diagnoses	Treatment	Mortality	Recurrence	Reference
1	Liver transplant	Spain	Diarrhea, abdominal pain, visceromegaly, and pancytopenia	Bone marrow microscopy and colon biopsy	Liposomal amphotericin B	0	-	Acosta et al.[5]
1	Liver transplant (pediatric)	Brazil	Hepatomegaly and splenomegaly. Bloody diarrhea	Bone marrow biopsy and terminal ileum biopsy (immunohistochemistry and PCR)	Amphotericin B desoxycholate followed by liposomal Amphotericin B	0	-	Araújo, Queiroz, Cabral[6]
1	Liver transplant	Spain	Enlarged lymph node (without fever, weight loss, or dysphonia)	Lymph node	Liposomal amphotericin B	0	No relapse after 36 months of follow-up	Campos-Varela et al.[7]
4	Liver transplant	Brazil and Spain			Liposomal amphotericin B			Clemente et al.[8]
1	Liver fibrosis (due to VL - ?)	Brazil	-	-	Glucantime®	0	Resolution of liver fibrosis in control biopsy 2 years after treatment	Corbett, Duarte, Bustamante[9]
1	Liver transplant (pediatric)	Iran	Fever, anemia, and thrombocytopenia	Bone marrow microscopy Gastrointestinal tract biopsy + tissue PC	Liposomal amphotericin B	0	No relapse after 2 months of follow-up	Derakhshan et al.[10]
1	Liver transplant	Georgia	Fever and digestive bleeding	Bone marrow microscopy and cecal biopsy. Serology (ELISA and spot IF) Blood PCR	Liposomal amphotericin B	0	Relapsed 1 year after treatment	Desoubeaux. et al.[11]

Continued on following page

TABLE 34.1 ■ **Clinical Manifestation of Visceral Leishmaniasis in Liver Disease Patients** (Continued)

Number of Cases	Clinical Scenario	Country	Clinical Manifestation and Laboratory Findings	Diagnoses	Treatment	Mortality	Recurrence	Reference
1	Non-specific inflammatory disease (liver and kidney)	Switzerland	Fever and fatigue. Bloody diarrhea	Colon biopsy and PCR	Liposomal amphotericin B	0	-	Eichenberger. et al.[12]
1	Liver transplant	Brazil	Fever	Bone marrow microscopy	Liposomal amphotericin B	1	-	Ferreira et al.[13]
1	Cirrhosis (?)	Italy	Hepatomegaly and splenomegaly, weight loss, pancytopenia *High serum levels of alanine aminotransferase	Bone marrow biopsy. Serology	Liposomal amphotericin B	0	No relapse after 14 months of follow-up	Giannitrapani et al.[14]
1	Liver transplant	Switzerland	Fever, splenomegaly, and pancytopenia	Bone marrow biopsy Culture (liver and BM) Serology	Pentavalent antimony and Amphotericin B	0	No relapse after 12 months of follow-up	Horber et al.[15]
1	Cirrhosis (HBV/HDV) and liver transplant	Italy	Fever, weight loss, and asthenia	Bone marrow microscopy Western Blot test	Liposomal Amphotericin B	0	No relapse after 14 months of follow-up	Lupia et al.[16]
1	Liver transplant (pediatric)	Turkey	Splenomegaly and anemia Cutaneous lesions	Bone marrow biopsy and PCR	Liposomal Amphotericin B	0	-	Ozcan et al.[17]
11	Cirrhosis	Italy	Fever, splenomegaly, and pancytopenia *Reduced serum albumin	Bone marrow microscopy and spleen biopsy Serology (immunofluorescent-specific antibody test—IFAT)	Liposomal-amphotericin B (N = 9) and Meglumine antimoniate (N = 2)	0	-	Pagliano et al.[18]

1	Liver transplant	Portugal	Fever, splenomegaly, and pancytopenia	Bone marrow microscopy *Negative serology	Liposomal Amphotericin B	0	No relapse after 18 months of follow-up	Pereira et al.[19]
1	Acute liver failure	Italy	Hepatomegaly and splenomegaly. Weight loss. Pancytopenia. Liver involvement *Increased-globulin serum level with a high polyclonal peak	Bone marrow microscopy	N-methylglucamine antimoniate	0	No relapse after 22 months of follow-up	Sagnelli et al.[20]
1	Hepatitis (Autoimmune)	Greece	Fever, hepatomegaly, and splenomegaly. Cytopenia and hemolytic anemia *Hypergammaglobulinemia and increased levels of aminotransferases	Bone marrow biopsy	Liposomal amphotericin B	0	No relapse after 6 months of follow-up	Sotirakou, Wozniak[21]
1	Hepatitis	Turkey	Fever, anorexia, malaise, weight loss, and joint swelling. Cytopenia	Bone marrow microscopy and liver biopsy	Liposomal—Amphotericin B	0	No relapse after 6 months of follow-up	Tunccan et al.[22]

*laboratory findings

present high sensitivity and specificity in both bone marrow and peripheral blood samples. Leishmanial antigens can also be detected in serum or urine samples with a wide range of sensitivity and specificity (rapid tests). The most widely used serological techniques are the indirect fluorescent antibody test (IFAT), enzyme-linked immunosorbent assay (ELISA), and rapid tests, such as immunochromatographic and direct agglutination test (DAT). Sensitivity and specificity vary according to the method, antigens used, geographical area, and type of patients (lower in HIV/AIDS patients, per example). In patients with chronic liver disease serological tests may be false negative due to clinical, immunological, and nutritional conditions.[2–4] Serological limitations are affected by the lack of agreement between methods, the inability to distinguish previous exposure from active infection, and the potential cross-reaction with other protozoa. Diagnosis based on positive serology without confirmation by direct examination should be supported by clinical correlation.[2,26]

When visceral leishmaniasis affects the liver and it is the only knowable site of disease, the diagnostic tools to establish the diagnosis may include parasite isolation by in vitro culture, molecular detection of parasite DNA, and serologic testing. Nevertheless, the current gold standard for diagnosis relies on the visualization of the amastigote form of the parasite within macrophages by microscopic examination of tissue aspirate, after Giemsa.[4]

Treatment

Treatment decisions are usually made on an individual basis. The choice of therapy depends on various factors, such as patient's age, immune status, and renal/liver function. The *Leishmania* species, disease extent, drug availability, concomitant infections, and previous treatments should also be taken into consideration. In this regard, patients with chronic liver disease and VL may have some limitations concerning treatment options.

Liposomal amphotericin B (L-AmB) is considered the drug of choice for severe VL or in immunocompromised persons. The recommended regimen is 3–5 mg/kg/day IV on days 1 to 5, 10, 17, 24, 31, and 38 (total dose of 40 mg/kg). Amphotericin B presents high tissue concentrations specially in the liver, spleen, and lung. There is no hepatic adjustment dose required, but hepatotoxicity has been described. It appears that the overall rate of hepatotoxicity is no greater for liposomal formulation when compared to conventional amphotericin B. However, fulminant hepatitis is a possible but exceedingly rare occurrence with the use of either drug.[27]

Pentavalent antimonials (PAs) are the first-line drugs for VL in many countries. Overall, they are the second most used drugs. These drugs require long courses of administration (up to 30 days). Patients should be evaluated for underlying conditions that contraindicate their use, before treatment. These conditions include renal or hepatic insufficiency, arrhythmia, and the use of beta-blockers or antiarrhythmic drugs. Adverse effects comprise acute pancreatitis, hepatitis, arthropathy, anasarca and oliguria, renal tubular acidosis, bone marrow toxicity and electrocardiographic changes, agranulocytosis, and neurological alterations.[2,28] It is advisable for patients to avoid taking other potential hepatotoxic drugs and also avoid drinking alcohol during treatment.

Miltefosine was approved by the Food and Drug Administration (FDA) for the treatment of leishmaniasis in 2014. It is an oral antileishmanial drug used for the treatment of visceral, mucosal, and cutaneous leishmaniasis. Miltefosine is effective, although its efficacy has been observed to decline. The drug can be used both on its own or in combination with other anti-leishmanial agents for various species. So far, there is no data concerning hepatic adjustment dose. Although currently licensed in Germany, India, and Central and South America, it is not that widely available.[29]

Visceral leishmaniasis treatment can be challenging, and the primary goal is to prevent mortality. However, despite being a treatable disease, cure requires an immunocompetent system to properly respond. All patients diagnosed should require prompt and complete treatment.[1] Response to treatment is observed through resolution of fever, decrease in visceromegaly, weight gain, and hematological parameters improvement. Immunosuppressed persons with VL who are coinfected with HIV typically have lower response rates to initial treatment and higher recurrence rates.[2] Increased mortality rate is associated with delayed diagnosis and underlying conditions (e.g., pregnancy, immunocompromised status). In some cases higher lethality is associated with the presence and intensity of thrombocytopenia or bacterial infection with impact on the outcome.

References

1. World Health Organization. *Leishmaniasis*. n.d. Available at: https://www.who.int/leishmaniasis/. Accessed September 20, 2021.
2. Aronson N, Herwaldt BL, Libman M, et al. Diagnosis and treatment of leishmaniasis: Clinical practice guidelines by the Infectious Diseases Society of America (IDSA) and the American Society of Tropical Medicine and Hygiene (ASTMH). *Clin Infect Dis*. 2016;63:E202-E264. Available at: https://doi.org/10.1093/cid/ciw670.
3. Clemente WT, Mourão PHO. Leishmaniasis in transplant candidates and recipients: Diagnosis and management. *Emerg Transpl Infect*. 2020:1-31. Available at: https://doi.org/10.1007/978-3-030-01751-4_54-1.
4. Van Griensven J, Diro E. Visceral leishmaniasis. *Infect Dis Clin North Am*. 2012;26:309-322. Available at: https://doi.org/10.1016/j.idc.2012.03.005.
5. Vargas Acosta ÁM, Belchí Segura E, Martinez Caselles A, Baños Madrid R, Pons Miñano JA, Parrilla Paricio P. Diarrea por leishmaniasis visceral en paciente con trasplante hepático. *Gastroenterol Hepatol*. 2013;36:271-273. Available at: https://doi.org/10.1016/j.gastrohep.2012.12.001.
6. Araujo SA, Queiroz TCN, Cabral MMDA. Colonic leishmaniasis followed by liver transplantation. *Am J Trop Med Hyg*. 2010;83:209. Available at: https://doi.org/10.4269/ajtmh.2010.09-0430.
7. Campos-Varela I, Leh O, Castells L, et al. Visceral leishmaniasis among liver transplant recipients: An overview. *Liver Transplant*. 2008;14:1816-1819. Available at: https://doi.org/10.1002/lt.21538.
8. Clemente WT, Pierrotti LC, Abdala E, et al. Recommendations for management of endemic diseases and travel medicine in solid-organ transplant recipients and donors. *Transplantation*. 2018;102:193-208. Available at: https://doi.org/10.1097/TP.0000000000002027.
9. Corbett CEP, Duarte MIS, Bustamante SE. Regression of diffuse intralobular liver fibrosis associated with visceral leishmaniasis. *Am J Trop Med Hyg*. 1993;49:616-624. Available at: https://doi.org/10.4269/ajtmh.1993.49.616.
10. Derakhshan D, Basiratnia M, Derakhshan A, et al. Concomitant BK virus infection and visceral leishmaniasis in a pediatric liver transplant recipient. *Pediatr Transplant*. 2021;25(8):e14100. Available at: https://doi.org/10.1111/petr.14100.
11. Desoubeaux G, Dominique M, Morio F, et al. Epidemiological outbreaks of Pneumocystis jirovecii pneumonia are not limited to kidney transplant recipients: Genotyping confirms common source of transmission in a liver transplantation unit. *J Clin Microbiol*. 2016;54:1314-1320. Available at: https://doi.org/10.1128/JCM.00133-16.
12. Eichenberger A, Buechi AE, Neumayr A, et al. A severe case of visceral leishmaniasis and liposomal amphotericin B treatment failure in an immunosuppressed patient 15 years after exposure. *BMC Infect Dis*. 2017;17(1):81. Available at: https://doi.org/10.1186/s12879-017-2192-4.
13. de Ferreira GSA, Watanabe ALC, de Trevisoli NC, et al. Visceral leishmaniasis in a liver transplant patient: A case report. *Transplant Proc*. 2020;52:1417-1421. Available at: https://doi.org/10.1016/j.transproceed.2020.01.069.
14. Giannitrapani L, Soresi M, La Spada E, Tripodo C, Montalto G. Progressive visceral leishmaniasis misdiagnosed as cirrhosis of the liver: A case report. *J Med Case Rep*. 2009;3:1-4. Available at: https://doi.org/10.4076/1752-1947-3-7265.
15. Horber FF, Lerut JP, Reichen J, Zimmermann A, Jaeger P, Malinverni R. Visceral leishmaniasis after orthotopic liver transplantation: Impact of persistent splenomegaly. *Transpl Int*. 1993;6:55-57.
16. Lupia T, Corcione S, Boglione L, Cariti G, De Rosa FG. Visceral leishmaniasis in a patient with active HBV/HDV co-infection. *J Infect Public Health*. 2020;13:306-308. Available at: https://doi.org/10.1016/J.JIPH.2019.07.026.

17. Özcan D, Seçkin D, Allahverdiyev AM, et al. Liver transplant recipient with concomitant cutaneous and visceral leishmaniasis. *Pediatr Transplant.* 2007;11:228-232. Available at: https://doi.org/10.1111/j.1399-3046.2006.00660.x.
18. Pagliano P, Carannante N, Gramiccia M, et al. Visceral leishmaniasis causes fever and decompensation in patients with cirrhosis. *Gut.* 2007;56:893-894. Available at: https://doi.org/10.1136/gut.2007.119495.
19. Rosenthal VD, Al-Abdely HM, El-Kholy AA, et al. International Nosocomial Infection Control Consortium report, data summary of 50 countries for 2010–2015: Device-associated module. *Am J Infect Control.* 2016;44:1495-1504. Available at: https://doi.org/10.1016/j.ajic.2016.08.007.
20. Sagnelli C, Martino F Di, Coppola N, Crisci A, Sagnelli E. Acute liver failure: A rare clinical presentation of visceral leishmaniasis. *New Microbiol.* 2012;35:93-95.
21. Sotirakou S, Wozniak G. Clinical expression of autoimmune hepatitis in a nine-year-old girl with visceral leishmaniasis. *Polish J Pathol.* 2011;62:118-119.
22. Tunccan OG, Tufan A, Telli G, et al. Visceral leishmaniasis mimicking autoimmune hepatitis, primary biliary cirrhosis, and systemic lupus erythematosus overlap. *Korean J Parasitol.* 2012;50:133. Available at: https://doi.org/10.3347/KJP.2012.50.2.133.
23. Bélard S, Stratta E, Zhao A, et al. Sonographic findings in visceral leishmaniasis—A narrative review. *Travel Med Infect Dis.* 2021;39:101924. Available at: https://doi.org/10.1016/j.tmaid.2020.101924.
24. Raeymaeckers S, Docx M, Demeyere N. MRI-findings of nodular lesions in an enlarged spleen, associated with visceral leishmaniasis. *Eur J Radiol.* 2012;81:2550-2553. Available at: https://doi.org/10.1016/J.EJRAD.2011.11.021.
25. Endale HT, Mengstie TA, Dawit DD, Mohammed R, Dessie G, Tesfa KH. Assessment of liver function test and associated factors among visceral leishmaniasis patients attending university of gondar leishmaniasis research and treatment center, Northwest Ethiopia. *PLoS One.* 2021;16(11):e0260022. doi:10.1371/journal.pone.0260022.
26. Van Griensven J, Carrillo E, López-Vélez R, Lynen L, Moreno J. Leishmaniasis in immunosuppressed individuals. *Clin Microbiol Infect.* 2014;20:286-299. Available at: https://doi.org/10.1111/1469-0691.12556.
27. Ellis M, Shamoon A, Gorka W, Zwaan F, Al-Ramadi B. Severe hepatic injury associated with lipid formulations of amphotericin B. *Clin Infect Dis.* 2001;32:E87-E89. Available at: https://doi.org/10.1086/319201.
28. Kato KC, Morais-Teixeira E, Reis PG, et al. Hepatotoxicity of pentavalent antimonial drug: Possible role of residual Sb(III) and protective effect of ascorbic acid. *Antimicrob Agents Chemother.* 2014;58:481-488. Available at: https://doi.org/10.1128/AAC.01499-13.
29. Sunyoto T, Potet J, Boelaert M. Why miltefosine—A life-saving drug for leishmaniasis—Is unavailable to people who need it the most. *BMJ Glob Heal.* 2018;3:e000709. Available at: https://doi.org/10.1136/BMJGH-2018-000709.

CHAPTER 35

Iron Overload in Sub-Saharan Africa

Victor R. Gordeuk

KEY POINTS

- Iron overload is common in rural areas where a traditional fermented opaque beverage is prepared from local grains in iron or steel containers and therefore has a high iron content.
- Gene by environment interaction: a genetic locus or loci plus high dietary iron in the form of traditional beer appears to create a high risk.
- Common cause of hepatic fibrosis and cirrhosis in certain rural communities.
- Contributes to the development of hepatocellular carcinoma along with viral hepatitis and aflatoxins.
- Diagnostic features include hepatomegaly, increased serum ferritin concentration and transferrin saturation, liver biopsy showing iron deposition in hepatocytes and Kupfer cells, bone marrow aspirate showing heavy iron deposition in macrophages.
- Management focuses on prevention by decreasing iron in diet and iron removal through phlebotomy therapy.

Introduction

Iron overload has been recognized in sub-Saharan Africa for over 100 years.[1] The condition is known as "dietary iron overload," for the consumption of a traditional fermented beverage rich in iron but moderate in alcohol content is strongly associated with its development.[2-4] The original 1929 autopsy study describing dietary iron overload in Africa reported high deposits of iron in both the liver and spleen.[1] Subsequent studies have been more specific, showing that iron deposits are prominent both in hepatocytes and in macrophages of the liver, spleen, and bone marrow (Figure 35.1).[5-9] This pattern of iron deposition differs from the distribution seen with *HFE* hemochromatosis, the predominant form of iron overload in Europeans, in which the macrophages are relatively spared of iron-loading compared to hepatocytes.[6,9,10] Dietary iron overload is distinct from alcoholic liver disease, as evidenced by the observations that hepatic iron concentrations[11-14] are frequently higher than those seen in alcoholic liver disease[15,16] and histological changes of alcohol effect are usually absent.[14,17,18]

Epidemiology

Dietary iron overload has been reported in 17 countries of east,[19-22] west,[23-25] central,[1,26-30] and southern[1,13,14,27] Africa (Figure 35.2). The prevalence of dietary iron overload may exceed 10% among adult males in some rural African populations where the practice of drinking locally

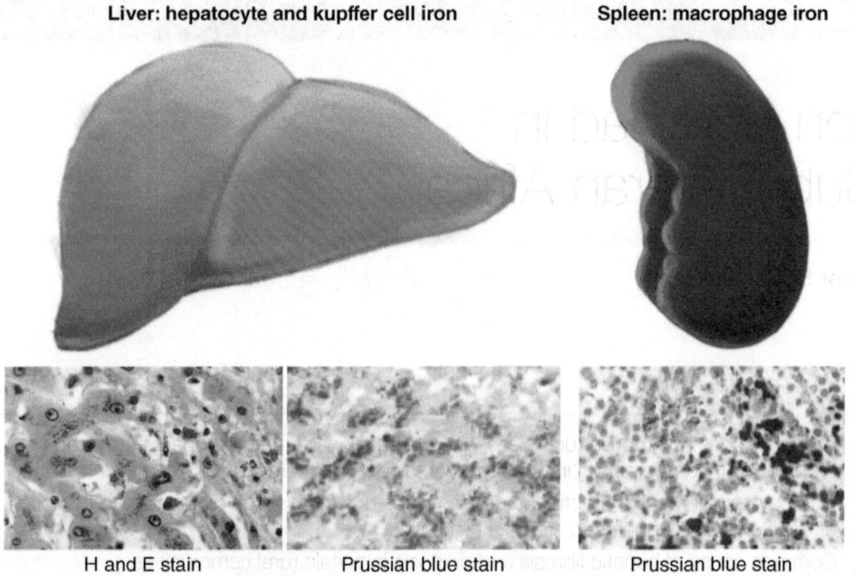

Figure 35.1 Dietary iron overload in Africa is characterized by iron-loading in both the liver (hepatocytes and Kupffer cells) and the spleen (macrophages). This is distinct from *HFE* hemochromatosis in Europeans, in which iron-loading occurs predominantly in the liver (hepatocytes) and in which spleen iron is not increased. (Image courtesy of Nadia Gordeuk)

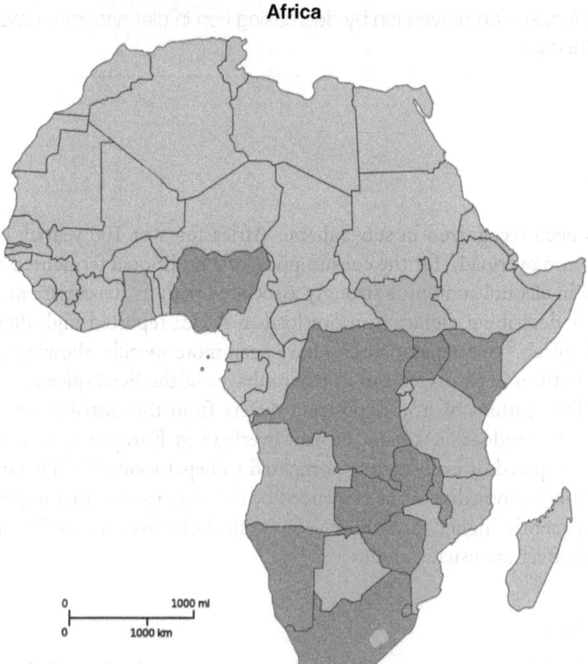

Figure 35.2 Seventeen African countries where dietary iron overload has been described. (Image courtesy of Nadia Gordeuk)

prepared beer is common.[31] In 1960, an autopsy study in urban adult black South Africans reported that 21% of males and 7% of females had extremely high hepatic iron concentrations (>360 μmol/g dry weight; normal range <30).[12] In 1979 an autopsy series at the same institution reported that 11% of males and 5% of females had similarly elevated hepatic iron concentrations.[13] The lower but still substantial prevalence of markedly elevated iron concentrations appeared to be due to a decline in the use of home-brewed traditional beer in favor of commercially prepared alcoholic beverages with lower iron content.

Studies in the 1980s and 1990s continued to show dietary iron overload as an important problem in Africa, especially in rural areas. In a Zimbabwe study of >500 rural community members 21% of traditional beer-drinking men older than 45 years had a high serum ferritin concentration and transferrin saturation of >70%,[17] a combination that suggests a risk for toxic iron overload. In a different rural Zimbabwe community 4 of 28 men (14.3%) who gave a history of the consumption of traditional beer had the same combination of elevated serum ferritin concentration and a transferrin saturation.[32] Based on similar criteria, the prevalence of iron overload was 16.5% among rural males in South Africa.[14] A high prevalence of iron overload was also found in an urban autopsy study from Harare, Zimbabwe, reported in 1999.[5] Few studies of the community prevalence of dietary iron overload have been done over the past two decades,[33,34] but in areas where traditional fermented beverages are prepared at home from local grain,[4,35] dietary iron overload is likely to be found.

The relationship between dietary iron and African iron overload was recognized in the 1950s, and for many years high dietary iron in the form of traditional beer was thought to be the exclusive etiology.[2] Traditional beer is prepared from locally grown grains in a process that requires up to 7 days. Typically iron or steel containers are used for the preparation (Figure 35.3). The concentration of ferrous iron in the supernatant of this opaque traditional beer is usually more than 40 mg/L.[3,32] In contrast, the iron content of commercially prepared clear beers is less than

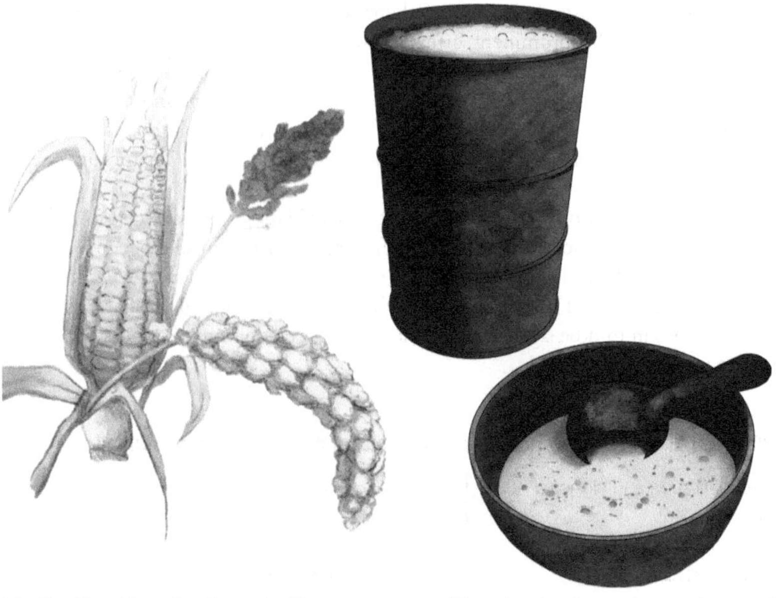

Figure 35.3 Traditional beer is a fermented beverage prepared from local grains such as maize, sorghum, or millet. The beverage is typically brewed in iron or steel containers by a process that takes up to 7 days. The opaque beer that results is high in iron and low in alcohol. (Image courtesy of Nadia Gordeuk)

0.2 mg/L,[3] and the total iron content of a typical western diet is 15 to 20 mg/day. The alcohol content of traditional beer in Africa tends to be low compared to commercially prepared beer.[14,17]

Considerable evidence indicates that iron overload in sub-Saharan Africa is related to both genetic variation as well as increased dietary iron. In a Zimbabwe community survey conducted in the 1980s, it was noted that only a minority of the traditional beer drinkers developed iron overload,[17] and this led to the hypothesis that there may be an inborn error of metabolism to explain the development of iron overload. Two studies conducted in central and southern African families have found evidence of an interaction between dietary iron and a genetic locus or loci in determining the risk for iron overload.[27,36] The postulated iron-loading locus in Africans with dietary iron overload is different from the *HFE* gene that is responsible for most primary iron overload in Europeans.[27,37] Potential candidates for the postulated iron-loading locus or loci in African dietary iron overload include *SLC40A1* (ferroportin, Q248H polymorphism),[33,34,38-40] *PIEZO1* (E756del polymorphism),[41] *TFR2*,[42] and *TP53* (P47S variant).[43]

Presentation

The typical presentation of African iron overload is a middle-aged or older adult with hepatomegaly and a history of the consumption of traditional, home-brewed beer.[18] In severe cases features of cirrhosis including portal hypertension and ascites may be present. Usually there is a history of greater than 1000 L of lifetime consumption of traditional beer. The serum ferritin concentration is commonly greater than 700 μg/L and correlates well with hepatic and marrow iron concentration[14,18,32] Ferritin concentrations up to several thousand μg/L may be encountered.[17,18] The majority of subjects with established African iron overload have transferrin saturations greater than 55%,[17,18] but the transferrin saturation may not be elevated in the early stages. Serum iron concentration and transferrin saturation may also be falsely low in the presence of ascorbic acid deficiency.[44] Clinical findings that may be associated with African iron overload are summarized in Table 35.1.

Portal fibrosis and cirrhosis are prominent hepatic findings in African iron overload.[8] These complications are especially prominent after a threshold hepatic iron concentration of about 360 μmol/g dry weight has been reached (normal less than 30).[12] Plasma non–transferrin-bound iron may contribute to hepatocellular damage.[55] All plasma iron is bound to transferrin under normal conditions, but a distinctly abnormal fraction of non-transferrin bound iron is found in patients with dietary iron overload and correlates with elevations in the hepatic enzymes, alanine and amino transferase.[55]

Large deposits of ferric iron in tissues accelerate the oxidation of ascorbic acid in African iron overload patients.[56] Clinical scurvy is an unusual finding, but subclinical biochemical evidence of depleted ascorbic acid stores is common in severe African iron overload.[14,18] Chronic ascorbic acid deficiency appears to lead to osteoporosis giving rise to the unusual presentation of vertebral and femoral collapse in middle-aged African men.[57] The exact nature of the disturbance of bone metabolism is unclear.

TABLE 35.1 ■ **Clinical Findings That May Be Associated With African Iron Overload.**

Hepatic portal fibrosis and cirrhosis[8]	Esophageal carcinoma[51]
Diabetes mellitus[45]	Infections:
Idiopathic heart failure[13]	Bacterial peritonitis[52]
Ascorbic acid deficiency[46,47]	Amebiasis[53]
Osteoporosis[46,47]	Tuberculosis[54]
Hepatocellular carcinoma[48-50]	

A number of studies indicate an association between African iron overload and hepatocellular carcinoma.[48-50,54,58] The incidence of hepatocellular carcinoma in southern Africa is high, and major risk factors include hepatitis B and C viral infections and dietary exposure to aflatoxin B1 and mycotoxin. In a case-control study that controlled for these known factors, the population attributable risk of iron overload in the development of hepatocellular carcinoma was 29%, while that of hepatitis B virus infection was 69%.[48] Another study raised the possibility that African iron overload poses a risk for hepatocellular carcinoma even in the absence of cirrhosis.[58]

Diagnosis and Management

Once African iron overload is suspected, the finding of an elevated serum ferritin concentration provides further evidence of the diagnosis.[18] The transferrin saturation may also be elevated[18] and circulating transferrin receptor concentrations tend to be low.[59] Because the serum ferritin concentration and transferrin saturation may be perturbed by inflammatory processes and hepatocellular damage, the diagnosis should be confirmed by liver biopsy or bone marrow biopsy if possible. Such direct measures of iron status demonstrate abnormally increased iron stores in macrophages[7,32] and, in the case of liver biopsy, hepatocytes.[18] Neither anemia nor erythrocytosis is a typical feature of African iron overload.

The differential diagnoses of *HFE* hemochromatosis, an inherited condition, and transfusional iron overload, an acquired condition, can be excluded fairly straightforwardly, despite the fact that both of these conditions are marked by increased serum ferritin concentration and increased transferrin saturation. *HFE* hemochromatosis almost always occurs in persons of European ancestry and there is usually not a history of increased dietary or medicinal iron. Transfusional iron overload occurs due to the accumulation of iron from red blood cell transfusions. It can be diagnosed in persons who have received more than 15 to 20 units of blood that were not administered because of blood loss.

Two methods for treating iron overload are available: phlebotomy and iron chelation therapy. Because African iron overload is not characterized by anemia, phlebotomy is the preferred method of treatment.[60] During phlebotomy therapy, one unit of blood (450 mL representing about 225 mg of iron) is removed once per week until a state of mild iron deficiency is induced as evidenced by a decline in the mean corpuscular volume and/or the serum ferritin concentration declines to <50 ug/L. Because of the association between African iron overload and the consumption of traditional beer, preventive efforts should be directed at reducing or eliminating the consumption of this beverage. Another possible approach is to develop methods to modify the preparation of the beverage to reduce its iron content.

Acknowledgment

I would like to thank Nadia Gordeuk for creating the Figures for this chapter.

References

1. Strachan AS. *Haemosiderosis and Haemochromatosis in South African Natives with a Comment on the Etiology of Haemochromatosis.* Glasgow, UK: University of Glasgow; 1929.
2. Bothwell TH, Seftel H, Jacobs P, Torrance JD, Baumslag N. Iron overload in Bantu subjects; studies on the availability of iron in Bantu beer. *Am J Clin Nutr.* 1964;14:47-51.
3. Saungweme T, Khumalo H, Mvundura EM, et al. Iron and alcohol content of traditional beers in rural Zimbabwe. *Cent Afr J Med.* 1999;45:136-140.
4. Cason ED, Mahlomaholo BJ, et al. Bacterial and fungal dynamics during the fermentation process of Sesotho, a traditional beer of Southern Africa. *Front Microbiol.* 2020;11:1451.

5. Gangaidzo IT, Moyo VM, Saungweme T, et al. Iron overload in urban Africans in the 1990s. *Gut.* 1999; 45:278-283.
6. Bothwell TH, Abrahams C, Bradlow BA, Charlton RW. Idiopathic and Bantu hemochromatosis. Comparative histological study. *Arch Pathol.* 1965;79:163-168.
7. Gale E, Torrance J, Bothwell T. The quantitative estimation of total iron stores in human bone marrow. *J Clin Invest.* 1963;42:1076-1082.
8. Isaacson C, Seftel HC, Keeley KJ, Bothwell TH. Siderosis in the Bantu: [ii] The relationship between iron overload and cirrhosis. *J Lab Clin Med.* 1961;58:845-853.
9. Brink B, Disler P, Lynch S, Jacobs P, Charlton R, Bothwell T. Patterns of iron storage in dietary iron overload and idiopathic hemochromatosis. *J Lab Clin Med.* 1976;88:725-731.
10. Valberg LS, Simon JB, Manley PN, Corbett WE, Ludwig J. Distribution of storage iron as body stores expand in patients with hemochromatosis. *J Lab Clin Med.* 1975;86:479-489.
11. Bothwell TH, Bradlow BA. Siderosis in the Bantu. A combined histopathological and chemical study. *Arch Pathol.* 1960;70:279-292.
12. Bothwell TH, Isaacson C. Siderosis in the Bantu. A comparison of incidence in males and females. *Br Med J.* 1962;1:522-524.
13. MacPhail AP, Simon MO, Torrance JD, Charlton RW, Bothwell TH, Isaacson C. Changing patterns of dietary iron overload in black South Africans. *Am J Clin Nutr.* 1979;32:1272-1278.
14. Friedman BM, Baynes RD, Bothwell TH, et al. Dietary iron overload in southern African rural blacks. *S Afr Med J.* 1990;78:301-305.
15. Chapman RW, Morgan MY, Laulicht M, Hoffbrand AV, Sherlock S. Hepatic iron stores and markers of iron overload in alcoholics and patients with idiopathic hemochromatosis. *Dig Dis Sci.* 1982;27:909-916.
16. Bassett ML, Halliday JW, Powell LW. Value of hepatic iron measurements in early hemochromatosis and determination of the critical iron level associated with fibrosis. *Hepatology.* 1986;6:24-29.
17. Gordeuk VR, Boyd RD, Brittenham GM. Dietary iron overload persists in rural sub-Saharan Africa. *Lancet.* 1986;1:1310-1313.
18. MacPhail AP, Mandishona EM, Bloom PD, Paterson AC, Rouault TA, Gordeuk VR. Measurements of iron status and survival in African iron overload. *S Afr Med J.* 1999;89:966-972.
19. Hofvander Y, Olding L, Westermark P. Liver changes in medico-legal autopsies in Addis Ababa, Ethiopia. CNU report No. 59. *Acta Med Scand.* 1972;191:167-170.
20. Senba M, Nakamura T, Itakura H. Statistical analysis of relationship between iron accumulation and hepatitis B surface antigen. *Am J Clin Pathol.* 1985;84:340-342.
21. Haddock DR. Bantu Siderosis in Tanzania. *East Afr Med J.* 1965;42:67-73.
22. Owor R. Haemosiderosis in Uganda: autopsy study. *East Afr Med J.* 1974;51:388-391.
23. Edington GM. Haemosiderosis and anaemia in the Gold Coast African. *West Afr Med J.* 1954;3:66-70.
24. Edington GM. Nutritional siderosis in Ghana. *Cent Afr J Med.* 1959;5:186-189.
25. Isah HS, Fleming AF. Anaemia and iron status of symptom-free adult males in northern Nigeria. *Ann Trop Med Parasitol.* 1985;79:479-484.
26. Gerritsen T, Walker AR. Serum iron and iron-binding capacity in the Bantu. *S Afr Med J.* 1953;27:577-581.
27. Gordeuk V, Mukiibi J, Hasstedt SJ, et al. Iron overload in Africa. Interaction between a gene and dietary iron content. *N Engl J Med.* 1992;326:95-100.
28. Buchanan WM. *Bantu Siderosis with Special Reference to Rhodesian Africans.* Faculty of Medicine Research Lecture Series, No. 1. Salisbury, Rhodesia: University College of Rhodesia; 1967.
29. Buchanan WM. Bantu siderosis: a review. *Cent Afr J Med.* 1969;15:105-113.
30. Buchanan WM. Siderosis in Rhodesian Africans. *Cent Afr J Med.* 1966;12:199-207.
31. Gordeuk VR. Hereditary and nutritional iron overload. *Baillieres Clin Haematol.* 1992;5:169-186.
32. Moyo VM, Gangaidzo IT, Gomo ZA, et al. Traditional beer consumption and the iron status of spouse pairs from a rural community in Zimbabwe. *Blood.* 1997;89:2159-2166.
33. Kasvosve I, Tshwenyego U, Phuthego T, et al. Serum ferritin concentration is affected by ferroportin Q248H mutation in Africans. *Clin Chim Acta.* 2015;444:257-259.
34. Katchunga PB, Baguma M, M'Buyamba-Kabangu JR, Philippe J, Hermans MP, Delanghe J. Ferroportin Q248H mutation, hyperferritinemia and atypical type 2 diabetes mellitus in South Kivu. *Diabetes Metab Syndr.* 2013;7:112-115.
35. Hlangwani E, Adebiyi JA, Doorsamy W, Adebe OF. Processing, characteristics and composition of umqombothi (a South African traditional beer). *Processes.* 2020;8:1451.

36. Moyo VM, Mandishona E, Hasstedt SJ, et al. Evidence of genetic transmission in African iron overload. *Blood.* 1998;91:1076-1082.
37. McNamara L, MacPhail AP, Gordeuk VR, Hasstedt SJ, Rouault T. Is there a link between African iron overload and the described mutations of the hereditary haemochromatosis gene? *Br J Haematol.* 1998;102:1176-1178.
38. Gordeuk VR, Caleffi A, Corradini E, et al. Iron overload in Africans and African-Americans and a common mutation in the SCL40A1 (ferroportin 1) gene. *Blood Cells Mol Dis.* 2003;31:299-304.
39. Masaisa F, Breman C, Gahutu JB, Mukiibi J, Delanghe J, Philippe J. Ferroportin (SLC40A1) Q248H mutation is associated with lower circulating serum hepcidin levels in Rwandese HIV-positive women. *Ann Hematol.* 2012;91:911-916.
40. McNamara L, Gordeuk VR, MacPhail AP. Ferroportin (Q248H) mutations in African families with dietary iron overload. *J Gastroenterol Hepatol.* 2005;20:1855-1858.
41. Ma S, Dubin AE, Zhang Y, et al. A role of PIEZO1 in iron metabolism in mice and humans. *Cell.* 2021;184:969-982.e13.
42. Majore S, Ricerca BM, Radio FC, et al. Type 3 hereditary hemochromatosis in a patient from sub-Saharan Africa: is there a link between African iron overload and TFR2 dysfunction? *Blood Cells Mol Dis.* 2013;50:31-32.
43. Singh KS, Leu JI, Barnoud T, et al. African-centric TP53 variant increases iron accumulation and bacterial pathogenesis but improves response to malaria toxin. *Nat Commun.* 2020;11:473.
44. Wapnick AA, Bothwell TH, Seftel H. The relationship between serum ion levels and ascorbic acid stores in siderotic Bantu. *Br J Haematol.* 1970;19:271-276.
45. Seftel HC, Keeley KJ, Isaacson C, Bothwell TH. Siderosis in the Bantu: the clinical incidence of hemochromatosis in diabetic subjects. *J Lab Clin Med.* 1961;58:837-844.
46. Seftel HC, Malkin C, Schmaman A, et al. Osteoporosis, scurvy, and siderosis in Johannesburg bantu. *Br Med J.* 1966;1:642-646.
47. Schnitzler CM, Schnaid E, MacPhail AP, Mesquita JM, Robson HJ. Ascorbic acid deficiency, iron overload and alcohol abuse underlie the severe osteoporosis in black African patients with hip fractures—A bone histomorphometric study. *Calcif Tissue Int.* 2005;76:79-89.
48. Mandishona E, MacPhail AP, Gordeuk VR, et al. Dietary iron overload as a risk factor for hepatocellular carcinoma in Black Africans. *Hepatology.* 1998;27:1563-1566.
49. Kew MC, Asare GA. Dietary iron overload in the African and hepatocellular carcinoma. *Liver Int.* 2007;27:735-741.
50. Kew MC. Hepatic iron overload and hepatocellular carcinoma. *Liver Cancer.* 2014;3:31-40.
51. Isaacson C, Bothwell TH, MacPhail AP, Simon M. The iron status of urban black subjects with carcinoma of the oesophagus. *S Afr Med J.* 1985;67:591-593.
52. Buchanan WM. Peritonitis and Bantu siderosis. *S Afr Med J.* 1970;44:43-44.
53. Bothwell TH, Adams EB, Simon M, et al. The iron status of Black subjects with amoebiasis. *S Afr Med J.* 1984;65:601-604.
54. Gordeuk VR, McLaren CE, MacPhail AP, Deichsel G, Bothwell TH. Associations of iron overload in Africa with hepatocellular carcinoma and tuberculosis: Strachan's 1929 thesis revisited. *Blood.* 1996;87:3470-3476.
55. McNamara L, MacPhail AP, Mandishona E, et al. Non-transferrin-bound iron and hepatic dysfunction in African dietary iron overload. *J Gastroenterol Hepatol.* 1999;14:126-132.
56. Lynch SR, Seftel HC, Torrance JD, Charlton RW, Bothwell TH. Accelerated oxidative catabolism of ascorbic acid in siderotic Bantu. *Am J Clin Nutr.* 1967;20:641-647.
57. Lynch SR, Berelowitz I, Seftel HC, et al. Osteoporosis in Johannesburg Bantu males. Its relationship to siderosis and ascorbic acid deficiency. *Am J Clin Nutr.* 1967;20:799-807.
58. Moyo VM, Makunike R, Gangaidzo IT, et al. African iron overload and hepatocellular carcinoma (HA-7-0-080). *Eur J Haematol.* 1998;60:28-34.
59. Khumalo H, Gomo ZA, Moyo VM, et al. Serum transferrin receptors are decreased in the presence of iron overload. *Clin Chem.* 1998;44:40-44.
60. Speight AN, Cliff J. Iron storage disease of the liver in Dar es Salaam: a preliminary report on venesection therapy. *East Afr Med J.* 1974;51:895-902.

INDEX

Page numbers followed by "f" indicate figures, "t" indicate tables, and "b" indicate boxes.

D

H

W